VERONICA STRONG-BOAG is a member of the Department of History and Women's Studies at Simon Fraser University.

Elizabeth Smith was a determined and ambitious young woman in Victorian Ontario, who set out to get a medical education against considerable opposition, and succeeded. The diaries begin when she was thirteen years old, in Winona, Ontario, and take her through the loneliness and dissatisfaction of life as a young teacher. They chronicle her battle for admission to the all-male medical school at Queen's University, and the discrimination she met there as a woman from professors and fellow students. The diaries end as she begins her career as one of the first woman doctors to be educated in Canada.

A cautious feminist and an anxious Protestant, Elizabeth Smith was often introspective, and used her diary as a way of recording her progress and as a mirror to create within herself a more perfect example of womanhood. She was typical of her period in her concern with life as a struggle against the sins of physical indulgence and moral laxity. Yet she was no stern, pedantic bluestocking; her anxiety and idealism were balanced by her wit and vivacity. Her overcoming of the obstacles that stood between women of her time and possible careers did not harm her chances for marriage and motherhood. In later life, married to Adam Shortt, she became one of the leading Canadian women of her time.

Elizabeth Smith's diaries are a rare expression of female experience, all the more valuable as the writer is articulate, sensitive, and outspoken. They cover a critical period in the 1870s and 1880s when Canada's first great feminist wave was emerging in response to inequalities in education, employment, and politics, and trace the development of a feminist consciousness in one outstanding individual. The passion and anger that were so much a part of this process remain alive for modern readers as they do in few other documents. The diaries will appeal to feminists and social historians as well as to those interested in Victorian life and letters.

ELIZABETH SMITH

'A Woman with a Purpose'
The Diaries of
Elizabeth Smith 1872–1884

EDITED, WITH AN INTRODUCTION,
BY VERONICA STRONG-BOAG

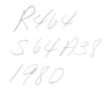

UNIVERSITY OF TORONTO PRESS
Toronto Buffalo London

© University of Toronto Press 1980
Toronto Buffalo London
Printed in Canada

ISBN 0-8020-2360-6 cloth
ISBN 0-8020-6397-7 paper

Canadian Cataloguing in Publication Data

Shortt, Elizabeth Smith, 1859-1949.
 'A woman with a purpose'

 (Social history of Canada ; 32 ISSN 0085-6207)
 ISBN 0-8020-2360-6 bd.   ISBN 0-8020-6397-7 pa.
 1. Shortt, Elizabeth Smith, 1859-1949. 2. Ontario –
 Biography. I. Strong-Boag, Veronica Jane, 1947-
 II. Title. III. Series.
 FC3072.1.S56A3   971.3'03'0924   C80-094406-2
 F1058.S56A3

Social History of Canada 32

The text of the diary is published with the permission of Mary E. Crowther.

This book has been published with the help of the block grant programs of the Canada Council and the Ontario Arts Council.

Contents

VERONICA STRONG-BOAG

Introduction

... I find myself displaying nervousness & the false timidity so inherent to girls of today that I must school myself to do away with nerves entirely and be a woman womanly in my strength ... (February 28, 1880)

The author of this earnest vow was the twenty-one-year-old teacher and medical student, Elizabeth Smith. The ardent denial of weakness and hypocrisy was characteristic of her. So too was her passionate espousal of the high ideal of a disciplined and responsible womanhood. Her sentiments in 1880 are echoed many times in the diary which is published here for the first time. Beginning in 1872 and running intermittently through to 1884, its pages represent the efforts of an ambitious woman and a liberal Victorian to come to terms with herself, her fellows, and her time.[1]

Few Canadian documents chart the development of an individual woman's dedication and ambition so well as this personal diary of Elizabeth Smith. To follow her from a farm girl of thirteen to a medical woman of twenty-five is to trace the emergence of the late Victorian feminist consciousness in a single person, a woman who went on to become one of the Dominion's female leaders. The transformation is a fascinating process. Elizabeth, or Beth as she was fondly called by her family, is well worth rescuing from the obscurity which cloaks much of the female experience in Canada.

The recollection of events was itself a minor concern. Elizabeth, like so many other nineteenth-century diarists,[2] viewed life as a near-constant struggle against the compelling sins of physical indulgence and moral laxity. The inspiring quotations and poetry, and the self-admonishments, which appear throughout her diary, were a means by which the thoughtful girl challenged herself to renewed endeavour. Yet for all her self-conscious seriousness Elizabeth was no sober-sides. Wit, humour, and a devastating self-mockery made her anything but the stereotypically stern and pedantic bluestocking. This honesty and liveliness won the young Elizabeth friends wherever she went. Readers of her personal journal will find it difficult to resist the same charm.

Fortunately, the handwritten originals of Elizabeth's diaries were preserved together with a great body of her correspondence. These now rest with the University of Waterloo. The complete manuscript runs some forty per cent longer than the present version: for the sake of clarity, interest, and space, repetitious passages, many of them devoted to religion and social chit-chat, have been eliminated, and several of the poems that headed certain pages have been silently omitted. Furthermore, since Elizabeth's own notebooks consist for the most part of a rather arbitrary series of entries, the edited version has been divided into ten sections on the basis of location, reflecting significant shifts in the author's life. Everything else has been kept as close to the original as possible. In all important respects Miss Smith of Winona has been left to tell her own story.

A cautious feminist and an anxious Protestant, Elizabeth was often intensely introspective, determined to examine, castigate, and occasionally applaud her own and her society's slow progress toward perfection. Employing her diary both as milestone and mirror, Elizabeth sought to create within herself a more perfect womanhood. This effort at human improvement is an essential ingredient in the feminism of the time. Challenging those who insisted that woman's place was the home alone, Elizabeth and her like-minded sisters in the women's movement proclaimed that a perfected womanhood would participate in the public sphere of politics and employment as well as in the private sphere of the home and family.

The pursuit of high standards and lofty goals was hard enough for any right-minded Victorian, but it was especially formidable for the independent female. Much of the accepted wisdom of the time tended to confine a woman's aspirations within domestic boundaries. Here alone womanly custodians of individual hearths should strive to reach the moral and spiritual heights. The perils and satisfactions of competition and combat in the wider world of politics and labour were better reserved, so it was felt, for the stronger male. To ensure that women, at least those of the middle class, did not too often venture beyond their allotted sphere, laws and institutions barred the way to women's easy progress in the realm that men had set aside for themselves. The breaching of such barriers required considerable courage and determination. Elizabeth had both.

She did not stand alone. There were large numbers of nineteenth-century women who determined to break male monopolies in education, the professions, and business, and demanded the right to live uncloistered lives. Elizabeth Smith had important precursors, but she and her contemporaries formed Canada's first great feminist wave. As one of a new breed of female professionals Elizabeth was living proof that women could seek careers without injury to their chances for marriage and motherhood. This apparent ability to combine successfully more traditional goals with new work patterns was essential to public acceptance.

Although the range of her experience would be unusual for a nineteenth-century girl, Elizabeth's origins in rural southwestern Ontario were not. The second daughter and third child of Sylvester Smith and Isabella McGee Smith of Winona, Ontario, was born on January 18, 1859. Her prosperous farm family, which developed the profitable E.D. Smith preserve business in the 1880s, was always an affectionate enclave, and would remain an inspiration throughout her long life. She seemed especially attached to her mother, her sister Gertrude, and her brother Ernest. Relatives sustained the young teacher and apprentice doctor in moments of despair and frustration. Cherished memories of family entertainments in the 1870s, for instance, gave special weight to Beth's dissatisfaction with the Speyside school in 1878 'far from friends and home – in an unknown part of the country' (January 18, 1878). Only in the friendships she made in the course of teachers' training and medical school did Elizabeth find a near-equivalent to family ties.

Isabella McGee Smith, a former schoolteacher and Nova Scotian who had come to Ontario in search of a husband, was the dominant member of the Smith family. While Sylvester attended to the duties of his farm, his wife raised her children with high standards and higher expectations. Elizabeth was especially influenced by her mother's championship in private conversation and in local newspapers of such feminist causes as temperance and higher education for women. The example of her mother may also have made her more critical of other less 'advanced' women. Elizabeth Smith was always uncomfortable with what she identified as frivolity or irresponsibility, especially in women. The female sex, owing to its purer, ultimately biologically determined temperament, bore a particular obligation to inspire and correct society. Moments of gaiety and silliness could be permitted occasionally, even in oneself, but they should never obscure or undermine women's influence for good.

Despite her mother's feminist sympathies and the fact that the family had domestic servants, young Elizabeth could not escape a girl's special liability for home chores. The birth of her sister Violet in 1872, for instance, entailed an interruption in Elizabeth's schooling while she stayed home to care for the new baby. The assignment of such duty to older female children helps to explain the lower school attendance rates for Ontario's girls in this period.[3] If spelling is any indication, Elizabeth's education, even when augmented by the instruction of a governess at home, was much interrupted before she graduated from the local rural school in 1874 at the age of fifteen.

During the years 1875–8, for which the diaries are largely incomplete, Elizabeth, as the daughter of a well-to-do farm family, 'came out' in society as her sister Mauritana had done before her. Like increasing numbers of middle-class girls, Elizabeth then rejected the option of remaining passively at home for a suitable mate to turn up. Without spurning marriage as a future alternative, she embarked on a search for economic independence and satisfying employment. Attendance at the Model School attached to Hamilton Collegiate Institute offered her a modest beginning.

The choice of teaching as first occupation was typical of thousands of young women seeking respectable work in nineteenth- and twentieth-century Canada.[4] To contemporaries there often seemed a veritable army of school-marms. The rapid replacement of male instructors by women in the nation's public schools, especially at the lower levels, stemmed from five main factors, all of which affected the Winona girl: the prevailing faith in women's special nurturing instincts; the absence of respectable job alternatives; the introduction of graded schools; the attractiveness for money-conscious school trustees of women's lower salaries; and the rapid expansion of the Dominion's school system at a time when male energies could be more profitably employed on new settlement and commercial or financial frontiers.

By the last quarter of the nineteenth century teaching had become a female occupational ghetto characterized by low salaries, poor conditions, and slight prestige. The custom of boarding out, for instance, with all the potential for supervision, gossip, and interference it entailed, not to mention the frequent absence of comfort and good will, was a special burden. Nevertheless, experiences like the teenage Elizabeth's may constitute one variation on the 'semi-autonomy' stage on the road to full adulthood which is now being documented as a common feature of nineteenth-century adolescence.[5] Viewed in this light a sojourn with a strange family introduced teachers who might well be adolescents to the disciplines, constraints, and expectations of the community while at the same time acknowledging their need for protection. As Elizabeth's entries suggest, the results might be either the discovery of new friends or bitterly unhappy associations. In any case the very fact of dependence would be increasingly at odds with the emerging sense of professional superiority which teachers like Elizabeth Smith were attempting to convey. In these years teaching professionals were just at the beginning of their long battle to win the kind of recognition which other experts such as doctors and lawyers had already largely achieved. The practices of boarding out and of employing very young teachers would eventually almost disappear in the course of the campaign for improved status.

Until the profession grew stronger, only a hardened, desperate, or extremely dedicated minority of women or men made teaching a lifelong commitment. Elizabeth's own loneliness and dissatisfaction suggest why the occupation frequently remained merely a way-station for either sex. It provided those like Elizabeth with a chance to study and save for a more attractive profession, and it offered others like Nellie McClung, some years later, an opportunity for economic independence before marriage.[6] Although Elizabeth argued rather self-righteously that the employment gave her financial freedom, many more women, lacking the buttress of family support during vacations and periods of additional schooling as well as Elizabeth's marketable musical talents, were less fortunate. The majority of female teachers had little cause for optimism about new careers other than marriage.

Although teaching was often frustrating and exhausting, Elizabeth was clearly popular with her pupils. Many continued to write letters and arrange reunions long after their ambitious instructor had left. Such affectionate loyalty gave her many happy moments in the classroom. Nevertheless Elizabeth found the duties of tutor and disciplinarian for the 'deplorably ignorant' and 'mischievous' a frequent hardship. Not even parents' praise and more personal flattery from the young men of the district reconciled her to teaching as a permanent outlet for her energies.

Although she was not always satisfied with her own progress, the diaries record advancing maturity and learning. Success with schoolteaching and the approval of trustees provided her with the self-assurance that would be essential in her medical career. The nineteen-year-old recounting her activities and her boredom in a small school was decidedly ambitious and consciously intellectual. She found little satisfaction in the restricted life of the small-town or rural teacher. Not even her intense religious faith could compensate for the perceived shortcomings of this environment.

Elizabeth's Anglicanism was essential to her sense of well-being. Faith in a benevolent but stern deity gave a moral framework to her life. Her principles rested on the confidence that the Protestant religion and especially the Church of England represented the surest guide to human experience. Such certainty did not always fall short of intolerance. Her fervent desires for a better Christian life often went hand in hand with a smug condemnation of the supposedly degenerate and vulgar rituals of Catholicism and Methodism. This association of high, almost unobtainable, spiritual ideals with a sense of superiority vis-à-vis other religions made Anglo-Saxon Victorians like Elizabeth earnest and energetic in the pursuit of the excellence which would dispel doubt and confirm superiority. It also made it very difficult for them to accept mediocrity, real or imagined, in others or themselves. The British Empire was built on such foundations.

Elizabeth also revealed that capacity for intense friendships – 'That is friendship where each puts implicit trust on the other – where congenial spirits dwell, where education is, where religion reigns supreme christianizing, purifying, making it sure, even unto death ...' (February 6, 1878) – which would always distinguish her. Friends' tested love helped compensate for the tedium of teaching and the hardships of medicine. Highly charged and persistent affection between women appears commonplace in the period.[7] Same-sex friendships offered the reassurance, sympathy, and intellectual stimulation which social custom rarely allowed between the sexes. Strong emotional ties among women were a powerful stimulus to the raising of feminist consciousness and the creation of co-operative endeavours to improve women's lot.

Other lifelong convictions were also observable in the young teacher; in particular Elizabeth's insistence on the heavy moral responsibilities of clergymen and mothers. Her visit to church on March 3, 1878, for instance, drew forth a typical condemnation of the drone-like preacher who deadened sensibility and sapped faith. The presumption that religious officials were properly the community's moral arbitrators was characteristic of traditional and conservative society. In the face of steadily advancing secularism and materialism, however, the churches' authority began to seem insufficient and unreliable. The social gospel of individuals like James Shaver Woodsworth and Salem Bland emerged in response to the predicament of the churches, but this was not the only solution to a 'moral vacuum.' A new feminist dogma based initially on a strong sense of spiritual merit was evolving simultaneously.[8] Christ's sacrifice had washed women clean of the sin of Eve. Women, as the bearers of the race and custodians of its humanity, had valuable moral qualities. Their instinctive purity, generosity, and high-mindedness made them essential social catalysts in a nation threatened by the false values of urban industrial capitalism. Elizabeth spoke for this feminist ideal when she criticized local mothers for their failure to meet women's important challenge, and she herself was determined not to be found wanting. Should it become necessary, she resolved to 'try to do my duty in that sphere as befits a mother's holy – mighty – office ...' (January 27, 1878). Like many others of her generation, Elizabeth came to feel that maternally-based sentiment supplied an important spur to individual and collective improvement. Her own life would be a constant struggle to bring this force to bear on the Canadian community.

Ready as she was to castigate the unreliable of her sex, the youthful Elizabeth was above all optimistic. Once educated, the responsible majority of women would improve the community and serve their sex. Every woman had this potential power. As early as 1877 Elizabeth was preparing to do her part.

Medicine was her chosen field. At this time no woman had been permitted to graduate with a Canadian medical degree. Elizabeth, however, was encouraged to believe that this discrimination might soon end. The registrar of the Medical School at Queen's University had informed her that there was no objection to women attending lectures and the editor of the *Toronto Mail* had written suggesting that the Toronto School of Medicine might also be willing to accept female candidates.[9] Cheered by such news the young teacher took the medical school entrance exam of the College of Physicians and Surgeons in Toronto in the spring of 1878. Her unexpected failure was the first in a series of setbacks which impeded her progress.

Elizabeth's chosen course was in fact particularly difficult. Medicine was one of the nineteenth-century's male monopolies. Despite many women's acquaintance with illness in their households and the ancient tradition of female midwifery, Canadian doctors, like those elsewhere, were frequently antagonistic to professional rivals of the opposite sex. Their objections can generally be grouped into two categories: idealistic and pragmatic. On the one hand opponents posed as defenders of their culture's view of women. Female aspirants were castigated as 'strong-minded' women and reminded pointedly 'that the noblest quality a woman can possess is modesty, and that the mingling of the sexes in the study of medicine is not calculated to preserve that female grace in its integrity.'[10] According to such Jeremiahs, precise knowledge of physical processes and close association with male physicians entailed heavy costs in coarsened sensibility. Nervous exhaustion was also considered a real danger for women in medicine or indeed in any field requiring great concentration.[11] 'Pretty girl doctors' guaranteed themselves early deaths 'in the hopeless endeavour to show that women can fill men's place in the world.'[12] Weakness and collapse were real possibilities because normal women were too frail to meet medicine's demands.

Such concern flowed from the middle-class preference for a pure, spiritual, and modest femininity.[13] Conservatives hoped that this superior womanhood would rule in the private sphere, 'exercising those qualities of mind and heart with which all bounteous nature has specially endowed her.' The admirers of this ideal argued further that 'In educating her we are educating wives and mothers, not doctors, and lawyers, and judges, and stump speakers, and engine drivers. We are educating her whose strength is her weakness, who is to rule by affection, who is to make the home circle the strongest attraction for her children and the soft antidote for her husband to the worry and bitterness of business life, by adorning it with the exceeding loveliness of womanly delicacy and refinement.'[14] Should woman's influence be compromised by having her energies directed into non-domestic channels, a major force for human betterment would be lost. Incidentally, of course, extra-familial commitments might involve some sacrifice of male comfort. Child-rearing and housekeeping might be essential but few men wanted any significant share in them.[15]

Male doctors had economic reasons, as well, for rejecting women. Professional journals regularly grumbled about over-crowding in the occupation,[16] and pointed to a surplus of male practitioners which already made it difficult for young doctors to secure a living. Furthermore, the continuing employment of midwives and the rising feminist movement made it very likely that many women would prefer doctors of their own sex for obstetrical matters in particular.

The male medical establishment would have preferred that women satisfy themselves with a nursing career;[17] but those women who insisted on becoming doctors were pointedly encouraged to devote themselves to the needs of the poor. In this way, women could be confined to medical practices of little prestige and less profit. As one wily guardian of male prerogatives explained, assistance to the underprivileged would supplement the work of male colleagues:

There are hundreds of cases of midwifery to attend which are now being attended by ignorant mid-wives, simply because they cannot afford the charges of the young male doctor. These poor working women pay about four dollars for the confinement and subsequent attendance. The young male doctor wont attend them for that price, and even if he would they prefer a midwife, for the simple reason that they cannot afford a nurse to wash them and the baby for the next few days, and this the midwife does. Now, if the young female doctor will take hold of the work there is plenty of it to do, and she will not only earn a decent living but also confer an incalculable blessing on her fellow women among the working class ... Then again, when the working-man's children are sick he does not dare to call in a doctor until the very last; a man with a large family, living on twenty-four dollars a month, cannot afford many dollar visits, which is the minimum fee that a young male doctor has been taught to take. The result is that his child dies for lack of attendance, or else is taken to the overcrowded out-patient room at the Hospital, where the poor mother is sometimes obliged to wait three or four hours away from the rest of her little ones. The young female doctor will find lots of work which is now going a begging, and if her education does not drive away the tenderness from her woman's heart, the possibilities for doing good are almost unlimited.[18]

If girls followed this advice, a 'woman's heart' in doctoring, as in nursing, would ensure a subordinate role and present no threat to masculine supremacy.

The suggestion that female doctors should replace midwives was significant. In Canada, as in the United States and Great Britain, male physicians were eager substitutes for midwives and bitter opponents of their licensing. Even when it was made illegal, however, midwifery continued to find a clientele, especially among the poor and the traditionally minded. Furthermore, feminist suspicion of the motives behind male 'intrusion' into the female 'mysteries' of pregnancy and childbirth added champions to the midwives' cause. For male doctors of course it was a brilliant ploy to propose exchanging the more numerous midwives for relatively few female physicians. Under the stern eye of dominant male practitioners, these professionals would pose little threat.[19]

Ironically enough, doctors' efforts to reform their profession in the nineteenth century tended to operate to women's disadvantage.[20] The setting of uniform academic standards for entry hurt women like Elizabeth Smith, who suffered because schoolgirls were offered a discriminatory training, and especially because they frequently lacked preparation in Latin.[21] Similarly, the increased costs of improved programs within universities were serious hurdles for women whose families were often more reluctant to finance a daughter's education than a son's. At the same time a girl's opportunities for earning tuition were generally inferior to her brother's.[22]

Concern for higher standards, together with criticism of 'irregular practitioners,' fostered an environment which was generally unsympathetic to variety of any sort in medical personnel. The frequent identification of women with such controversial healing practices as electro-therapy, homeopathy, and Christian Science only injured the feminist cause as the regular doctors tightened their control over the profession. Yet female interest in alternative methods of curing was hardly surprising. Unorthodox medicine, fighting a rearguard action against the advancing ranks of modern professionals, welcomed even female allies. At the same time the reform-minded of both sexes found the holistic remedies of the unorthodox more relevant to their concern for the general betterment of the community. The fact that unorthodox medicine laid less stress on formal educational requirements added further to its attractions. Some women, however, were not satisfied to remain on the periphery of their chosen profession.[23]

Allegiance to the regular practitioners and their code was never easy. The male medical establishment constantly blocked female advance by its 'defence in depth.' Once a single obstacle was overcome, the enemy re-formed to the rear. If women won entry to the medical schools, the hospitals remained barred. When the latter finally opened, internships and residencies were often refused. Even when medical women at last scaled every barrier, male physicians declined to consult with them and sometimes obstructed their entrance into prestigious medical societies. In the United States the situation was depressing enough,[24] but a multitude of degree-granting institutions and a stronger egalitarian tradition opened some medical schools there to women from the 1850s on. In the Dominion fewer schools and more conservative traditions made conditions much more unwelcoming. Canadians like Dr Emily Howard Stowe and Dr Jennie Kidd Trout had little alternative but to travel south for professional training.[25] In 1879 Elizabeth Smith herself was seriously contemplating attending medical school in Ann Arbor, Michigan, as a solution to the problems of obtaining a degree in her own land. Nor was this remedy ignored by women's critics within the Canadian profession: an exodus of female students to the United States could be regarded as infinitely preferable to establishing suitable programs in the Dominion itself.[26] Indeed the prospect of training in the United States drained off the most determined female claimants for some time and allowed Canadian doctors to sustain their resistance a little longer.

By the late 1870s, however, the conservative position was crumbling under assault from women demanding useful activity, decent employment, economic independence, and the right to serve their sex. As with most feminist causes there were male sympathizers, but women were their own most ardent champions. The most important feminist salvo in the public debate was provided by the anonymous 'Agnodice'[27] mentioned in these diaries. This partisan replied to women's critics by insisting that female modesty was not so frail that medicine undermined it; nor for that matter were household duties threatened by study. As for women's alleged incapacity, 'Agnodice' pinpointed the source: 'The want of nerve, and the inaccuracy ... I believe to be chiefly due to the education they receive, and to the inherited effect of generations passed under circumstances carefully calculated to prevent habits of self-control and strength of nerve.' Women's condition would change when 'little girls are encouraged to lead the same outdoor life as little boys, to take the same interest in beetles and dormice, tame rabbits and guinea pigs.'[28] Until that day the social existence of the middle-class female would be essentially meaningless and parasitical. Like her young admirer teaching in Speyside, Agnodice called for 'a purpose, a life-work, a determined end in what I undertake.'[29] Allegiance to a 'vocation' would release women from 'Society's' bondage.

This passionate advocate was echoed by a chorus of other feminist voices, who reminded readers that women were already labouring in coal mines, fields, and factories. In reality the decisive difference between employments was not, they insisted, the

degree of difficulty but the rate of remuneration.[30] Other parti-
sans added that employment was not only women's right but
their need. What else could succour those who found no male
provider?[31]

On a number of occasions the claim was put forward by
feminists that men had usurped women's traditional role in
healing. One female doctor spoke for the majority in asserting
that 'By right of inheritance, the care of the sick is woman's
province.'[32] Elizabeth Smith herself always laid stress on the
'special inheritance' which made the mothers of the race its natural healers.[33] Since faith in women's distinctive nurturing qualities was widespread, such reasoning had powerful appeal. The
natural ability of women was, however, finally insufficient for
the best care of the nation's children; knowledge of modern science was needed to upgrade women's traditional skills. Only
with access to medical schools or training could women properly
fulfil their historic function.[34] For most girls basic instruction in
health care would be sufficient, but a few could legitimately
demand to become professionals. As such they could assist all
women in the better performance of their duties.

Not only youngsters would profit by the presence of female
physicians; women themselves desperately needed better treatment. One prominent Montreal champion of her sisters made
this very clear:

Good authorities assert that only one woman in ten is in absolutely
sound health. What of the other nine? The three worst will go to a
medical man, adding to the unavoidable suffering of their ailment the
uncalled-for suffering of an experience painful even to the rich woman
who sees a first rate specialist in the presence of relative and nurse, and
doubly painful to the not less modest poor woman, who goes alone to
an inferior practitioner, or is the subject of a clinical demonstration to
men students in a hospital. Three suffering less acutely will resort to
some mischievous patent 'cure all', whose apparent efficacy is due to
the opium it contains. The importunate and repulsive advertisements
of these horrid drugs and the statistics of their enormous sale prove
that women are doctoring themselves every day with the worst results.

The three remaining sufferers will go through life with permanently depressed health, joyfulness and usefulness alike unknown to them. We could all name such women, many with gifts and graces above the average, whose health is vaguely described as 'delicate', not a few of whom would never have become invalids had they sought medical advice in girlhood, or in early married life, and who would have sought such advice could they have had it from a woman.[35]

These observations would have been familiar to a Hamburg-trained doctor who found plenty of demand for her services in Canada. This immigrant identified still another critical concern when she condemned 'male-midwifery' as 'a practice ... revolting ... contrary to all ideas of morality and refinement.'[36] Such assessments not unnaturally led to the claim that not only health but modesty would be guarded by female doctors. Elizabeth Smith was well aware of the unmet needs of her sex.[37] She understood and shared a fellow student's anxiety 'to do anything I can to hasten the much needed reform in the medical treatment of our own sex ...'[38] Women must be spared the ignorant, often insensitive, treatment of male physicians.

Women doctors' sensitivity to the plight of their sex did not stop at Canada's borders. Many of Elizabeth's contemporaries and successors were still more shocked by reports from China and India. There infidel women, lacking even the solace and protection of Christianity, suffered concubinage, purdah, widow immolation, and slavery. Feminist sympathies then combined with Christian and imperialist sentiments to send these young Canadian doctors to serve in foreign fields.[39]

While some sister doctors heeded the call from the Orient, Elizabeth Smith chose to dedicate her efforts especially to Canadian patients. Whatever their field of service, most female physicians saw themselves allied with the reforming forces of the age. Wherever they ministered these women would strengthen their own sex for the assumption of a more active role in the community. Medical education, like woman suffrage, was designed to increase female influence over social developments. A professional's skills and knowledge would go far toward building a better future. By identifying social problems and proposing scientific solutions physicians would win recognition, approval, and power for their sex as a whole. Thus women would be important participants in the coming 'Age of Reform.'[40]

Doctors Jennie Kidd Trout and Emily Howard Stowe were two early Canadian exponents of women's right to medical training. Refused entry to Canadian medical schools, both had turned to the United States. Dr Stowe graduated from the New York Medical College for Women in 1867; Dr Trout finished some eight years later at the Woman's Medical College of Philadelphia. On their return to Canada they faced a chill reception from male professionals. Angered by their own treatment and critical of Canadian medical practice, these pioneers became anxious sponsors of younger women. Recruits would both reform the occupation and benefit female patients. Although Dr Stowe became the more famous, both Toronto women were models for girls considering medical careers. The Winona student was Dr Trout's special disciple. Despite her rejection of the older woman's advice in 1879 to choose Ann Arbor, Elizabeth Smith 'left her resolved to go through my profession and do in what measure I may be able the work that she had done,' and added, 'But never will I be able to do what she as a pioneer has done.' (April 22, 1879) Elizabeth successfully rewrote the medical school entrance exams that spring.

Elizabeth's efforts to secure medical education did not cease there. Hoping to encourage Queen's to admit women she ran this advertisement in Toronto newspapers for several weeks:

Ladies wishing to study medicine in Canada will hear something to their advantage by communicating with Box 31, Winona, Ontario P.O.[41]

Well over twenty letters arrived asking advice, seeking encouragement, and offering suggestions. Augusta, Emily Stowe's daughter, was one correspondent, but she was not to knock at the doors of Queen's. Although the Kingston school agreed to create a summer program equivalent to but distinct from the men's winter course in 1880, Emily Stowe rejected this solution for her daughter, noting:

... there is every objection to a 'summer course' – No person can study as well then as in cold weather, you cannot dissect, and by the profession generally they would never be recognized as of equal value with the winter courses. There is [sic] never the same hospital advantages in summer as winter. With regard to the excessive value of a Canadian degree, it is more imaginery than real, & if obtained from separate or summer courses its value would fall.[42]

She recommended that Elizabeth apply to schools in the States or like Augusta chance the storm at Toronto. Dr Stowe's daughter did indeed secure entry to Victoria University that fall. The lone female, she fought her way to graduation from the medical program in 1883, a full year before Elizabeth would claim a Queen's degree.

Despite Dr Stowe's warning, Elizabeth seemed confident of her prospects at Kingston. To prepare herself financially she continued upgrading her teaching qualifications in Hamilton and returned to teaching, this time at Nelson, until the end of 1879. Her generally cheerful frame of mind was sustained by the succession of flirtations which accompanied her progress anywhere. So attractive were these passing fancies that she played with the doubt that she 'could be content to live with one man for life ...' (September 5, 1879). At no time did passivity or disinterest characterize Elizabeth's relationships with men.

Elizabeth's descriptions of her sojourn at Ottawa Normal School in the first months of 1880 reveal the same high spirits, even in face of the school's attempt to segregate the sexes. Despite her good intentions, Elizabeth was soon increasingly involved with another student, Charlie Roberts. The growing intimacy of this relationship, and later its mounting despair and disillusionment, would form major themes in her diary from this point. In fact many of the journal notations were recopied from regular letters to Charlie. The origins of these entries may help to explain the number of flirtations mentioned in them: was

Elizabeth reminding her absent lover of his eager rivals? In any case the emotions some passages reveal are an unusual survival from the nineteenth century. If Elizabeth's later preoccupation with Charlie's spiritual state is difficult for the modern reader to appreciate, her other feelings are easier to understand. Such personal concerns were not, however, allowed to interfere with her medical ambitions. In fact 'education' was all the more prized as it offered the 'independence to be able to marry for love & not for mercenary motives.' (May 21, 1880)

At Kingston in April she was joined by three other female candidates, Alice McGillivray, Elizabeth Beatty, and Annie Dickson. All four would finally graduate, three in 1884, and Annie Dickson, who was forced to leave school for a time, in 1886. The close ties between the 1884 graduates led them to title themselves, only somewhat facetiously, Shadrach, Meshach, and Abednego. Their relationship would be essential in supporting the three through the 'fiery furnace' of first surgery, medical examinations, and male hostility. Elizabeth was fascinated with the program and satisfied with her fellow scholars. By the close of the first term the future looked bright, both for love and for medicine. Despite proposals of marriage and protestations of love from others, Charlie had won Elizabeth's heart. At the same time she and the other new female students compared favourably with the men the faculty already taught.

The vibrant young Mrs McGillivray reflected the prevailing confidence when she outlined plans to spread the good word of women's medical mission in the newspapers:

Now my dear, we must awaken Ontario, this winter to a sense of the needs of her young daughters. We must hurl the 'Fiery Cross' through hill and dale, and startle something to life, either dissent or assent, the first better than nothing, because then we can have the satisfaction of exposing the meanness and small-mindedness of some of our *modest* fellow-creatures.[43]

While it is unclear what happened to this proposal, the students' feeling of accomplishment was confirmed by Dr Trout herself:

I thank God that a few noble women are preparing themselves to work in that part of 'The Master's' vineyard which needs their services so much. I rejoice that you are so devotedly earnest in the work. I am glad that it is a matter of principle with you for it is the most noble work on this His Foot Stool, yes more noble than the ministry in one way. I believe in the old Christ-like apostolic way of healing the bodies and saving the souls of men by one and the same person. It is not necessary to 'preach' in order to do this niether [sic] is it requisite to be what is nowadays called 'pious'. If we accept Christ as our Master, Teacher – look to Him as our pattern Physician we will without making ourself a pious bore, say and do many things that will help and elevate humanity. You all have my blessing and heartfelt welcome to the profession.[44]

As this pioneer made clear, medical women were specially consecrated to service. In large measure the Kingston students, good Christians, accepted their mission.

With her first summer session completed, Elizabeth took up teaching again in the fall of 1880 at Aldershot and in the spring of 1881 in Hamilton. The hard work and frequent boredom of these months were relieved by letters and visits from Charlie, family entertainments, and brief holidays. In April of 1881 she returned to Kingston only to discover that as there were only two new female students the course would be postponed to the following winter. Since a winter session was preferable, for the reasons outlined by Dr Stowe, the students were not entirely displeased. Inevitably, however, they were upset that the decision had not been taken the previous fall.

During this enforced break in her training Elizabeth again taught. Again this proved no substitute for the challenges of medicine. In the fall Queen's offered a partially coeducational program to Elizabeth and her friends. Separate dissecting, cloak, and waiting rooms, and special classes in jurisprudence, obstetrics, anatomy, and part of physiology safeguarded women's modesty. For much the same reason the women entered lectures before the men. In this way the first somewhat coeducational experiment continued, good will predominating among the men and dignified earnestness among the women. By the close of the session Elizabeth was all the more resolved that her sex must 'seek nobler things than the creature comforts, of idleness or the inactivity that nonentity brings ...' (March 11, 1882). Yet such sober thoughts did not exclude amusements. Throughout the year Elizabeth continued to tantalize her 'swains' and develop her friendships with Elizabeth Beatty and Alice McGillivray, although political differences were emerging as a problem with the latter, evidently an outspoken Liberal.

The summer dampened their high spirits. Anxious to increase their practical experience, Elizabeth and Alice elected to go to St Thomas to work with Dr Corlis, the husband of a new student. Both girls had high expectations which were bitterly disappointed. By July each was eager to leave, Elizabeth fortunately to be welcomed as an apprentice by a doctor cousin. The change was beneficial, but in the period before her return to Kingston Elizabeth began to be dismayed by Charlie's smoking and his religious doubts. The former offence may seem trivial now, but for many a reformer of the period smoking was more than an unhealthy habit – it was a sign of moral weakness. The spiritual doubts were more serious, causing Elizabeth considerable unhappiness.

With the opening of College in the fall, however, she faced more pressing problems. The session of 1882–3 was the most formidable the women would endure. Antagonism from new students and one lecturer, Dr Fenwick, jeopardized their entire program. By November, as Elizabeth's frenzied notes suggest, the situation had deteriorated drastically. When the female students were driven to march out of the offender's lecture, charges and counter-charges flew. Dr Fenwick insisted that mixed classes forced him to garble his delivery; in this he was supported by the male students. The College journal spoke for the latter, condemning the women for 'the unwarranted and uncomplimentary fashion' in which they disturbed the professor, and concluding that coeducation was a failure.[45] Fortunately Elizabeth and her friends were upheld by the majority of the faculty. The male students, however, were determined to press the issue, insisting that the female 'intruders' be ejected. Issuing a collective ultimatum, they threatened to take up an offer from Trinity Medical College, a rival school in Toronto. Salaries and positions on the line, the medical staff reluctantly agreed to refuse other women and to offer separate classes to those already enrolled.

During the course of this confrontation the women were cheered by frequent notes of support from the public and the press. As Elizabeth indicates, one student was hailed as a heroine in her home town. Elizabeth was herself comforted by her family, especially her brother Cecil who was championing her cause among students at Montreal's McGill. Such sympathy strengthened the women to endure continuing slurs and threats. In the New Year courses settled down somewhat, but bad feeling persisted, reducing Elizabeth to a near breakdown by term's end. Not even encouragement from the new boarder in her rooming house, Adam Shortt, a student at Queen's, could do much to bring her out of her despair.

Except for a brief note in 1884 the College diaries end in 1883 with Elizabeth's hope for a separate woman's college of medicine. News of this had been circulating for some time. In Toronto the always active Dr Trout, in association with Dr Stowe, had been endeavouring to bring about the creation of a new institution by offering financial inducements. Her sole stipulation required the inclusion of women on the faculty and the Board of Directors. For a time these requirements were rejected. Disappointed, Dr Trout next turned to a similar project being promoted at Kingston. On June 8, 1883 women's defenders met in the Kingston City Council Chamber. There prominent citizens, among them Sir Richard Cartwright and Principal George Grant of Queen's, came out in support of a special female medical institution. Grant, one of the Dominion's foremost educators,[46] set the tone by asserting that 'He thought the study of medicine one of the things for which woman was specially adapted, and as in England and the United States, every facility should be given to her to ratify her reasonable ambition.' Perhaps in an effort to reassure male physicians, he added that he did not foresee an immediate rush into the profession, nor did he expect that there would ever be as many females as males. Grant concluded with a letter from Dr Trout guaranteeing two hundred dollars per annum for five years on condition that women shared in the management of the institution and taught on the faculty as soon as a suitable appointment could be made. The principal agreed to these conditions and in turn offered one hundred dollars a year for the same period.[47] Guided by such champions the Kingston Women's Medical College was ready to open in October 1883.

Unfortunately for the prospects of the Kingston institution, the Toronto situation had changed markedly by June. At a meeting called by Dr Stowe's Women Suffrage Club and chaired by the Honourable Justice Patterson, previously recalcitrant male doctors accepted a Board of Directors composed of both sexes. Mindful of her bitter experience with these same men, Dr Trout denounced the change of heart as unfair to Kingston.[48] Despite this repudiation, the patronage of Dr Stowe and Toronto suffragists was enough to guarantee a second institution. A fundraising committee was set up and by October of 1883 the Toronto Woman's Medical College was also admitting students.

By creating separate medical schools for women, Canadians were joining a well-established trend. The Woman's Medical College of Philadelphia (1850), the New York Medical College for Women (1863), and the London School of Medicine for Women (1874) were some of the leading representatives of the separatist impulse. Between 1850 and 1895, Americans alone founded nineteen medical schools for women.

Of the two Canadian establishments the Kingston institution was the weaker by far. Although Elizabeth, urged by Dr Trout,[49] decided after considerable soul-searching to remain, the Toronto program with its more elaborate facilities and greater public support attracted more students. The unequal rivalry was confirmed when the Queen's school folded in 1893, leaving the field to its Toronto competitor. Before its closing, however, dedicated students had gone out on the medical mission proposed by Dr Trout.[50] Elizabeth Smith with Elizabeth Beatty and Alice McGillivray formed the first graduating class in 1884. Elizabeth Beatty went on to become a Presbyterian medical missionary in India, and Alice McGillivray, the class's valedictorian, to become professor of practical anatomy at Queen's. Elizabeth Smith herself first applied for an appointment at the Toronto school but, not unexpectedly, Augusta Stowe was hired there. Elizabeth then returned to Hamilton to enter general practice.

By the time she left Kingston Elizabeth's relationship with Charlie had come to a disillusioning close, as the last entry indicates. Rarely at a loss for new admirers, she had also become increasingly involved with Adam Shortt,[51] the boarder who had been so supportive during the crisis of 1882–3. Just as with Charlie this intimacy was expressed in countless letters which passed between the two lovers. Adam's graduate work in Scotland and his difficulty in finding a university appointment on his return to Canada postponed their longed-for marriage until Christmas 1886. Only his acceptance of a post in Queen's Department of Philosophy and Elizabeth's employment as a lecturer in Medical Jurisprudence and Sanitary Science in the Kingston Woman's Medical College ended their unhappy separation. Since they appear to have received no significant financial support from either of their families, two incomes were a prerequisite to reunion. Just as Elizabeth had prophesied, employment did permit her the freedom to make a love match.

When the closing of the College in 1893 ended her teaching career, Elizabeth devoted herself to her growing family. She found the responsibility for bringing her two daughters and son 'up in innocence & purity' both time-consuming and exhausting.[52] Housework and children drained even her abundant energies and reduced the scope of her outside interests. Although the medical profession was unusual in that women often continued in it after marriage and childbirth, Elizabeth did not choose to do so. Throughout her long life she made diagnoses and recommendations for relatives and friends but at no time did she resume practice. An explanation is difficult to find, especially as the Shortts were seriously strapped for funds at various times. One can only suppose that the social requirements of Adam's position first at Queen's and then in the Civil Service and Elizabeth's growing participation in voluntary work militated against her resumption of the vocation for which she had struggled so hard.

Despite her self-consecration to maternity, however, Elizabeth appreciated her need for regular escape from domestic duties, acknowledging, 'I take housework & children so seriously it becomes a mill of constant exactions till [I] get worn & blue – If I go out & talk awhile with bright women I come back ever so much brighter and more ready to go on ...'[53] Even with good servants, and her letters indicate that these were almost impossible to secure, she complained that 'My life is not only one constant uphill effort to keep the house clean & in order but a constant fight to keep from making unnecessary work.'[54] Such frustration no doubt made involvement in the woman's movement all the more attractive. Her activism was also a response to her sympathetic yet fearful observation of the poor, the unemployed, and the degenerate. The mounting dilemmas of a modernizing state appeared to call for professional and feminine attention if they were not to become deadly threats to social peace and individual happiness.

Nor was Elizabeth's anxiety alleviated by her opinion of contemporary politicians. Like other reform-minded women she discovered that 'Every election gives me the blues [and] men go down in the balance of my estimation & it takes quite a while for me to get the taste of it out of my mind ...'[55] Accordingly, despite recurring physical ailments, Elizabeth Smith Shortt assumed an increasingly active role in community life as she grew older. As a member of the executive of the local Young Women's Christian Association she put her talents to use investigating and ameliorating the unwholesome effects of city life on young girls. Such efforts, together with her work for the Local Council of Women, offered her the additional advantage of contact with potential servants,[56] yet despite such selfish considerations she expressed real concern for the moral and physical state of women left alone in the city's harsh confines. Elizabeth trusted that girl members would indeed receive immediate benefit from 'uplifting' contact with 'ladies' in the YWCA and the individual middle-class home.[57] This faith in the power of individual example typified reformers of many kinds during the period. In some cases it undoubtedly degenerated into little more than paternalistic camouflage for social control. Certainly the pioneer doctor desperately wished to stabilize Canada's rapidly developing community under middle-class direction. She firmly believed this class to be uniquely qualified for leadership by reason of superior morality and industry.

While always resistant to revolutionary change, Elizabeth was receptive to a wide variety of proposals for improving the health and morals of the underprivileged. As a supporter of Adelaide Hoodless,[58] she campaigned to convince school boards to adopt domestic science programs for female pupils. She insisted that, deprived of such training, girls, particularly factory workers, were 'ripe to spoil foods by abuse of cooking & to ruin the digestion of this generation & the next & create abnormal tastes that make for the destruction of good citizenship.' The safeguarding of the home depended on the practical relevance of girls' education for their future as wives and mothers.[59]

A loyal Kingstonian, Elizabeth was also especially attentive to the situation of older students enrolled at Queen's or the local nursing school. A women's residence for the university and better accommodation for the nurses, for instance, would enable girls to reach the high standards that should distinguish educated womanhood. These young women were essential social elements. It was up to them to create and maintain the lofty ideals by which Canada would be reformed and purified.[60] Settlement houses such as Toynbee Hall in London and Hull House in Chicago were particularly recommended to college graduates as examples of ways in which their superior principles might be concretely expressed. There assistance to the poor and the immigrant would unite the 'classes and the masses' in a joint endeavour at social betterment.[61] Elizabeth Smith Shortt's daughter, Muriel, did in fact follow her mother's advice and served at Evangelia Settlement in Toronto.

The Shortts' removal to Ottawa in 1908 when Adam was appointed Civil Service Commissioner did not reduce the number of Elizabeth's commitments. As in Kingston, her medical training was often applied to appraisal of community problems. Sickened by the human costs of tuberculosis, she issued a pamphlet, 'Some Social Aspects of Tuberculosis,' and took an active role in the Anti-Tuberculosis League. Through this association she campaigned for more treatment facilities, TB testing of herds, pasteurization of milk, and anti-spitting by-laws. Presidency of the Ottawa Local Council of Women and the Women's Canadian Club also involved her in crusades for reduced hours for nurses, better garbage collection, female police officers, children's playgrounds, school medical inspection, baby health clinics, additional female factory inspectors, and improved care of the insane. Even before going to the nation's capital she had concluded that the franchise was essential to the achievement of her goals.[62] Like other female activists she believed that the full weight of women's influence would only be felt at the ballot box.

By World War One Elizabeth Smith Shortt's activities had won her recognition as one of the Dominion's female leaders.[63] In her sixties during the post-war decade she did not retire to rest on her laurels. From this time on her two major preoccupations were mental hygiene and mothers' pensions. Her long-time concern for the feeble-minded, like that of another woman doctor, Helen MacMurchy,[64] intensified after the war's heavy toll among the physically and mentally sound. Speaking as Convenor of the National Council of Women's Committee on Mental Hygiene in 1926 she pointed out 'the very serious menace to our standards of life and living [posed by] the uncontrolled multiplication of the defective minded ...'.[65] The increase in custodial institutions which the Council had traditionally recommended was no longer a sufficient response. Like Helen MacMurchy, Elizabeth Smith Shortt turned to the consideration of sterilization and sex education as possible solutions. Such remedies often seemed very close to eugenics, the theory that human beings should be selectively bred for improvement. Certainly they would help guarantee that the numbers of the economically and intellectually marginal would remain manageable, and therefore that social problems would be more subject to control and the nation itself reformed. In no way was sexual liberation of any citizen the goal. Restraint not licence was the key to these programs.

Although support was at best uncertain for sterilization procedures, Elizabeth Smith Shortt discovered more agreement on the subject of mothers' allowances in the post-war period.[66] Although she had at first advised the National Council of Women that 'Mothers' pensions in too many cases would put a premium on degraded women getting rid of their husbands, while it would also relieve careless men of the responsibilities of providing for their progeny,'[67] she renounced these views after a 'dispassionate' survey in 1915.[68] Her interest in this form of state assistance and her stature as an activist were acknowledged in 1920 when Ontario appointed her Vice-Chairman of its Mothers' Allowances Commission. With this measure authorities gave symbolic and practical recognition to the mother's value to the entire community, a value long stressed by female reformers like Elizabeth Smith Shortt.

By the 1930s, and indeed until her death in 1949, old age and poor health combined to decrease sharply Elizabeth's activities. Disappointment with her own marriage, scepticism about ultimate reform, and pain from recurrent illness had left their marks. In the light of the Freudian-based psychology which permeated much thinking about social roles in post-World War One Canada, women found it harder and harder to reconcile a maternal nature with a professional or public career of any sort.[69] Even before the post-war decades Elizabeth's failure to resume medical practice suggests that, courageous as she was, she too may already have found the difficulties of this reconciliation overly burdensome. With each passing year her bitterness and disillusionment grew.

In this souring of mood and loss of confidence Elizabeth was not alone. Early in the 1920s feminists and reformers of all stripes began to lose the essential optimism which had armoured them in their demands for social change. Experience had demonstrated that neither woman nor the world was easily transformed.[70] Indeed it is difficult to know how this beneficial transformation was to occur so long as neither class society nor biological determinism was called into question. As farm girl, teacher, doctor, and activist, Elizabeth never advanced substantial criticism of the basic ideological structures of her society. Instead she helped forge the fabric of a modern and middle-class-dominated community in which women would be directed by the facts of physiology to a distinctive but rarely equal share in the community. Faith in an education and a womanhood defined by middle-class morality was not sufficient finally to the task of social redemption. The world was after all a rather more complicated and intractable place than Elizabeth or the majority of Canadian feminists imagined.

Even her initial harmonization of the more traditional goal of marriage with new work patterns allowed Elizabeth, like many other pioneer professionals, to avoid asking basic questions about the double shift of wage-earning women, first in the workplace and then in the home. Many of the early professionals could take on this burden because like Elizabeth they were exceptionally strong and ambitious or because they possessed the financial reserves to hire domestic substitutes. Their understandable desire to equal or better male achievement also made them reluctant to admit a predicament largely peculiar to their sex. In any case the dilemma of their poorer counterparts, so central to the modern oppression of women, went unexamined.

It is difficult to avoid a sense of disappointment when assessing the course of Elizabeth's life after medical school. One regrets the disappearance of the vivacious, warm, and sensitive girl of the diaries. Yet her transformation into an uncompromising and even embittered campaigner is hardly surprising. The long brutal struggle to win entry into medicine followed by a still lengthier battle to secure social reform and women's rights exacted their toll. Elizabeth and other feminists paid dearly in the hard coin of temper, health, and confidence. The full costs of their sacrifice are clear when we remember the joyful courage of the young Elizabeth in these diaries.

NOTES

I would like to thank Michael Bliss, Alison Prentice, Douglas Ross, and Susan Trofimenkoff for their helpful comments on this introduction. My thanks too to Mrs Doris Lewis and the University of Waterloo Library for their generous assistance.
1 For an excellent discussion of Victorian attitudes see W.E. Houghton, *The Victorian Frame of Mind* (New Haven 1957).

2 For perhaps the most famous Victorian example see M.R.D. Foot, ed., *The Gladstone Diaries* vols. I, II (Oxford 1968).

3 I.E. Davey, 'Trends in Female School Attendance in Mid-Nineteenth Century Ontario,' *Social History/Histoire sociale* VIII (Nov. 1975), 253

4 See Alison Prentice, 'The Feminization of Teaching' in A. Prentice and Susan Trofimenkoff, *The Neglected Majority* (Toronto 1977).

5 For Canada see the pioneering study by Michael Katz, *The People of Hamilton, Canada West* (Cambridge and London 1975). The urban focus precludes attention to the boarding arrangements of the rural schoolteacher. Nevertheless, Katz's description of 'a stage of semi-autonomy, which provided not only a convenient living arrangement for young people away from home but also a supervised environment in which to take the first step toward the independence that would arrive with marriage' (257) appears an apt characterization of the situation facing many young instructors. More research needs to be done, however, before the relationship of the life cycle to teachers' housing patterns can be fully appreciated.

6 See N.L. McClung, *Clearing in the West* (Toronto 1935).

7 Nothing is yet available on the importance of friendship networks for women in Victorian Canada but Carroll Smith-Rosenberg's 'The Female World of Love and Ritual: Relations between Women in Nineteenth-Century America,' *Signs* vol. 1, no. 1 (Autumn 1975), 1–29 may be usefully consulted together with Nancy F. Cott, *The Bonds of Womanhood* (New York and London 1977), ch. 5.

8 On this development in the United States see Barbara Welter, 'The Feminization of American Religion: 1800–1860,' in Mary Hartman and Lois W. Banner, eds., *Clio's Consciousness Raised* (New York 1974) and K.K. Sklar, *Catharine Beecher: A Study in American Domesticity* (New Haven and London 1973). In Canada the relationship between feminism and Christianity has yet to be fully explored, but a pioneering study by Wendy Mitchinson, 'Canadian Women and Church Missionary Societies in the Nineteenth Century: A Step Towards Independence,' *Atlantis* vol. 2, no. 2, pt. II (Spring 1977), 57–75, offers valuable insights.

9 Queen's University, Douglas Library, Adam Shortt Papers, Box 9, J. Webb to Elizabeth Smith, April 13, 1877 and F. Fowler to E. Smith, June 21, 1877.

10 'Female Physicians,' *Canada Medical Journal* (Montreal) VI, (June 1870), 570

11 See, for instance, 'An Ontario High School Teacher,' 'The Average Health of Our Girls,' *The Educational Monthly of Canada* IX (May 1887), 208–10.

12 'Girl Doctors,' *Canada Medical Record* (Montreal) vol. 16, p. 349

13 For a description of this ideal see Barbara Welter, 'The Cult of True Womanhood,' *American Quarterly* XVIII (Summer 1966), 151–74.

14 'The Education of Women,' *Queen's College Journal* Feb. 10, 1871, p. 5

15 See Martin Meissner, 'Sexual Division of Labour and Inequality: Labour and Leisure,' in Marylee Stephenson, ed., *Women in Canada* (Toronto 1977).

16   For example, 'Medicus,' 'Over-Production of Medical Men,' *Canada Lancet* XXIV (Dec. 1892); 'The Overcrowding of the Medical Profession,' ibid., XXV (Jan. 1893); 'Overcrowded Professions,' *Canada Medical Record* vol. 23 (1894–5), 142–3; 'Overcrowded Professions,' *The Canadian Medical Practitioner* XVIII (Feb. 1893).

17   See 'Female Physicians,' *Canada Medical Journal* VI (June 1870), 570.

18   'Co-Education,' *Canada Medical Record* (June 1890), 215

19   See Noel and José Parry, *The Rise of the Medical Profession* (London, 1876), ch. 8, for a discussion of the relationship between midwifery and female doctors in the British context. See also Jane B. Donegan, 'Man-Mid-Wifery and the Delicacy of the Sexes,' in Carol George, ed., *'Remember the Ladies' New Perspectives on Women in American History* (Syracuse 1975).

20   For a discussion of professionalization see Elizabeth MacNab, *A Legal History of Health Professions in Ontario* (Toronto 1970), ch. 2, and W.G. Rothstein, *American Physicians in the Nineteenth Century* (Baltimore and London 1972), ch. 16.

21   See M.V. Royce, 'Arguments Over the Education of Girls – Their Admission to Grammar Schools in this Province' *Ontario History* LXVII (Dec. 1975), 1–13.

22   The difference between salaries of male and female teachers is typical. For a sample of the relative wages see Prentice, 'The Feminization of Teaching,' p. 58.

23   Jennie Kidd Trout, for instance, operated the Therapeutic and Electrical Institute in Toronto between 1877 and 1882. For a useful examination of the irregulars which calls attention to their attitude to women see Joseph Kett, *The Formation of the American Medical Association* (New Haven 1968), chs. 4 and 5. Unfortunately the only analysis of the Canadian situation is John A. Lee, *Sectarian Healers and Hypnotherapy* (Toronto 1970) which despite often useful information concentrates almost entirely on the 1960s.

24   See Carol Lopate, *Women in Medicine* (Baltimore 1968) and Kate Campbell Hurd-Mead, *Medical Women of America* (New York 1933). The best study of women in U.S. medicine is Mary Roth Walsh, *'Doctors Wanted: No Women Need Apply'. Sexual Barriers in the Medical Profession, 1835–1975* (New Haven and London 1977).

25   For a useful description of these women see C. Hacker, *The Indomitable Lady Doctors* (Toronto 1974).

26   See 'Medical School for Women,' *Canada Medical and Surgical Journal* (Montreal) XI (March 1883) 508.

27   Pioneer Athenian woman doctor whose right to practise medicine was defended by the women of her city in the fourth century B.C.

28   'Agnodice,' 'Letters on the Education and Employment of Women,' *The Educational Monthly of Canada* (May–June 1879), 275

29   Ibid. (April 1879), 292

30 See the argument in 'The Place of Women in Society,' *Queen's College Journal* (Jan. 24, 1883), 95.

31 For a typical example of this argument see Agnes Maule Machar, 'Ladies' Corner. The Higher Education of Women,' *Queen's College Journal* (Feb. 14, 1890), 115–17.

32 Mrs H. Cleland Mackenzie, M.D., 'Women in Medicine,' National Council of Women of Canada *Yearbook* (1900), 174

33 University of Waterloo, Elizabeth Smith Shortt Papers, Elizabeth Smith Shortt, 'Inaugural Lecture on Being Appointed Lecturer on Jurisprudence.'

34 See Mrs Dr Felton, 'A Woman's Sound Plea,' *British Whig* (Kingston) April 11, 1890.

35 Mrs Ashley Carus-Wilson, *The Medical Education of Women* (Montreal 1895), 19–20

36 Ch. Fuhrer, *The Mysteries of Montreal. Being the Recollections of a Female Physician* (Montreal 1881), 7

37 See Smith Shortt Papers, Maggie Dixon to Elizabeth Smith, Feb. 5, 1882. This letter describes the writer's fear of childbirth and includes the only half facetious remark, 'I hope when you graduate you'll invent some means of bringing children artificially into the world.'

38 Smith Shortt Papers, Elizabeth Beatty to Elizabeth Smith, Jan. 5, 1881. See also the condemnation of male obstetrical practices in Herbert M. Little, M.D., 'An Address on Obstetrics during the Past Twenty-Five Years,' *Canadian Medical Association Journal* XIV (Oct. 1924) 903–8.

39 For a contemporary's account of female medical missionaries see H.B. Montgomery, *Western Women in Eastern Lands* (New York 1911). See also Strong-Boag, 'Canada's Women Doctors: Feminism Constrained,' in L. Kealey ed., *A Not Unreasonable Claim* (Toronto 1979).

40 See the claim in 'Higher Education,' *British Whig*, June 12, 1883.

41 Queen's University, Douglas Library, Adam Shortt Papers, Box 9

42 Adam Shortt Papers, Box 9, E. Stowe to E. Smith, July 2, 1879

43 Smith Shortt Papers, A. McGillivray to E. Smith, Oct. 24, 1880

44 Smith Shortt Papers, J. Trout to E. Smith, Nov. 9, 1880

45 'Medical Co-education a Failure,' *Queen's College Journal* Dec. 21, 1882

46 For a lengthier presentation of Grant's views on female education see Grant, 'Education and Co-Education,' *The Canadian Monthly and National Review* III (Nov. 1879(509–18, reprinted in *The Proper Sphere*, W. Mitchinson and R. Cook, eds. (Toronto 1976), 124–35.

47 *British Whig*, June 9, 1883

48 'Woman's Medical College' (Toronto *Globe*), *British Whig*, June 14, 1883

49 Smith Shortt Papers, J. Trout to E. Smith, May 29, 1883

50 For an analysis of Queen's graduates together with those of the Toronto College see Strong-Boag, 'Canada's Women Doctors.'

51 For a revealing examination of Adam Shortt which concentrates on his role as a 'prototype liberal empiricist' but largely ignores his personal life see

S.E.D. Shortt, *The Search for An Ideal* (Toronto and Buffalo 1976), ch. 6.

52 Smith Shortt Papers, Elizabeth Smith Shortt to mother and sister, April 14, 1895

53 Ibid., undated (probably April 1898)

54 Ibid., May 7, 1899

55 Ibid., May 17 (?), 1898

56 Ibid., May 27 (?), 1904

57 For an excellent discussion of the faith in such association see B. Harrison, 'For Church, Queen and Family: The Girls' Friendly Society 1874–1920,' *Past and Present* (Nov. 1973), 107–38.

58 See R. Stamp, 'Adelaide Hoodless,' in R. Patterson, J. Chalmers, and J. Frieson, eds., *Profiles of Canadian Educators* (Toronto 1974).

59 For a typical expression of Elizabeth's faith in this education see Smith Shortt Papers, 'Domestic Science' (longhand) speech before the Kingston School Board (n.d.).

60 Ibid., 'My Dear Girls,' Talk to Queen's Students, Jan. 18, 1899

61 Ibid., 'Education and Responsibilities' (undated speech)

62 Ibid., Smith Shortt to mother and sister, July 9, 1905

63 For an indication of her influence see 'Mrs. Adam Shortt Leads Canadian Women in National Thought,' *Everywoman's World* 8 (Jan. 1918), 12, 19, and 'Canadian Women in the Public Eye,' *Saturday Night*, Nov. 29, 1919, p. 25.

64 See Dr Helen MacMurchy, *Sterilization? Birth Control?* (Toronto 1934).

65 Smith Shortt Papers, 'Open Letter to National Council of Women,' c. 1926

66 For a detailed examination of this legislation see Strong-Boag, ' "Wages for Housework": Mothers' Allowances and the Beginnings of Social Security in Canada,' *Journal of Canadian Studies* 14, no. 1 (Spring 1979), 24–34

67 Smith Shortt, NCWC *Yearbook* (1913), 95–6

68 Smith Shortt, 'Report on Mothers' Pensions,' NCWC *Yearbook* (1915), 225–8

69 See Jill Conway's provocative and enlightening discussion of the failure of professional women in the United States to stem the wave of Freudian-influenced thinking, 'Women Reformers and American Culture, 1870–1930,' *Journal of Social History* 5 (Winter 1971–2), 164–77.

70 For a discussion of the less optimistic post-war mood and its results for one woman's organization see Strong-Boag, *The Parliament of Women: The National Council of Women of Canada* (Ottawa 1976), ch. 8.

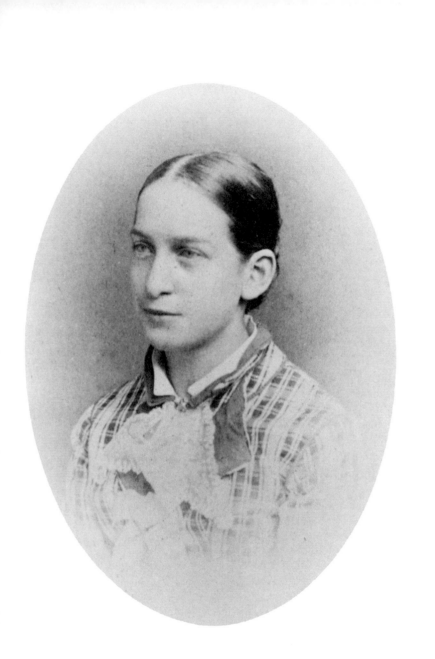

Elizabeth Smith, age sixteen

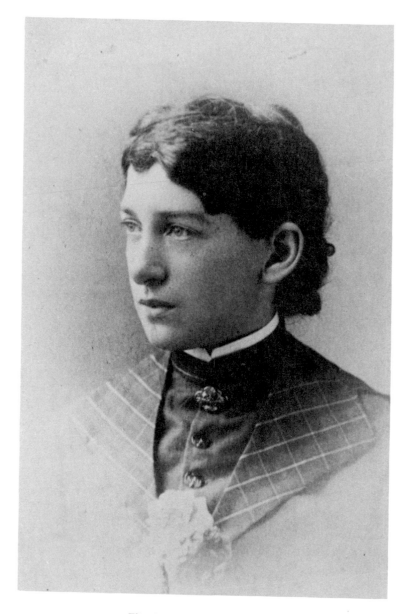

Elizabeth Smith, about 1880

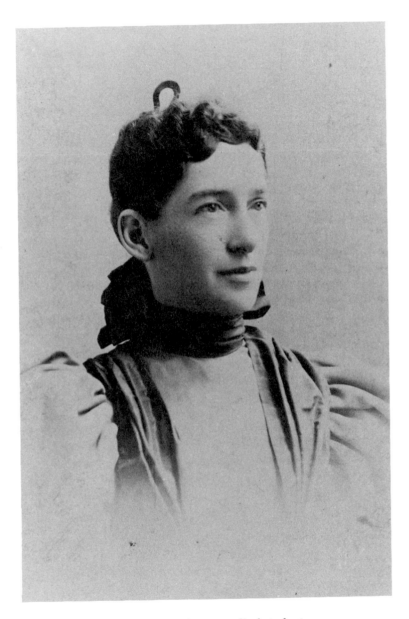

Elizabeth Smith as a medical student

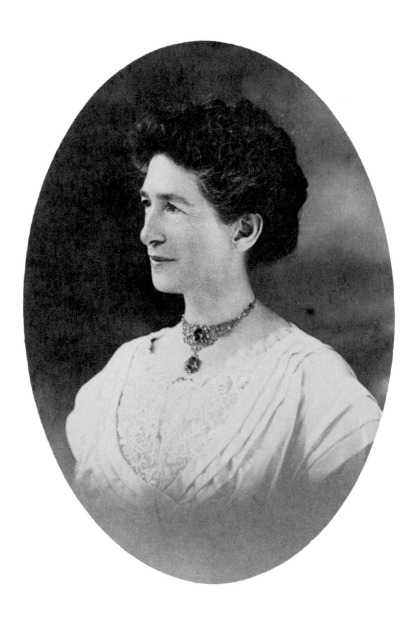

Elizabeth Smith Shortt, about 1912

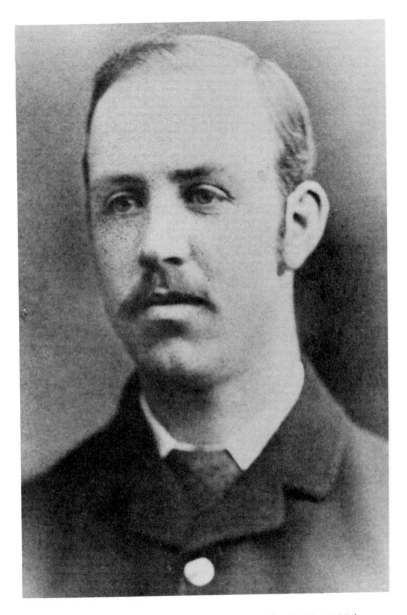

The young Adam Shortt, date unknown (probably 1880s)

'A WOMAN WITH A PURPOSE'

1

Winona, Ontario
June 1872 to January 1875

The diaries of Elizabeth Smith begin on her family's farm in
south-western Ontario. After a series of intermittent entries characterized often by youthful errors of spelling and style, they
first end just after the author's graduation at fifteen from the
local school. Like so many other diarists, Elizabeth is preoccu-
pied with family and local concerns: the death of a grandfather,
the visits of friends, the tedium of school, and the illness of her
brother. Only very occasionally are there hints that the high-
spirited girl looks beyond her own small community. The solid
prosperity of the Smiths, which is evident in their ownership of
a piano and in the education given their eldest children, Mauritana and Ernest, provides the essential foundation for Elizabeth's
future exploration beyond the rich fruit-growing lands of her
parents' farm.

1872

Elizabeth   Elizabeth   Elizabeth
My Diary Elizabeth Smith

June 2nd.

We were down at the Fifty Church today it was not full. I sat
with two of the Magill gents. Martins are very glad to see us now

since we've got the piano & house. One would not care much for such friends, as 'Grace Glen' says its Pa's money that makes the friends. Mary Lawrence was to visit Ellen today, they think that dress is all that is needed to dress in the height of fashion is their highest ambition & to catch a bean [beau] is all they want. Pshaw! Cecil[1] is a good boy sometimes but a bad one more often. I am afraid he will be the black sheep of this flock I better stop writing for Cecil is tormenting me.

June 4th

I was so sleepy I could not write last night. I was to School yesterday and I was chief cook & bottle washer. Pa's money again, Baby's name was registered today Violet Smith[2] why it looks good in writing. It rained today & only Gertie[3] went to school.

June 6th

A man was ... here again today they are working the roads today. Pa has ten days [of work on township roads] this year I have not much use of a diary now it is the same thing over & over same day & every day.

June 6th [sic]

What will I be doing a year from now, today I made Luthé a calico skirt & was watching the baby. They are now working the roads tonight. I wish Pa would get us a set of croquay.

1 Cecil Brunswick Smith, 1865–1912, civil engineer
2 Violet Bernice Smith, 1872–1954
3 Gertrude Smith, 1861–?, teacher

5 June 1872 to January 1875

June 9th

We (that is M.[4] G. Pa & I, ma seldom goes) were over at St.
Georges today & there was a baby christened Angus Mentfred
Muir son of Mr Watson Muir. Good night young diary, your
more a note book than a diary.

June 10th

Victor Harvey commenced working here last monday, it don't
take long to make a hired man or boy forward now when he
came here he would stop in the kitchen but now he goes straight
to the dining room & sits on the sofa what is the world coming
to; there must be a change, somewhere. We have plenty of rain it
has been very showery today. I think I will try & write better
tomorrow night. good night night night

June 11th

Aunt Hannah (that is Pa's Aunt) came here today she is now 76
years of age what a great many things she has seen in her lifetime & what will I see if I live to that old age

June 13th

It has been raining very hard today. It is the same routine of
washing dishes every, three times a day as I am staying home
this spring & the other girls go to school.

June 14th

... Pa was to Hamilton today & Ma got the curtains for the parlor ...

4 Mauritana Smith, 1856–1946

June 15th

The children came home this forenoon & said there was to be no school for a week. Jane Redelle's birthday is on the 12th of this month. We were up at Mount Lion yesterday. Mr MacIntire preached for the last time.

June 17th

Ma finished my brilliant dress today & Pa took Aunt Hannah & I down to grandpa's. Aunt was here nine days. Gertie has been quite sick today with a break out on her legs and they were swelled.

June 20th

I was to tired to write last night & night before & day before yesterday. Gertie was sick & the doctor was here & I went to stay with Rebecca while Mr & Mrs Harvey went to Hamilton. Yesterday Grandpapa brought Miss E. Rymal & Miss Mary Smith after tea they are nice girls. My long promised company was here today that is J.A. & S. Bedell & James Talman came after dinner. Jamie & Adah staid more than five hours the first time in two years they are queer children. Thomas Talman is a nice boy to my notion

June 21st

Pa Mauritana Miss Smith & Miss Rymal went down to the Fifty [Church] in the forenoon & they & I went up to Mount Lion in the afternoon.

7 June 1872 to January 1875

June 23rd

Miss Rymal & Miss Smith went home on the eight Oclock train
& Miss Lily Maggie & Fannie Wray were here this afternoon
they are lively girls they flatter & blarnie.

June 30th

Dear me! I've not written for five days. Last Wednesday I was
down to Mr Wesley Smiths in the afternoon alone & Friday I
went to Hamilton to go to the Examination they could not get
the Hall that night so they had it in the School. Ernest[5] won the
scholarship of twenty dollars last Thursday. Pa got the large hay
fork at Grimsby & today Pa & Ma went down to Granpas to pay
them a visit. George Rilet is here now.

July 10

We went to a temperance picnic on dominion day yesterday Pa
went to Council & brought home the Smiths & Ernest [with]
them the same day & I went after Pa up as far as the shed.

July 11th

Ma hung the curtains today

July 21st

Dear me I have not written any since the 11th. Mauritana &
Ernest went to the Menagerie on the 12th of this month. Ernest
has been sick for about 2 weeks with the sore throat

5 Ernest Disraeli Smith, 1853–1948, Conservative M.P. 1900–4, 1905–8, Senator
   1913–46, and founder of the E.D. Smith preserve business.

25 August

We (that is Pa & Ma G & I & Violet were down to St. Catherines on the fifth of this month & Ernest went back to school the 20 of this month & the rest EXCEPT ME ME are going to start to school tomorrow. I have to stay home to take care of the baby. We were down to the Fifty church to day & I saw some for the first time in a long while

Sep 4th

I was to visit the school today & saw Jessie Beemer for the first time queer girl & Ma & G went down to Wesley Smiths to tea

Sep 29

Pa & us girls were at the Exibition in H[amilton] last Friday. Mr & Mrs Hiram Dewitt & two Mr Mulhollands from Toronto in the evening Miss Rilet & Miss Le Pollard came saturday Grand Pa & Grandma & Mary Pettit came. Mary went down to church with us at the Fifty. Mauritana & Mary stayed down to grandpas & went down to Henrys in the afternoon & M went to school Monday

Oct 10th

On the first of this month Aunt M L & Uncle Jonathan Jensen Williams & wife & Pettit & baby & Aunt Hannah came here John & wife staid all night & that night Mary Michael & Lizzie Cartier came here & staid a little while. boys can see the tavern manners on her she talks so low & laughs so boisterously. That night when pa came home from Hamilton he brought home with him an hired man he is a queer man. Mrs Bedell & Mrs Johnson have a little baby girl. This Bedell was born on the 23 of september.

9 June 1872 to January 1875

Ma & M to town last Saturday & bought M's party costume & *fixens* –

Nov 3rd

the party is over & done with there was about 65 here Pa went after E that day & Dunnings was here for the first time & stayed till Monday. Mary was here also & we had a splendid time. Dick is so funny. M's trimming were pink.

1874 March 8th

Oh, me. Oh me what vast space of time has passed since I last wrote here. Well to commence where I left oft that was a famous winter in the C[hristmas] Holidays. M & E were down at Uncle Johnathans to a party of course they had a good time while gone they got a letter from Dick saying he would be down on the 3 Oclock train but dident come till about the last of Jan & Mary being back from St. Catherines we had a jolly time but previous to this we had a few friends in among which were the Henrys we had a passable good time then. On the 3 of Feb Mauritana & Mary & Dick & Ernest & Pa went to H.; E & D back to school & M & M[ary] to Rymals from there to Uncle Isaac Smiths & then to Marys where Mauritana staid 6 weeks & had a splendid good time going to parties & such like. After she came home we went to school that is G. C. & I of which came of except our little likes & dislikes. On the 23 of May our Aunt Eliza of Buffalo was brought home to be buried at Grimsby & in the fall Aunt Amanda was laid in the mould at Bartonville. Pa went to the Central Show with the rest & from that time has been ailing last November M went away to the W.F. College[6] and came home on

6 Wesleyan Female College: Wesleyan Ladies' College, a Methodist institution founded in 1861, the first college chartered for the separate education of girls

the 7 of Feb only one term. Ernest went back to school after Christmas but his eyes failed him & so he went to Dr Bethune in Toronto twice & keeps puting leeches on his eyes & has to stop at home & doctor them. Dick has not been here since last Easter when he & Pierce Aniles came down & we had a good time. Last fall we had a small Croquet party & since then L. Hagar has wedded a fair country rustic L. Biggar & also Murray Petit has doubled himself by means of E.H. Fuller of Grand Rapids M[ichigan]. D. Burkholder married R. Walker and he went to Texas but came back as poor as he went. Martins have gone to H. to live. Grand Pa died on the 25 of Febuary at his own home, at his funeral all his children were present after he was buried the same day Aunt Henriette & Aunt Hannah came here & the day before Uncle & Aunt Emmet were here & today we expect Aunt Catherine & Uncle Dan from Grandpas ... Pa has been gone since friday and to H. as he is one of Grand Pa's E[xecutors] ... Ada's Grand father died about the same time as Grandpa did he left $500 to buy a bell for some church we haven't heard the rest of his will. ...

March 20th

Pa came back on Tuesday and a while after Aunt Catherine was here she is a fine looking woman for her time of life certainly, she said Ransom was coming here in the spring. I was to Hamilton last Saturday with Pa & Ma & got our summer dresses 11 yds for my dress & will have to send for more & I also got my tooth filled which was awefull awefull he had such a dreadful machine & almost killed me it hurts yet. Ma & Pa were up at Glovers today & the roads were very bad, but are drying quite rapidly. This is the most remarkable springtime. For [how] many remember no snow in March, hardly any this winter. They are preparing for an examination down at our school on the last day of M[arch] I expect to go and after to go to school if the roads will permit. Ellen has gone to H. I dont know what to do. Ernest is

sick now & his eyes are bad bad. I do so hope they will get
well. ... I hope all will be well at last. Oh! dear. Oh! dear. Oh!
dear dear a b c d e f

...

March 22nd

Sunday evening quiet & peaceful within doors but lately without
it was terrific. A storm of snow & rain passed over & after the
sun came brightly out. Robbie didnot come as we expected. We
did not go to church today for we lacked our mourning costume.
Silly Silly Simon

March 25

The day before yesterday Mr & Mrs W. Smith came here about
halfpast twelve & about 3Oclock went home taking M & I along
with them to play on their new piano which is a Thomas & the
price was 600$ but they got it for 500 for paying cash it is a mag-
nificent one beautiful toned & such a beautiful outside, such
carving. Mr T. Pettit brought us home about 8 or 9 Oclock having spent a nice afternoon. ...

27 of March

... In to play with V. Ernest's eyes are a little better to day, I am
very glad of it. Another acquisition to our house hold in the person of (Old Dave) Two men servents now wish we had another.
I would like to see somebody[7] very very much has been a long
time since I saw him nearly a year.

7 Dick

March 28th

Saturday night the work done & a quiet long evening before me. The Accessors were here to day they were Mr Carscallan & Mr Tinesdale.[8] Ernest was assessed for the first time. John Brown went away to day for he said he had sore hands but I offer different reasons for the acessors said he was a worthless drunkard as is also his wife part of the time in jail & drunk, enough said. Ma sent by James Pettit for the remainder of my dress & got it, if I may use so homely an expression. Mr Sweet was here to hire to night but they made no bargain. I am more than half through *Peviril of the Peak*[9] & like it exceedingly how determined must have been Sarah's will to remain mute so long & how sad not to have her love returned while Alice B. loved & was loved through all dangers & became happy at last. How great & large must have been Scot the novelist's genius, good night & hope of warmer weather & better writing.

March 29th

Sunday night. We did not go to church today dresses not done or any one to take us. I invented a plan of making a small album today of small heads or pictures. George Rilet was here this evening to tea was up at Harveys to send a letter to the post. Quite cold yet without snow I really did resist the temptation of reading *Peveril* today although it went against the grain. Had no quarrels to day & kept in good spirits which I would like to do all the time if possible but it seems almost impossible so many crosses during the day. Vio is a perfect little beauty is perfectly lovely stop stop all has given out pen ink & brain

---

8 County tax assessors
9 novel by Sir Walter Scott

March 30th

Nothing of importance has happened to day or anything at all worth saying over. Ernest eyes are better but Pa seems worse to night. Mr Harvey was here to night for a call. Well I think (there tis again now telling what I think) I had better not have written tonight for if any one should see it (Which I hope to Goodness will never happen) they would think but never mind what they would think there now stop stop. Adieu A−L−A−S

...

Good Friday 3 of April

My dress is finished & Gertie's begun. Joel Lee was here to day to play with Cecil & a man was here requesting lodging for the night. Mr & Mrs Bedell called here to day he on business ...

Easter Sunday April 5th

P[a] M. G. & I were down at the Fifty to the Methodist meeting. Hatie Marlatt was there & Hettie Martin, a large number present it has snowed since we came home & now the ground is completely covered quite a depth almost sleighing. There is four day meeting now. We all wore our new dresses today ...

April 8th

Ma & Cecil were up at Thomases today & this after noon G & I went after them. they have a new organ 'princes' Gusta is going to take lessons as soon as they get a teacher ...... teacher, bah.

April 26th

It has been hoyty toitie since last I wrote I have been going to school for two weeks when I could. G & I are taking music lessons of Miss Van Wagnor & so is Gustie. We just take lessons on saturday. Last night we had an awful fright the first I knew 1 Oclock was M. standing at running at the door yelling murder & help & then we yelled at Ernie awful till we woke him & M told him to get the gun for robbers were killing Pa & he have about 3 leaps down stairs & no robbers to be seen but Ma had fainted & fell out of bed & Pa leaped out to help her ... my pen runs scratching new events

Nov 29th

Ma G & Ernest were at H. yesterday & Ernest was to see Dr. Roseburgs & he gave him no hope But said they would get worse but that he would get him a pair of Spectacles at Toronto for about 10 dollars. Ma got a set of dinner dishes & knives & silver forks & our present to make for Christmas. Oh! the long long summer what joys & sorrows, fun & quarrels especially at school but now it's all right there for I have it as I like most of the time. Aggie Geddes had Jessie & Jane Gertie & I there all night last week & we had a splendid time. The last day of school Friday (this is Sunday) we had a game of ball Levi Stewart Levi Dean & a Biggar boy were there we had fun fun fun & we had a spelling match Egbert & I chose I had altogether the best side had his all over have not finished it yet four up on our side 2 on theirs. Oh the summer summer in the beginning of the Holidays I had a party of school scholars & before May Allen staid a week & was here then. They are not of much account, scorn the country people except to sponge on in summer. And after the party who should be here one night when I came in but Master Dick & oh the good good times we had we went to the White Church's quarterly meeting Sunday & this fall Oh my one night when we came home from school there laid Dick's hat on the table how he

surprised me I thought him in Toronto he had been there &
passed an examination but came back to learn the result & after
he found very successful while he was here Him M & I went to
Johnsons & Station after Amanda & Mary from Falkland he went
away the next day & the next Uncle & Aunt Pettit brought cousin Jane & two children from Buffalo dident we enjoy ourselves
Manda is a dear good girl but Mary is I think a little affected
with laziness & seems to take the place of their darling Anna that
died, she is to be a teacher. They went to the central fair with us
& then to the station. We were at two picnic this both at the
same place although the last was the best by all means, staid in
the evening at Mr P. Van Wagners till about 3 in the morning we
got home safe & came after having spent a gay evening. This
month or last, Eddie & Addie Rymal were here came on Sunday
& staid till Tuesday Ed took Gertie & I to school that morning I
was so disgusted with them. He likes kissing in the dark better
than anything, I think & she well she's a well almost a fool as far
as boys are concerned & such a know nothing. Him & I together
broke a croquet mallet. Murray Pettit has a young heir to his
property so has Andrew Carpenter a daughter. Oh alack I had
near forgotten My cousin Anna Pettit has married John Muir a
lawyer of H. & she is living there now. Oh such a grand wedding
as she had & did not ask M or Ernest but Pa & Ma & they dident
go. She had two coachs from town for to drive to the church for
her & bridesmaids. Lizzie Mayhore married William Thomas last
week & she is about 16 near 17 years of age such folly such igno-
rance such nonsense he two years older I think I heard

Catilena

There's not a song that trembles
    Around my heart tonight
But thrills with untold gladness
    And eloquent delights
For I have cast the shadows
    Of sorrows all aside

To let hopes joyous music
  Through all my being glide
To let hopes joyous music
  Through all my being glide

Then sweetly dream
Dream on.....Dream on   } Chorus
Nor breathe a single sigh }
To wake the gently zephyr
That fans the starlit sky
To wake the gently zypher

And there is not a tearstain
  Upon my eyelids now   Mine
Nor yet a shade to ruffle   Yes I love you
  The spirits sunny flow   Yes I do
Life seemeth Oh! so joyous   Yes I love you
  So blithsome & so light   This is true
Like some long dream of summer   Beth
  That haunts a winters night
Like some long dream of summer
  That haunts a winters night

Like rosy childhood playing
Among the early flowers
My happy heart is straying
On sunny footed hours
Perhaps I may be dreaming
When I my ills forget
Break not this blissful seeming
Oh do not wake me yet
Break not this blissful seeming
Oh do not awake me yet

...

Confirmation was held in Stony Creek school house & there were about 15 confirmed among them there was Edith Van Wagner & Miss humble self. Mr. Wadleigh was our vicar at the time & is still & is likely to before some time. They are buying an organ for St. Georges church him & Miss Taylor I hope they will succeed with all speed. Snow lies about 8 or 10 inches in depth the first snow of the season of any account.

Dec 6th

Another week has gone very wearily to me for I have had a cold the entire time, & now am just able to keep up. I was poorly yesterday but worked at the Xmas present I have three done & last night in the evening I composed this piece of poetry if it can be called by that name

On Leaving School

Oh goodbye friends & schoolmates
How happy I have been
Here among desks & books & slates
How many hours I have seen

How many errors have been made
Within these dear old walls
How many lessons wrongly said
And many mistakes by all

How many changing joys and sorrows
Here known to both girls & boys
Good resolutions made for tomorrow
Breaking, finding more sorrows than joy

And our right true & worthy teacher
That has taught so long & well

Comes extremely near to Mr Beecher
For eloquence (If I may tell)

Remember me you dear old scholars
When you & I are far from here
If beyond this world of cts & dollars
Then drop for each a kindly tear

Once more goodbye old friends & schoolmates
In things of life we'll mend
And in appointments being never late
Will ever cling closer to friends

By *Beth*

Tired Tired Tired Tired
And needing a straight
Jacket I remain
yours in a
        Nutshell

1874   oh my   1874   beloved

Dec 20th

Well, let me see. I suppose any person seeing this would say
'greatest event of her life was leaving school & stirring her up to
this trivial pice of poetry.' well I say, I don't expect to let any one
see this – so no matter. Well I have done going to the district
school & left kind thought I think behind me well I'm careless
and well there I go again I do believe I've said well 5 times since I
commenced. I had a good time the last day I went Sarah T. was
not there. Jessie is a loving little duck, almost cried, she did.
There I'm getting silly never mind ...

19 June 1872 to January 1875

New years day. 1875

Xmas is past once more I enjoyed it. I got a book, ribbon bows, music, apron (nice one) two pictures, cuffs, nice pen & candy of course & all the rest got accordingly after we had looked at our presents we went as we were invited to Mr William Smiths to dinner & staid till dark. Mr W. Rent & two sisters Miss Grant, Mr Pettit & Mr Tyneck & we had a jolly time. Miss Grant & the Rents were [from] Hamilton & he is a splendid player on the violin & took quite a fancy to me there! I hope your shocked I want you to be. We had a splendid dinner roast turkey & beef, honey cakes pies fruit, of different kinds in plenty. The Rents are very rich but not wonderful handsome especially the girls. Last Sunday Josephine Carpenter came home from the Fifty Church with us & staid to dinner & we went to church in the school-house in the afternoon & she went home from there she's a queer specimen of human nature appears mixed up in the upper story of her cranium. Wednesday Aunt Martha & Ambrose & Herbert were here first time. Brose has been since Myrties party Oh by the way Dick had a party on Xmas eve & invited Ernie there but he did not go on account of misunderstanding & last night we got a letter from D & said he was going to London till the ninth of Jan. ...

Jan 3rd

Sunday morning Ma & M & Ernest are gone to Mr Gersham Carpenter's funeral (Franklin's father) at the Fifty [Church]. Snow on the ground but not sleighing drifted yesterday. On New years day Uncle R was here also Mr & Mrs Talman in the evening. Mr James Smith left Mr McNeilly 25 acres of land by virtue of his wife being his daughter & to Lib $300 beside a lot of household stuff. Mary wrote if we would come up & me to stay awhile she would come home with us. I do hope ma will let me. I write this kneeling by the table & Vio jogging me. I will build castles in the air now.

Jan 10th

I am, well yes, that's so too, that's so too, he is that's a fact too as far as I know. I wish could see that third person singular. hmm! ha! yes! Aunt Hannah came here last Sunday & staid till Friday & Ernest took her home & brought Ellen up & she is here now. I read a story by the Margeret Catchpole a Suffolk girl, fearful cold day today froze even oil in a lamp last night. Adieu

Jan 22

Wonder! Monday E Henry was here in the evening and we expected Ida Mercy & Albert but they did not come. Myrtie & Edgar, oh, la, such fun. And Tuesday E. M. & I went as appointed to Hugo Carpenters & met Mr W. Walker & Blanche Laura M & Miss Howland there (sister of Mrs Kings & we had a nice time. Gab. Tuesday we Ernest I mean got a letter from Dick he is at Toronto University talks of being a lawyer Oh dear & asked if Cecil had fallen asleep again oh the fun we had that day playing Croquet enough said bye bye.

Jan 24th

Sunday. It is snowing now & we have good sleighing. Friday Mr A. Lee & wife & Maggie were here & Saturday Mr & Mrs & Daisy were here last night were invited to a party at Hugo Carpenters to be on Tuesday next I am to wear a long dress for the first time. I think I guess Ma will go to Hamilton tomorrow. We have finished reading 'Jappet in Search of a Father' one of Cpt Marryat's,[10] a very silly book. he shed so many tears & talked like a schoolboy. Oh goodbye old diary forever. I will not lose you though ...

10 Frederick Marryat, *Japhet in Search of a Father* (1835)

2

Speyside, Ontario
January to December 1878

At age nineteen, now an ambitious, religious, and sometimes self-righteous teacher at a small rural school, Elizabeth resumes her diaries. The problems of boarding with strangers and coping with an ungraded class fill up the days of the inexperienced Elizabeth. The strain of such a life regularly exhausted and discouraged female teachers who had few occupational alternatives. As the entries indicate, the homesick girl fluctuates between moments of satisfaction with her social and professional successes and despair over slights, real or imagined, by friends and the examiners of the Ontario College of Physicians and Surgeons. Both flirtatious and introspective, she frequently seems very much a teenager, but she has moved a long way from the young girl who last wrote in Winona. Her determination to leave her mark beyond small-town Ontario and her growing recognition of woman's special predicament are now setting the stage for a more unconventional second career.

Jan. 18th. 1878

'The hopes that dance around a life
Whose charms have but begun'

Yes that's it, although I have breathed the air of this mundane sphere for the space of nineteen years this day; yet life has but

fairly started in the true meaning during the past few months. I
am now as it were but learning to go alone, to rely on my own
efforts to make or mar my 'shroud of sentient clay' always be it
understood subservient to a higher – a Supreme Being. Placed as
I am – far from friends and home – in an unknown part of the
country – teaching a country school with the dreariest of dreary
weather – where everything conspires to point with home-sick
finger to the homelike past – as a mid-night wanderer to the
faded glory of the recent sunset – is it probable that I should
write those words in wilful hypocrisy – no never it is but an
inkling of what I feel. I thank God for my religion – it is my rock
of strength it has never failed me yet – it never will. Crying is as
great a mystery to me as dreaming – I can't understand it.

Men, I believe abhor it, they feel decidedly queer when they
see it. They imagine it to be effeminate nay babyish as to themselves. Though why we should all be so prone to give way to
tears when moved to gentle moods by the misery of others, our
own hopes and disappointments and the knocking of the Holy
Spirit in shape of religion at the door of our hearts. – I cannot
tell. When alone among strangers – in trials of mind and body
when the mind flashes homeward thinking 'how they would feel
for me now', then the floodgates of my eyes want to open no
matter where I am. Now I have about as much disgust for that
pusilanimous piece of conduct – crying as any male monster
could well have and yet, if I must I must and – well. I've cried
once since I've been in this wilderness of discontent but twas of
short duration and before I was nineteen ... So I'll cut for a new
deal and if I commit any such nonsensical thing in a twelve-
month I'll surely have to record it.

Jan. 20th.

Better than grandeur better than gold
Or rank or titles a hundred-fold
Is a healthful body a mind at ease
And simple pleasures that always please

23 January to December 1878

Yesterday Miss Brown[1] and I took a walk up to the village of
Speyside. The day was beautiful – so warm and hazy – one of
those delicious spring days which get lost by some manner of
means and show themselves in midwinter – Winter has been
most immoderately moderate so far – fitful of mood one day cold
and cross the next relaxing into such warm smiles that they
would charm a griffen into good humor. At the foot of the hill
stands 'patience' (my school) the needful. Whether to battle with
the world or to live secluded from the world the true companion
of ambition – we gradually ascend – after the top of the first hill
is gained – and pass through a long beautiful avenue with cedars
on either side o'er a level road – on still on as tho' we momentar-
ily expected to reach by the next turn a glimpse of some 'castle
fair' in the midst of a princely domain, on still on till we find our
terminus – such a disappointment ... Is not this an emblem of life
our youth all stretches fair as fairyland before and hope points
ever onward to a beautiful future – which if not laid on the basis
of Christianity will inevitably turn to dross – The end will be
blank dispair. And on our return we viewed the paths by which
we came with much diminished fervor and the way was shorter
grown. This was like looking back from old age over the way we
had come which seemed to have been short & uneasy to the
peace which enfolds them now.

Jan. 22nd.

Nothing much to write tonight. This life like most others will
become in some way monotonous. There are some things which
will always prove a mine untold in depth which makes me content. There is no truth like God's truth and no comfort like His.
Experience is a rough master but It proves a sure one of which to
learn that God helps those that help themselves, and if you want
a thing well-done do it yourself. They say a self made man has a
rough fellow for his teacher but they might add a strict one and a
sure one.

1 another teacher at Speyside

I have read of one saying to another in trouble 'go home you have God and your work.' Now that means much – it means all the consolation one needs. It means the best means of forgetfulness. I get through the morning toilet and desultory remarks with the family – and go to my school with the blithe consolation that it is the beginning of another day – that the last has gone and forever. With a quavering voice I go through the opening of the school and I'm sure my voice is very broken and my eyes moist when I finish the Lord's Prayer and raise the desk-lid to conceal my face while I steady my nerves. But duty once begun I hardly know where the minutes have gone when school is done for the day and I am free to my own inclinations, which have not a very bountiful chance of being fulfiled and so the days pass on and they do not know me here and perhaps never may. Perhaps after I quit my teaching here they may never know ['or care to' has been lightly crossed out] my destiny – my kismet –

'Tis only noble to be good.
  Kind hearts are more than coronets
  And simple faith than Norman blood'

Jan. 27th.

Another week has rolled away into the countless weeks of the past. They are slipping away those sweet, swift, days.
Like a leaf on the current cast
With never a break in their rapid flight, flow
We watch them as one by one they go
Into the beautiful past ....
I am truly glad when a day closes & there is no use to deny it to myself for it is so, ... it is a good maxim. 'Be good and you will be happy' and if we could be pure and sinless it would be a 'beautiful past' to look back upon through the vista of by gone years, when I attain to the dignity of gray hairs. And I try – will try to be good as far as in me lies so that whatever the future may have for me I will not regret the past. Though experience is an expert teacher and if we could live our lives twice over we could make it

better if we would but how many would? 'Put not your trust in
princes' nor in any man when money is in question. Yesterday
Mr. McNaughton took me to Georgetown – where I purchased a
clock and rented a Melodeon – as I had some pupils promised but
when I reached home the instrument was an old useless thing
that roared continually – It was at the man's house not at the
store or I should have tried it before bringing it. ... Well when I
see mesdames with the children – two boys & a girl regular pests
gradually worrying out their mother's life – of course She is to
blame together with le pere for bringing them up in such a fro-
licsome fashion, I think 'this 'tis to be married ...' and conclude
that my name shall remain what it is unless *strongly* induced and
then I should try to do my duty in that sphere as befits a
mother's holy – mighty – office not bringing them up to be a
thorn in my old age, and an evil to society but a noble mind,
with a brave unfaltering nature to uphold truth for truth's sake
and walk according to God's laws and their own conscience. It
would be worth living for to leave such behind.

The years are creeping slowly by
The winters come & go
The wind sweeps past with mournful cry
And pelts my face with snow.

Jan. 30th.

Yes this year but just begun one twelfth has passed away. Well
thanks to Mr'ssrs McNaughton and McLaughlin who fixed my
melodeon I'm not in such a bad fix after all. The instrument goes
alright now. It is bitter cold tho' there's no snow nor has been
none

Feb. 5th.

Snow now lots of it. Came on Feb. 1st. Went to Milton on Saturday with Miss Brown, had a good – sleigh ride, & talked lots of

nonsense. I do feel less respect for myself after such escapades of folly, but then Better than grandeur better than gold
Or rank or titles a hundred fold
Is a healthful body a mind at ease.
And *simple* pleasures that always please.
Well scandal is truly 'hell-born' as someone said and if there's anything that scalds & sears a woman's spirit it is that dreadful monster scandal Now because I prefered to board for cheaper board – and nearer the schoolhouse the family with whom I boarded at first have notwithstanding their soft-speeches to me about their good-will and perfect indifference as to whether I left or not set the whole neighbourhood in a stir with my name. I wouldn't care one bit but that it may influence some of my music pupils in expectancy. The clash of a lot of ignorant country people, prejudiced & conceited should not trouble a mind of better culture and it shall not mine, tho' tis hard to be talked of where you will never go in a derogatory manner, when it is undeserved –

Feb. 6th

Received a letter from Alice today. It's a truism that friendship is rare but hers is sure and dearly sweet, – One on whom I can trust, One to whom I can confide and be sure of being understood of being sympathised with, dear dear Allie. That is friendship where each put implicit trust on the other – where congenial spirits dwell, where education is, where religion reigns supreme christianizing, purifying, making it sure, even unto death – How I should like to see her, but that's a poor wish as its not likely to be fulfilled very soon and with me must a contented spirit dwell ...

Feb. 16th.

How the time flys the days go by on eagle wings and I am each day coming nearer to the end, that end which some hail for the blessings of immortality others dread as the end of mortality for them no hereafter, no hope, how dreadful the thought! But what a holy happy thought – there will be no more sorrow there, for we shall have all tears wiped from our eyes. What an eager, furious & joyous fight ought we to wage with the world, the flesh and the devil while this probation lasts. What joy to know that at the last we should enter in to everlasting glorious life and hear our Master say Well done good and faithful servant enter thou into the joy of thy Lord. ... My school still goes on in its quiet monotony and my duties are a tread-mill that keeps me from escaping – a spur to keep me going My letters are a source of great comfort to me – rays of sunshine which penetrate through the barriers of distance and make my life more sunny. It is the greatest encouragement for one to have viz, loving friends who are satisfied and take an interest in your well-being & well-doing.

Feb. 24th

Well we are jogging on together 'time and I' and the days we have lived will never be lived by me again. How well we should live them the first and only time we ever may. Went to Milton with Mr. Hampshires today in order to hear once again the loved service of the church. There's another deprivation to be undergone here. No Church of England within 6 or 8 miles & so I go to the Presbyterian, but I love our own church ordinances the best by far. Here's another phase of my *checquered* life riding over bleak country roads with this ruddy cheeked farmer & family – far from any one of my friends and relatives, in order to get to the church of my choice but I hardly think I will do so much again. They are all very kind to me but blood and water will not mix and I cannot, do not wish to forsake the tenets which I have always held since instilled in me by mon mere. Her opinion is a good criterion.

I hope to have courage to *live* my life and not dream it although 'tis sweet to rest in those scenes of life which seem to be provided as resting places along the wayside of life. When I look back to the past at them they seem to have brightened and brighten still with the space time puts between And the future looms up before me holding these bright spots to view as temptations to lure me on and not wish that 'all was ended *now* the hope the joy & sorrow All the aching of heart and restless unsatisfied longing All the dull deep pain and constant anguish of patience' Yes the future seems *very* bright sometimes seems a flowery road to mad ambitious heights and again the way seems long and dark and dreary and all seems wrapt in impenetrable darkness of trouble and toil and pain where the pleasures disappear in the sea of difficulties which overwhelm, & destroy them. But the first – I think is the true the right way and I should be more especially glad that my way is smoothed by a Divine Fatherly care and the help of earthly friends. When I retired for the night and lay dreaming of the future listening to the patter of the rain on the roof then I *can* think and plan best of anywhere. When I think that I am here alone in the midst of many by the world forgotten and the world forgot that at that very moment there are beautiful belles queening it over social gatherings in silks & charm on its the nobility – the ton of the counter or the country house – the laughter and love in bright eyes. The glitter of jewels fair and stirring of satin sheen where all seem happiness with the hidden asp beneath, The robber at his mid-night work. The felon in his cell, the ruined and the lost to honor, love and everything pure and good, The student at his plodding task, the idle the gay the sick the rich & the poor the saved and the lost are all mingling about me, are all hurrying on on in the upward or downward way. That the spark of life is very dear to all no matter how situated, that the little little world on which I live is but a speck in this great world – that the world is wide these things are small they may be nothing 'tho' they are all. ... Oh I cannot express my thoughts they are wild & imaginative they are so quick I cannot follow them And life is all similarly strange. Sometimes I pinch myself to be sure that tis not all a dream here and I will wake to find myself in my dear old home one among the old familiar faces. And my dreams are so real so lifelike they help me to like the rest of the night more than if it

were mere oblivion. And that oblivion is another strange
unaccountable fact we could not live without that sweet entire
absolution from care and things of life In fact were that oblivion
less than oblivion we could not exist and tis all a fabrication that
'by manly mind not even in sleep is well resigned.' And such
will be the last sleep only dreamless unending to this weary body
and a new life of untold unspeakable joy for the soul.

'Whether tis nobler in the mind to suffer
The slings and arrows of outrageous fortune
Or to take up arms against a sea of trouble
And by opposing end them – to end
The heartache and the thousand natural shocks
That flesh is heir to, tis a consummation
Devoutly to be wished.'

March 3rd.

Time does pass in some unaccountable manner and 'dat ish
goot.' A letter from home does have a decided tendency to cheer
me up. Life seems more endurable when there are persons taking
an interest in your welfare, in your every movement and 'tis
more than stimulating to love some one whose approval you
desire and will struggle to attain as more valuable than money. I
wrote a long letter home and to Ella dear spirituelle little Ella
What a strange girl she is and how touching her words of depreciation of herself 'I can't be good' 'I don't want to be' Was at
church today but behaved very badly. I really did try to get
interested in what he was saying but it was no use and the best I
can say is that I did not go to sleep. Why cannot ministers of the
Gospel put some life into their words and not be talking at cross
purposes all the time. If they cant do this, if they do not feel their
words why do they mar the chance of some one else doing good
in the pulpit which they fill I know we cannot expect eloquence
in all but we can and do expect a teacher of the people, one who
should by his preaching and in his life lead the people on to bet-

ter things teach them how to meet and over come difficulties and to throw that earnestness which their feeling it alone can put into their words. Do you think that people are in any degree freed from the burdens which they bore on entering the church when they only hear an automaton pouring out syntactical essay on Paul saying he wrote this epistle with his *own* hand. No I really think they go away hardened with a dread of going to church to be kept in the uncomfortable situation of balancing between an inclination to sleep and a sense of decorum to keep awake –

'For those that wander they know not where
Are full of trouble and full of care
Weary and homesick and distressed
They wander east they wander west
And are baffled and beaten & blown about
By the winds of the wilderness of doubt.'

Mar 10th.

Every day brings its own troubles and its happiness. Last week was very commonplace and very busy. The Inspector visited my school. I don't think he was very well pleased with it no more was I. Putting it aside that they are deplorably ignorant, what little they did know flew out of the window when he came in at the door, I'm sure I felt like beating them some of them at any rate. If they would only remember what they learn but I guess it never troubles them anymore when they get a new lesson. When I think of the case I was at school and then to think of some of them being worse I do not [wonder] that the masters sometimes got off the balance. I'm sure they did well to keep their temper as well as they did. Schoolgirls are about the most mischievous specimans of the animal kingdom. Received letters from Alice, Maud & Lou the other day. The dear old girls. They are at the usual amount of pranks. Poor miserable teachers of the H[amilton] C[ollegiate] I[nstitute] how my heart bleeds for them.

Among all my friends I find that Alice grows ever the highest in
my estimation. I trust her and tis mutual but I cannot say what I
would for a promise comes back to me viz: to let her read this,
and she might think I did it purposely. The iron chains of winter
lost a link and substituted a golden one, a week of delicious
Spring weather. The frost is all out of the ground and the roads
are drying on top. So we could not go to church today. ...

'Hope rules a land forever green
And all who serve the brighteyed queen
Are confident and gay
Points she at aught? The bliss draws near
And fancy smooths the way.'

Mar 17th.

Yes I have abundance of hope and it is well, for whether I ever
attain what fancy hopes and points or not there will have been at
least the 'pleasures of Anticipation.' The past week has been one
of those uneventful ones that will come to all. There was the
same routine of constant employment, Chiefly, the office of
school-teaching heads the list. Then my music pupils, and my
studies, but the little things thrown in keep me [from] rusting.
The other morning one of the neighbours barn's and sheds were
burned. I was awakened by the cry of fire, and rushing out saw
the lurid flames licking up the buildings with ravenous rapidity
and in one half hour what it had taken years to earn had vanished, so quickly indeed did it burn that some stock was burned
with the buildings. Thus it is that our treasures upon earth take
wings and fly away. And if the wealth of the Indies were thus
subjected where would these boasted possessions be? ...

'A feeling of sadness comes o'er me:
That is not akin to pain
But only resembles sorrow
As mist resembles rain'

Mar. 22

Though I had thought myself secure from the intrusion of 'the world' I find myself once more taking a share in the busy bustle of mundane affairs. Last night on an urgent invitation I went home with one of my scholars, Nathan Moore (also a music pupil) of whom I think a great deal. They had a new organ in the house a first class article valued at 210 and I was to test its qual. I was the lion of the evening. Several of their friends in. My scholars are becoming very fond of me and I like them too. I am planning planning constantly, more for the exam, of my school which I think I shall give in two or three wks. now for Sunday my first induction as organist at Dublin. My visit at Dunns, Robertsons, Spears tomorrow, my studys preparatory to my exam, at Easter at Toronto. My music pupils, my day pupils, the intended visit at the exam of the other school, the meeting of friends at Easter and the going home. ... My own minor affairs and my correspondence keeps my brain active that at no corner I may run afoul of one plan with another. To guard my speech has become so onerous ... Oh! The roads are in a most elastic state, almost impassible with vehicles and – and – its all over town. Received French grammar from home, & more things are said in the receiving of that book than you would surmise – ...

'Times aren't now what they used to be then
Folks don't know now what they used to know then'

Mar 24th

Well I shall try to describe the last two days. Finished my little duties for Mon morning, gave a music-lesson and went up to Mr Dunns. The day was very very fine, warm as July, and t'was a beautiful walk only too warm. Reached Mr. Dunns sat for a while by an open window with balmy air playing upon my brow reading serials. After dinner we set out for quire-practice as I had conceded the point of being an organist for Acton R.C. Church.

Well you may say what you please but t'was no joking matter
after putting a hearty dinner under your belt to be jolted in a
seemingly iron vehicle (so springless did it seem) over rough
country roads. Well t'was over at last & Susie & I reached the
church where several damsels & the priest had preceded us. The
priest is a young man & I half believe he knows he's making a
goose of himself by the glances he gives me to see if I'm appre-
ciating the joke. Well now! I know its dreadfully, awfully wicked
but I'm going to flirt with him. There sat father,(?) at the instrument with a number of 'female women' in a half circle around
him. Presently I was installed at the rig and the old (young) fellow standing over me or sitting by which every you prefer. And
then 'oh! Shades of murdered Hamilton' how I laughed in my
sleeve at the picture I would make if my friends had an eye to
pierce distance. *Mr.* Nolan smirking & smiling such spaniel like
'eh's'! What I could have whipped him then and there. Well we
returned across the fields and waited at a log cottage for them to
come for us with the carriage. Such peculiar people & surroundings. An old old grey-headed Irish couple in such old fashioned
habits, in an antedeluvian house. Log-small & scrupously clean
& I could not but feel it in my heart to pity the zeal backed by
elbow-grease that had kept things in such a spotless condition.
Table, chairs, tins, floor all polished to perfection of water &
soap. An enormous thrifty Shamrock in the window. We waited
till evening and then they came and with them rain and a dark
dark night. Well after jolting, splashing, rocking, roaring, and a
regular wake of a time we reached home none the worse of the
ride. For the evening nothing less would serve but that I should
sing. Well tis useless to put in the flattery, the praise I've received
for my musical talents (?). ... Next morning lo! the face of terra
firma had changed so woefully from concerts of frogs, birds and
all depth of sunshine to dreariest, windiest March – nay – Jan.
day. ... Early we started and then I took my place after some confab with Nolan at the instrument in the gallery. I was to lead the
singing & with two others to sing the main part alone. All joining in the chorus. The church is very Catholic & I could not but
be amused at the performance especially the after part when he

put little pictures of the Virgin Mary fastened to a string around some old peoples neck's. To see the great old grey headed loons come snooking down the aisle with a little picture strung to their backs, really twas too ridiculous, but I preserved my gravity & am very hypocritical.

...

'And then – and then – ye gods
That I had still naugh but my
Shuddering and distracting thoughts

April 4th

This has been a beautiful day and the day of my examination. Well I have surely done my duty in this school business. I have drilled without ceasing, late & early and they did credit (in most things, to my trouble). There were about 30 persons there & I am placed on a pedestal of fame, become a shining light and I am glad to give satisfaction, glad to have praise, for that is a failing of mine- love of praise. I always did try hard for it and when it came t'was very sweet. This is not so bad a life after all and when I get through my studies I think I shall be quite 'sans souci' quite a bore – This is the beautiful side of spring, these days warm, cloudless, birds without, no, and now there's smooth sailing for two weeks. Steady, study, school and music. ...

...

April 12.

Ah well things don't go as we think sometimes. Monday morning started off to school, beautiful morn[ing] birds singing, grass growing, in good health, happy as a king but I made a misstep and sprained my ankle badly, hobbled up to school by the aid of Miss Brown and taught – but suffered the while, by night I was in great pain & two of the scholars helped me back home. Next day I could not teach and my foot got worse, black. Next day no school & next I taught but made it worse, and today, Friday no school. It is getting better. People are very kind & try to help me –

'A prayer of earnest heart
That I my pilgrimage would dilate
Whereof by parcels she had something heard'

April 26th.

Yes I have been home. Thursday I taught school went through the usual regime and more. I was more than elated at the thought tho' I did limp a little. I got on the train at the crossings, picked up out of the field as it were. A whole bevy accompanying 'comitante cateria'. They were more than kind. Well who should I meet but Irene Page, my former chum at the Model and had a lively chat as far as Milton where she got off. For the remainder of the journey I was alone and if all the thoughts that went racing tearing through my brain had been consigned to paper they would have been long and varied. I was happy yet sad and – and – well

There is e'en a happiness
That makes the heart afraid

When I reached Hamilton found Mrs Cummings and Ma & Cecil to meet me. As I could not remain in H. that night as I had decided I called & saw Alice a few minutes – long enough for a hug and a goodbye kiss. Went home and was nearly demolished but I think there never was one so glad to get home before. ... It was late Thursday night when I reached home and *very* late when I fell asleep. I was not half myself for the time I was home. I was beaten & blown about by the wilderness of thought. I wanted to talk freely and confidentially to them and felt it my bounden duty to visit Edith — to make her enjoy her visit and the exam[2] looming up before me made me about useless, going around with a book in my hand talking to anyone who happened to be in my way. Good Friday night 'twas fearful, such crashing claps of thunder. It seemed that God had felt the base ingratitude of mankind in sacrificing the Paschal Lamb and was about to rend the earth into fragments on this anniversary of that Awful day. ... Monday Ernie & I drove to H— before we reached the fair city it began to rain & eventually rained in torrents. Paddled up town to make some purchases. Went over to see Alice had a partial comfab. very unsatisfactory time. Alice & Ernie went to the G[reat] W[estern Railroad] Station with me and saw me off for Toronto. Ernest would have gone had I insisted, but I knew he wanted to stay to the party & his business matters so I let him off. Reached Toronto at a little after four. Sat a few seats from Herridge going down. When at the G.W. Station in T— I saw a young gentleman come in the car. He looking as one seeking for someone and I thinking it might by some possible chance be my cousin Dan (whom I expected to meet me) gave him a pretty good look but as he seemed satisfied in sitting down and talking to Herridge I said nor thought nothing further of him. Well I waited at the G.W. Station quite a time and finding no one come for me I took the st. car for Beach St. & arrived there all right, after a great deal of worrying as I knew nothing of Toronto & st. car did not go to Beach St. 52. Arrived at my destination found Dan had just arrived a few min. before me & was the gent. who sat with Herridge. No wonder I did not know him for he had whiskers (a new importation) & the only excuse I can find for him is that I had not such a rustic look as a year ago when I saw him last at Hamboro. Next morning Dan went up to Jarvis St High School, where the Matriculation exam took place and left me in Mr. McMurchys[3] room to wait for the appearance of him. He did not come but presently a nice young fellow ushered me down stairs and after uncloaking I took my place. The observed of *all* observers, the centre attraction to about 70 or

2 matriculation exam of the Ontario College of Physicians & Surgeons
3 Archibald MacMurchy, Principal of Jarvis Collegiate and father of the future doctor, Helen MacMurchy

more young men. Of course had the best seat, every thing done for me before I could express a wish almost. Succeeded in answering all serene, the only thing not to my liking was the short time we had to write. At the close of the forenoon session, Andrew Panton steps up with 'Well you are a brave lady' and I was very glad to see him. Walked down with me & had a good chat. He was very nervous through his exam, said 'he'd no idea he was such a fool.' Mr. Campbell a nice young fellow boarding with Dan & studying for a lawyer walked up with me at noon, he's real nice! Made great friends with McMurchy junior, & had lots of fun. Enjoyed the thing immensely. Excitement is intoxicating & I was dissipating to a great extent. Dan and I went up through the museum part of the Normal [School] & ; I enjoyed it very much, the pictures & busts especially. One of Mary the beautiful but unfortunate queen of Scots left a lasting impression, as she was at her execution. ... Like Dan better than ever had such nice talks. Next day at the exam all went serene but Latin it was unfortunately out of my range in either Virgil or Cicero. So I donna ken how I succeeded. Young Mc. seemed to attach himself devotedly to me promises to write on first knowledge. He's nice too. Thursday morning got up pretty early. Dan came with me to G[rand] T[runk Railroad] Station put me safely aboard reached Georgetown about nine & had to wait there about 3/4 hr to connect. Such a time changing from one track to another. Such anxiety when I had to depend on myself. Andrew Panton came down with me, he's very nice. Uh I think I said so before. Was deposited in the crossroads about eleven, left my trunk there & came on worse & worse, such a time to get through the mud but I got here at last & taught school in the afternoon. After having well verified Miles Standish when he says

　　If you want a thing done do it yourself

for Lou failed to go with me as she had promised, failed even to send me word and I don't care for anybodys help. I'm quite able to help me self – when He is still Above.

...

Mayday – 'Springs delights ect – – –

Beautiful, warm sunshiny day! The cherry & peach trees out in
bloom the grass very long the swallows sailing swiftly by, and
tonight a whip-poor-will sings his pitiful wail, spring grain an
inch & a half high. The wild flowers past their prime. Saturday
went as promised to Dunns, from there to quire practice, stayed
with Susie Dunn at McCanns all night. Mr. Nolan staid there too
had quite a convival time. Not so bad as some may think they
are. Sunday saw J[im] Dunn for 1st time, 'twas arranged for the
day grew well acquainted in a short time. Driving home to
Dunns had a nice chat & then he walked home with me, & that
was another [story]. By strong invitation I agreed to go back with
him if he called for me at four on Tuesday. Well with Tuesday
night came *he* and another walk. Suffice to say that *I* enjoyed
myself that night well for when Greek meets Greek then comes
the 'tug of war.' Came for a walk this morning and said Au
Revoir. So endeth the first chapter in which he figures, medium
height, coal-black hair & moustache, slender build, good voice
and regular features altogether quite a beau ideal. Sings raptur-
ously, talks sensibly, nonsensically, wittily and altogether well,
dresses like one of [G?]rebles models & reads much. I really truly
enjoyed myself last night, because I cast aside my reserve and
was a joyous girl once more & it was so nice. Beside they all flatter & pet me there and whatever I do is approved of by applause.
There I've written sufficient for one night for I am getting too
'fanfarade.' [fanfaronade] ...

Beautiful! how beautiful is all this
visible world, How glorious in its action
& itself –

May 8th

Oh yes all nature is beautiful now. The fruit trees in bloom. The
sweet fragrance of their blossoms filling the air, the gently play-

ing breeze tossing the newly bursted leaves, above all a summers sun, & a blue sky, & over the face of terra firma the many shaded mantle of green decked with a profusion of spring flowers. As I walked along a roadway bordered with cedars & beheld all this in a serene state of mind & thought that heaven was more beautiful than this, how could I but think of the hand divine which overruled all. Again as I write the clouds lower, a sudden darkness o'erspreads the earth, the thunders distant roll becomes more near, the lightnings flash more vivid, until a blinding sheet of water is dashed with swift strength along o'er vale o'er hill, madly wrenching the boughs & making all things living stand in dread awe. Oh it is beautiful it is grand, glorious & worthy the Master's hand. We seem too unspeakable, small ... , so basely aspiring if trying to throw off the guidance of our Maker. ...

It is May it is May
And all earth is gray
For oh, it is May it is May

May 16th

To think that I've neglected for so long to write. Well Monday night went home with one of my pupils to stay all night; not a pleasure but a necessity, as I don't wish to be at enmity here. Tuesday & Wed nights gave the accustomed music lessons. Thurs, paid a visit to Mrs Anderson, ... old Scotch person, well off, accumulated by toil & industry, well read & the — lawgiver & pattern giver of this community, the father (she is) confessor of them. Lends me Sunday magazines & I like to talk with her. ... Next day gave my music lessons & went with Miss Brown to her aunt Leslies where her sister is. Went with them to church & in afternoon went to Dunns & from there to choir practice. I drove & thats the best part for the horses are very wild. I felsh goot then, jockey like. This week was passing away very monotonously until I rec. a letter from home & from T— saying I failed Latin & French. I am much, very much surprised at the

French for I translated it all, but I expect it was the oral exam that broke the camels back. I was not surprised at Latin ... I know they will not feel pleased at home no more do I, tho' I'm trying to be sanguine, trying to see if my boasted complacency that all's well so long as I carry all to Him & I think I succeed. Those around me do not notice anyway, even when reading the ill fated news I could keep up the life of a game of cards, but yet it carries itself around with me like the dyspepsia, a hard lump some-where. I have been very busy lately fixing up the schoolyard. Two rockerys and a flower bed & the grove cleared up so that now it presents quite a satisfactory appearance. The last week has been very cold, frost so hard that the pond was frozen over. I'm sadly afraid the fruit has been nipped in the bud, and I've caught a nasty cold. How egotistical is youth. Their pangs & doubts & fears are to them the one vital topic which, must necessarily interest everyone else.

...

May 25th Saturday

Thursday night went with the Browns to a party at Mr. Duffs. Quite a number there, & I danced all night. Although a perfect stranger I was almost the Belle of the ball ... Some of them made such an ado to get an introduction that it was quite laughable. Mr Cooper of Waterdown quite so so. Had a lively chat almost a flirtation with the egotistical youth. About two Oclock it began to rain heavily so they concluded to dance all night and so we did and came home in the morning light. Slept till about nine and as they all went away the 24th but Miss Brown and I. We had a day quietly to ourselves. I enjoyed yesterday very very much one of those quiet peaceful resting places on the road of life. It was a beautiful day, warm balmy winds and *all* that makes a spring day delightful. Oh, I did enjoy it.

May 31st

Quite warm today; for the first Friday night and I am free till
Monday. I like this life I'm quite a Bohemian. Well the party of
which I spoke & of which I may call myself the Belle although
quite a stranger when I went there, oh! 'tis trés laughable, such
a furor as I made I have found out since. The gentlemen are
ready to fall down ect & the girls, oh my. I can hardly contain
myself, when hearing bout this & that ones remarks until I get
alone. One poor deluded wretch flies from one beholder to
another trying to get an introduction which on his fifth trial he
succeeded in doing & then 'after the opera is over' is in quite a
bad state of affairs as to his susceptable organs, asks this one that
one 'what's her first name' 'was that all her own hair' 'do you
know her' ect and by the medium of Elsie B I've sent him (tho'
he does not know) my card viz Cassandra Smith, he has read
Virgil. Last night I visited Mr Moores had a very pleasant time.
They have a good organ, b'ot it of J. Rymal of Waterdown.
Thought him *quite* a *great* personage, a superior kind of man
because forsooth his business seemed to sell instruments rather
than to farm bah! people are so verdant. I know more of him
than they and he's *very very* common. Well I do have fun
observing especially at school. ... I like my scholars. I like my
domains and altogether life is quite endurable.

June 9th Sunday morning

Beautiful morn after about a wk of freezing cold weather and I've
a nasty cold. Yesterday I gave 2 3hr music lessons, got over about
60 lines of Virgil and did a lot of marking – ...I shall be so glad
when this is over for I hate this Sunday afternoon business. I
hate going up to choir practice – it takes my Sunday afternoons
and I would so much prefer a quiet rest then, a perfect calm. ...
First of June I rented an organ a very good one 8 stops, a large

one & new. I like it and so do my pupils, [of] whom there are three now. Well I guess I'm pretty near home sick. I keep planning thinking about future pleasures for the summer. Counting the days, wks ect till I shall be free, so often that It seems really to lengthen in time. Only nineteen more teaching days think of that think of that, and then 'I shall hold to them the hands the first beheld to show they still are free Methinks I hear a spirit in your echoes answer me & bid your tenant welcome to my home again.'

June 17th

Last week was more than usually busy. Besides keeping them late at school every night, I taught a music lesson every night – beside quite an ironing of starch cloths my first troubles in that line – which took up a good bit of time, practising a little – studying a little. ... I was very wrothy at the idea that when Andrew P was successful [in the examinations for medical school] after the poor answering he made that I should be so used because I was a girl, not a boy forsooth! For I nothing doubt that if my answering had been given by a boy & the explanation that he would have been styled a successful candidate – uhg – Mars guide us – Jupiter help. Sunday went that dreaded round to Dunns from there to choir practice and back at night to Hampshires to start a sunday School & I have started one. The first for next Sunday at 4 oclock. Again if I was a *boy* – they would make me superintendent – talk of it anyway. But I will note the progress of my affairs that way as they progress. Today Monday – I employed a travelling artist to sketch my school and flock – a daguerrotype – quite a day for Dufferin School, quite excitement long to be remembered by them & I'm glad to have the pictures of the little shrimps. As I view the fields the hills trees & valleys the homesteads and far away blue sky from my schoolroom door I cannot but be less stern, less rebellious to the things of life as I find them. They are great softeners of surly mood. ...

June 20th

One year ago what a lengthy entry I made in my diary and how diff. was everything then – then 'the blush of dawn' was on my cheek. Everything around me conducive to happiness, friends, comfort, happy school days – and yet I now remember I was *not* happy I was not content and the great craving for something I had not – I hardly knew what my eager haste to set the world at defiance to paddle my own canoe to some fairyland of fame – kept me discontented – I am more content now with a patience to 'work & wait' – but not content to remain as I am oh no no no – day by day as time speeds on I am more resolved – as I hear of some disagreeable remark – cynical – of some that are false as — I set my teeth *resolved* to win laurels if nothing more. 'Now the dust and the toil of noon day check the words I fain would speak.' If health – if life endures, I am confident of success for God helps those who help themselves

Tell me ye winged winds
That round my pathway roar
Do you not know some spot –

June 22nd

Saturday morning awoke with the dread of the two following days on my mind. Telling as tho' rest and peace & love were far from me and nothing remained but the toil & the din & the strife. Went through the usual morning routine, finished my mending ect & gave two music lessons. Then went after eating dinner to Dunns and from there to church. And as it ever is if I can only forget myself and seek to please someone I am happiest. Miss Dunn walked up to Speyside with me and that kept me from a meditation which would have made me 'blue.' Then the Dunns are so *kind* & jolly that I can not but be pleasant. And if I

have done wrong in being organist for the R.C.'s then I'm sure
theres some good in the love & kindness I have won from so
many – perhaps I have done good too. I hope I have. I think they
will be some better for my having gone among them. Tis strange
as it may seem I was in wilder spirits than common. Thus it is
that extremes meet – from sad despondence to flighty gaiety –
Sunday morning raining hard and yet I kept up my spirits –
going through rain & mud to finish the task begun of – organist.
The sermon was on transubstantiation. There were a number of
boys & girls taking their first communion & so the old priest
Dunart [?] preached to them that the bread they ate was indeed
the body of Christ and the wine His blood – that is the worst yet
that I have heard – that and making the Virgin Mary to be a deity
are the most glaring differences between them & protestants as
far as I have seen. ...

I'm tired of all tonight
Tired of the toil & din
Tired of a life so little bright
Tired of a world of sin.

June 27th

As the end of the daily routine comes nearer it is more intolerable – The days seem weeks and yet the wks glide past like days.
Yesterday Jennie Martin called at the school to see me I was very
glad to see her – she is very fair to look upon and I like her. It
was such a nice surprise, the first mixing of the old life with this
present tired existence. I needed something to cheer me for I was
so disappointed at not getting a letter from –[?], I was so sure of
it. & then it failed to come – and – Alice & Ella they have kept me
so long waiting for their letters it is unkind – it might not be so
bad for them as they have plenty of congenial company but as I
am situated they might give a thought to that & be punctual as
some others. But there now how childish I am to complain. It
makes it easier, to unbosom myself but not to mortals, only

paper. All things work together for our good, my good, is to be made a cynic – stone heart and ironed willed.

> Give me a rest unending
> A calm so sure and sweet
> Joy and sadness blending
> And rest for the weary feet

July 1st

I had thought to have had such a good rest today and that is all the good it is to say I will do this or that. Sunday yesterday went for the last time (I hope) to Choir practise at Dublin. Came back to Speyside got dinner & Came down to Sunday School through the most oppressive heat. Came home to tea & found two gentleman in J. McN & Mr Sinclair. I can so far flatter myself that they came to see me – partly, talked till eleven Miss B & I & they & I guess they would have talked all night but that is not my way I don't see through those spectacles. ... I gave two music lessons & then went with the family to Mrs Leslies & staid till six, got a letter from Maud too & have since looked over 30 lines of Virgil & am writing this in the twilight. So that is the rest I had laid out to have – no rest here, not here not here my child.

...

> No storms to cloud my sunlit sky
> No glimpse of friends untrue
> If none are there then none will cry
> Let us give the devil his due

July 28th

Yes, no rest – no staying the tide of human affairs which sweep & whirl me on on forever on Wed night I gave music lessons &

they (Dunns) came for the organ – Thursday I made several
calls – Mrs Anderson's who were very jovial and kind – Mrs
Stewart also as nice as she may be, she forcibly reminds me of
that brutal old adage –

'A woman a dog and a walnut tree
The more you beat them the better they be'

Went on to Dunns & staid all night played ball & enjoyed it –
played the organ & *they* enjoyed it – went to school next morning and went through the duties of the day feeling a glad sadness
that I should so soon bid them all goodbye – for I love my scholars and they me. Friday night bade them all goodbye and set sail
with all my belongings for Hamilton staid all night with Alice &
had a nice talk and next day she went with me to see Mrs
Lawson where I waited for ma and she did not come till 2
Oclock. Had a good talk with Mrs L & she said she could not go
to Clifton this year as she had no one to keep house for her. After
dragging myself around town shopping with Ma we started for
home – I never came to Mountain Hall[4] with such a sense of
wearisomeness – such a glad to die feeling such a craving for
rest – I came home to rest glad to see them all glad doubly glad to
be free from care & give my nerves the the relaxation they
needed – None of them can know the wearisome cares, the duties
I left behind – the duties of that last wk were trying and now
they are as tho' they had never been. ... Wed morning Pa & Gerty
went to the station with Mary & I. Many went West I East to St.
Catherines. After waiting an hour for my train I arrived in St
Kitts about 10 Oclock & had the satisfaction to see Uncle drive
away without me – having missed me – not recognising me – So I
waited in the station till the next train came in – two hours after,
and got a hack & reached Uncles about 1 Oclock. had lunch &
rested the afternoon & went out in the evening next day went
down to the farm in forenoon and evening up town. Friday
afternoon made several calls. ... Tuesday went down to Port Dal-

4 the Smith home in Winona

housie to Alice. Went down on steamer Persia & came back on a small boat, Alice & Lizzie Porteous accompanying me. Had a very pleasant chat with them. Had tea at the Manse. Arrived at Uncles weary and happy too. Wed at Aunt Carries to tea & met Mr Biggar & Msses Hill – the former a poor lunatic body – *very* amusing – the latter, no distinguishing point neither above nor below the average. Thursday Uncle & I started bright and early in a beauty of a buggy & a beauty of a beast to draw it from St Catherines out through Homer & St Davids villages not far from the City of Saints by the road past the cemetery – I noticed one monument in particular, that of a dog chained & watching the grave of the departed – very touching but how misapplied. They are not there souls have flown far far away & all that remained for any to watch over was but 'dumb unconscious clay.' Past the villages of Homer & St. Davids on, on till Brocks monument rise in midair before us. On a prominent rock of Queenstons' Heights stands this memorial of a departed brave. Queenstons Heights faces the dark Niagara – Opposite the village is Lewistown a much larger place. We gazed for a time on, the river, the two collections of houses facing each other like arrant foes. The time honored Brocks Monument the spot where he bit the dust – and past on – wiser if not sadder – but it does bring a sorrow for the departed, when we see all that remains of them to be a tradition – a monument – to stand on the spot where years, & but a few, before there was naught but bloodshed, where soldiers fought & fell where man slew his brother man & all for a nations love. ... We drove on till we came to the 'whirlpool' by driving across a field we reached the river & looked down a height sheer 60 ft on that eddying whirling pool of dark green waters. After looking well, on this wonder of nature we retraced our steps for a short distance & then drove till we came to Suspension Bridge. Here all was bustle from the great number of trains owing to the different lines connecting there, Gt Western, Welland Canada Southern & [others] We rested at the hotel & got dinner there. The first persons I laid my eyes on, on entering the parlor of the hotel, oh hear ye martyrs! were easily seen to be but recently united in the bonds of matrimony. Why will people make them-

selves ridiculous. Its all fun for those who see & are not concerned. it vastly amuses me, to watch the varied specimens of
humanity which cross my checkered life (!) There a huge girl
with red face & a dress full of dignity & a seedy looking chap –
solemn as an owl to an observer but very deferential to her –
bending so close – both *dumb* in the presence of others – and void
of hunger so much so that it quite amused me. After dinner we
went up to the falls of Niagra. Before leaving the bridge we
looked well around the famous bridge & down the river ect. As
we drove up the left bank of the river, Earth & its vanities
seemed vanishing but when the full splendor of that mightly
cataract burst upon my view, when the thunder roll of waters
dashing in mad fury from its rivers bed to roll & foam & writhe
in such awful chaos, the mighty sublimity of that grandest spot
of nature touched my very soul & struck me dumb. Pen cannot
write it; Words cannot describe it; Only the eye the ear all outward & inward sense can make to feel mightiness of our Maker.
There if never else might be felt the nothingness of mortals and
omnipotent might of our God. That any one should commit sui-
cide there above all places this world affords is strange. There
where we seem face to face with an awful Judge it might well
strike remorse to the conscience ... Sat night I went up on the
five Oclock train to Hamilton. The first person I recognised was
Dick who told me Alice would come home on the 11 Oclock on
Tuesday morning. I staid with Mrs Lawson that night & we
went to hear Mr Carmichael but he did not preach. In the evening we went to C Presby Church but did not hear Mr Lisle.
Saw & walked with Miss Hurd a very nice womanly girl, also
several familiar friendly faces. Monday morning called on Maud
... Maud & I had a real good time. Such a day brings back the
days gone forever, to our minds in vivid imagiary. We, Mrs L.[5]
Mrs Smith, Tiny Maud & I had lunch & ice cream & lots of
fun. I enjoyed the day very much very much. Tuesday called on
Mary Turnbull & Anna Troup. Had very pressing invitations to
go to Oaklands with the picnic – Called for Alice in the afternoon

5 Lawson, an old family friend in Hamilton

& she went with Mrs L & I up to Dundurn Park. Had supper at
L's & enjoyed the jaunt very much. Stayed with Allie that night.
Next day ... after dinner Alice & I set out on the st car towards
home went to 'the jumping off place' off it & then scrambled up
to the H[amilton] N[orth] W[estern] R[ail] R[oad] track &
walked down to Lacys through the scalding heat & holding my
parasol, satchel, parcel & tram, very pleasant, very. ... Next day
Alice & I went for a long ramble in the wood and had a good
time talking & reading – Just before as we were lounging before
the door on the lawn, who should make their appearance but
Dan & George. We had a nice quiet evening rather too long & a
game of croquet – in which Alice & George were successful. Next
day the morning slipped away in some unaccountable way, in
the afternoon we went for a drive and fishing & to get the mail.
Expected Van W's but as it rained did not come. Had another game
of croquet & Dan & I won. Commenced another but could not
finish owing to the rain. Spent a pleasant evening. Next morning
Sat (Oh ages ago) Pa, Ernie, Mr Laefy Alice & I started early for
H. ... I said goodbye to Ernest at Alice's and although my feelings
were somewhat spasmodic I managed to keep up. The girls actually chaffed me on my sphinx like face – as tho' it were quite
natural that such a griffin as I should have no feelings, as tho' it
were quite the thing to part from all one holds most dear – perhaps forever – and go on with the gibe & jest as tho' made of
dust without a heart. If it had been needful I might have put on
the Spartan cloack of mobility but it's all nonsense – they were
only thoughtless – Maud not Alice for she rebuked Maud & I
could na' say a word for chokin' ... Alice & Mag Stewart took me
for a row – in a boat, not with a club. Had a lovely trip over the
deep green waves of Lake Ontario. Came back, strolled down the
sands & back. Met Titus & Maud with whom I walked & started
the scheme of the parasol – *thereby* hangs a tale. ... Next morning
went to C. Pres. Church – In the afternoon was happy with Alice,
a book, sweet skies, easy chair & shade of trees – read, laughed
talked. In the evening went to St. Pauls & heard Mr Laidlaw
preach. After church walked home with Maud & said – 'sister
part in peace' Went back with Alice & arranged for the morning.

It is partially arranged for Alice to come & stay a couple of wks with me here & that will be jolly for me. Monday morning, this morning – got up, breakfasted & got aboard the North bound train before I was hardly aware of it, by seven oclock & here I am – was set down – the platform over there in a sleepy state of mind –! (perhaps they thought so) & found Mr Moore & Nathan waiting to receive my trunk. Came here, found that owing to a giving way & repairing of the schoolhouse there would be no school for a few days – Ah! – if I had but known, but then 'alls for the best' The only pleasurable feelings I have experienced since being lunch, dinner & supper & what will the end be.

August 21st

Well, yesterday did move off to make room for today. In the forenoon I wrote letters & posted five. After dinner went over to Mrs McNaughtons & had tea – Everyone seems overjoyed to see me – to hear the welcomes I get reminds me of the prodigal child. Took tea there and called on Hampshires & visited the schoolhouse, to find there would be no school next day – as the room was dirty & floor covered with shavings. Went on to the post office. As I was passing McPhersons, a child was running out but on seeing me came to a decided stand still – indeed much the same appearance as tho' it had seen a ghost. After gazing for about the space of a minute it suddenly bolted for the door calling at the top of its voice 'maw' & so on everyone opened eyes & mouth to gaze at the invading monster. I reached Dunns about dark & was very warmly welcomed – staid all night & gave Lizzie a lesson. ... I feel quite settled & happy impossible as it may appear, but if I could but look down at the bottom of my heart, through the plans and cares of the present I would see the homesickness I *will* not let come to the surface. There is the patience which perfect faith in the future gives – that of hope of plans being fulfilled & that only – then when I think how swiftly the last six wks have passed it gives me courage for the future. I expect Alice tomorrow joy & doubt.

Aug 22nd

Taught today and found it just the same old story. No Alice came
as I almost expected for I knew she had no great liking for coming out here where the only attraction was myself & she had
seen me so recently but to spare my feelings she would not give
her objections until after my departure; for a' of that I was very
much disappointed not to have her with me today. ...

Aug 25th

... After the rain the morning broke with a clear cold sky and
sunshine over all the fields. I am enjoying this morning in a
quiet rest as they do not go to church today. Yes all are where –
Pa in Burgesville, Ma & Vio at home the others at church, I here
and Alice where? Maud at Gross Isle, and the world goes on
apace shifting us now here, now there. The Sunday school has
prospered sometimes over 40 there – indeed all the countryside. I
wonder if I were an old maid if they would cast such a wall of
greatness and public favor about me. I doubt it for there seems
such a romantic or mysterious halo to be thrown about a single
man or woman if not beyond a certain age. Oh Jove aid my pen
to describe this afternoon. Started early for S.school. Mina & I
called at Mr Hampshires for keys & Nancy went on to school &
waited for all to come. They came & still they came, bearded
one[s] & robust women, trouping along. Oh what a *gay* sell!
Such an army of young men, moustached brawny boys meager
expectation! I Fancy they thought I was the teacher but I shipped
the young men to Mr Dregde. What would I have given to have
faced & looked at the audience when I played & sang oh for one
moment, one till I could have sketched the look on their faces in
my imagination. Well who should I have in my Bible class but
Miss Fletcher a former acquaintance & modelite,[6] and that was
enough to teach the Bible class with her in it, who knew my
former jolly rattlebrain self, to hear me expound the gospel to

6   an acquaintance from Hamilton Collegiate Institute

them oh dear, when I had thought to have laid down the law so cooly. Miss Fletcher came home to tea with me & we found Mr Campbell – a bachelor – a neighbour – a farmer there also. Now mark ye that's *twice* he's been here in the evening since I came. What's that mean, o dear if I only had Alice here he would make a days merriment. Indeed my risibility is enough to control when alone but then – more's the help. I can't put it all down in black & white. Had news of the modelites of Miss Fletcher & of Milton folks too heyday – one week gone!!

Monday Aug 26

A letter from Alice to say she is not coming as I prophesied but still to my great disappointment. Well I did feel better this morning than I have for long. Went to work with a will – and made a thorough drill of it. A load of young men – I think from Milton on their way to Acton saluted me by bolting an apple at the door. I donna ken whether any acquaintance of mine was among them or not. After school gave Lizzie Dunn her music lesson and returned through the fields at sunset reading 'Colonel Dunwoddie Millionaire.'[7] Found the 'open Sesame' to a youngster's speaking machine. This is the third or fourth day she has trod the way to school & yet never before could be induced to open her mouth organ – neither by coaxing – tricking – shaming or threatening till today on putting a threat into execution – When the strap struck the first time it struck fire and she blazed forth right *through* the lesson. Well I am almost homesick. Shame on Alice. I am weary waiting for the news from home. I wish they could drop down at school & see me in the midst of my family – with order, cleanliness, flowers & music ect.

Sep 1st Sunday

... It is indeed too true, mankind alone mars the beauty of harmony. We are not ourselves but must needs ape somebody who

7   William Mumford Baker, *Colonel Dunwoddie Millionaire* (1878)

we think possesses superior attractions. Each in their diff spheres try to imitate, but how many set up inferior models for copying. Here the jaunty miss of sixteen summers, labors under the delusion that she has made us believe that she is fit to and does rule in society – Man & boy bend the knee before such a queen, so she would have you think – and in so doing belies her better self – her own thoughts – which like Banquo's ghost rise up before her; disdaining anything verging on sacred ground or if spoken of at all by them, very slightingly, because forsooth she thinks it is fashionable so to do. Again we see her with upturned nose pouting lips & defiant eye as she meets her gentleman friends, smoking perchance a cigarette to confirm their wavering opinion that *she* is not a sensible girl – but only a shallow – viz sham belle of the nineteenth century talking more nonsense than a phonograph could repeat & feeling an inward consciousness all the time that she is not what she seems & feels that life is *not* an empty dream. And her gentleman friends are they not equally false to their nobler natures. There goes a gentleman in his teens with the never failing *something* in his mouth; with dangling cane & hands filling his pockets he struts in batlikeform through the principle streets. And thus from the child of three years imitating its parents to our preachers in their pulpits who not free from the inspection must needs try his powers of imitation in trying to be a Beecher, or a Talmage[8] until this perverted generation finds itself acting a continual farce. Another species of this affectation is the petty plagarisms of society where continual forgeries in speech are being made. One more clever or witty than the rest may haps say'es something to create a laugh, straightway one or more hearers book it for a future occasion & passes off for quite an original genius or worse trys to pass off something seen in the writings of others. Would it not be far better to do as others of a similar class viz: – keep a collection of good clippings & *read* them for the benefit of the hearers? It would at least be more honest than appearing in borrowed plumage, quoting is good & therefore praiseworthy but plagiarism is abomnible.

8 Henry Ward Beecher and Thomas DeWitt Talmage, prominent American preachers

Would that each would be true to himself – true to nature, would cultivate the germs of nobility slumbering in every breast tho' in every stage of development. They might expect the millenium to come if they firmly believed that

'Life is real, life is earnest
And the grave is *not* its goal
Dust thou art to dust returnest
Was not spoken of the soul' –

Monday Sep 2nd.

The morning dawned bright and clear o'erhead but necessarily *rather* of a clinging tendency underfoot. I could see it was going to be warm, so dressed accordingly, wended my way cheerily to school, with scholars about me. Mr McNaughton hailing me to give me some ½ dozen apples, luscious, going up by the hopyard I beheld first a cluster of men *on* the fence, then oh! shades of womanhood – about twenty women young to old, *roosting* to all appearances, on the fence to keep out of the wet. Well it was a very warm day – but beautiful to look from my observatory over the farmhouse's, the bright green fields and *the hopyard* – how picturesque to see the sunbonnets – (prevailing colors of which are red and yellow) – the blue jackets and diff colored dresses glancing up & down in the vines indeed it is very very pleasant to the eye – and resembles a vineyard or better a hopyard with poppies of rare size, sprinkled among the vines. ...

Letters are already mailed
Which will change your life for you –

Sep 8th

Sunday night – beautiful beautiful moonlight – clear etherael blue with fleecy white clouds & I am listening to the water – rip-

pling falling with its musical echoes toward its destination.
Listening – and wondering how many years from now in that
unknown future I will look back over the vista of bygone years
and pause to think of tonight as a long past time, an almost forgotten drama. When the people around me now, my daily meet-
ings with them will be never more never more, When I shall
have passed out from among them as the leaves from the trees in
Autumn. When the things that I now do and others say will
have less or as little interest for me as they now do. As they
expected company back with them they took the buggy & the
democrat[9] & as the old folks took the buggy that would leave me
to go with Grant & of course that did not suit so I pilfered
Nathan too. The sheeps eyes cast at me in church by the young
pupils & the jealous, sly ones by the girls was the most of interest. A *very* prosy sermon on the woman cured of her infirmity of
eighteen years: The aspect of that woman was not pleasant to
behold. Came back with the old folks had dinner and prepared
for S.school. Mr Campbell came to go with me and that tickled
me immensely for Mrs T.M. was here and her sister would have
given her best bonnet to have been in my shoes. Its awfully
wicked of me I know but thats the extent of my liking for C.C. I
first love to see the black looks of those girls – dreadful, dreadful,
& I do try so hard to be good – to be like the good Samaritan &
do good on the sly as it were the oil the springs of this workaway
life of some about me. And I did try to be successful in my Sunday School teaching and I did not do badly today, I hope but I
am tired – tired –

Sep 23.

Well it is possible that I have left you, old diary so long. To begin
where I left off, the first of the week went quietly along raining
most of the time & I got a most undesirable cold – the rain ended
in a flood which did considerable damage throughout the coun-

9 a type of carriage

try carrying away dams & bridges at an unheard of violent storm
for Fair Canada. Sunday we did not go to church but went to
Sunday School. Mr Campbell going & coming with me & taking
tea here also I like him better, much better in fact – we had a
good talk coming home from S.S. and he seemed to sympathise
with me thoroughly – through the contact with such peculiar
people. Monday I began at sundry things for entertainment,
made two cedar anchors with colored maple leaves for rope
about it. ... Wed night we had a rehearsal at Schoolhouse, lots of
fun Jim is quite comical. Thursday another rehearsal (dress) Friday night the night. Well I had fixed up the Schoolhouse one end
curtained off for dressing room the other for grub and centre for
stage. The stage was carpeted – a centre table an organ a rocking
chair – flowers, curtains & window, clock & two small black-
boards made into mottos: Nil desperandum, faith hope & charity. About 7 Oclock the clouds gathered up from somewhere and
finished a beautiful day with rain – so that I had some idea of
postponing it – but people came & so we carried it out & made
$17 but there was not more than ⅓ as many there as there would
have been had it been a nice night. Well Myrtie came, the dear
old girl. Just as Jack's name was called he put his head at the
door & someone said there were ladies with him. I went to the
door & beheld Myrtie. I made one dive for her and clutched her
bearing her triumphantly too the dressing room and Jim, for we
were just having a *small* flirtation when I left him to go to the
door. I heard murmurs of – it's her sister – her sister's come. Well
I did well that night I am sure and am very glad for Myrtie can
tell them at home what a woman I've become. Well I enjoyed the
evening very much till I got tired – came home throught the mud
about 2 Oclock – with the crowd & had good fun for all. Myrtie
staid that night & went home next morning – it seemed like a
dream to me that she was here & I actually had here my own
flesh & blood relation. Went out with them in the morning &
saw them off & went to schoolhouse & put things to rights
considerably – came back to dinner – dressed for Sunday & went
away up to Dunns as they coaxed me too & went to Acton with
them back & staid all night & went to Church next day. Poor
Jim – its too absurd – to ridiculous but when Greek meets Greek

then comes the way and it is a well understood fact that neither
are in earnest. Came down to S.S. and had a very large one, tho' I
declare I nearly went to sleep singing. ...

Sep. 30th

Monday passed quietly away – with teaching and music lessons.
Friday morning Mr Moore took me up to Acton to the teachers
convention ... Mrs Moore went up with me to the school where I
listened till noon to Mr Little's dessertation on teaching Geo-
graphy ... I was billetted with Minerva Howson a former modelite & as we came down she introduced me to Mr Moore editor of
Free Press & I struck up a flirt ... Jim [Dunn] was there too, came
all the way from Speyside to get a glance at my happy [face] only
to be disappointed for I was at the front & he came late & Mr
Moore was filling his place. Next morning Irene came round for
me & we had another walk & talk etsotera till four when coming
down from school with Irene & Moore I saw Jim watching for
me & so I left Irene & took to Jim. ... Such a jolly time as we had
at the station seeing the crowd of school teachers off. ... we went
down town & then he took down to Speyside where I staid till
Sunday afternoon & then went down to Sunday school and
through that – a large attendance too. Mr Campbell came home
with me, so between them all I don't know what the *gossips* will
do I'm sure & more. I don't care – for I do & that's enough –
Jim's nice, Moore's nice & Campbells nice but thats neither here
nor there to me – 'They may call me cruel-hearted' but I care not
what they say for I'm just the same old girl [not in] love no matter what they say.

October, 1878

Monday passed off very quietly as the general run of days here
do. Tues Jim came down for me at four and we had a lovely walk
back up to Speyside. We got a nice long vine & brimed my
hat – some cedar & all the rest of it – had 5 games of croquet – all

to ourselves – they seem to have it understood among themselves that we enjoy ourselves very well alone – had tea & went for a walk with the Misses Powell – came back by moonlight – played euchre – lots of repartie & fun then visitors came & we had what I call a singing bee (not a bumble bee) for it was an incessant turn about first myself then Jim and apples for accompaniment – next morn he came down to school with me and then we said *adoo adoo* and that is the last of Jim except a note – perhaps the last time we'll ever see one another again – tho' I do miss him just now – he was so jolly & saw so much of him – but now I sigh (!) ... Well when the letter I expected from home today did not come I felt about as lonely as an orphan chicken – just like having a good cry but then you know I have gone out of the business and I don't have time anymore to indulge anyway – I am working myself and the little beggars harder than ever this week ... I work hard enough in the day to be glad of the night – tired so tired & longing for a home face and homenews – Oh these beautiful beautiful days – They will be gone too soon, too soon, but the sooner they give place to dreary winter the sooner winter will give place to summer & then, then this phase of life will be over I think will the next be more congenial. I think it will be that at least – not so quiet anyway – not that I dislike quiet – for I know I can be a better girl – a better Christian here where I am in comparative quiet where no one crosses my way and that does not say much for my Christianity, for to be *in* the world but not *of* the world is the better nobler way to fight against wrong, to resist temptation successfully – to uphold the right for rights sake to do good to weak humanity this is to live and not in vain. Well more fun – Jim & I spent the greater part of a day over making up a description of my entertainment – he wrote and I supplied data – but he did put it on thick – and so in turn I took the pen & soft soaped him a clear case of 'you scratch my back & I'll scratch yours – Well we had immense fun writing it but I am having the fun all alone now – for I had a Free Press sent me from Acton today with the whole rigmarole in it – enough to make a *pig* laugh – and then I face them all and wonder *who* on earth put it in (!) I wonder if it is wicked to have

such sport and to be so deceitful over such a little thing – conun-
drum – as Jim says – well received a letter from home which
apprises me that they will have a full dress party on Oct 18th
and I guess I will go home on Thursday night – joyful joyously.
Also a letter from Alice the dear girl – how I would like to see
her,ock, Alice darlin never fear you're still my own dear girl – I'd
kiss you fifty times or more I'd never get my fill.

Oct 10.

Well well. what next. Was at Agnes Browns wedding today –
such a dry affair – went there – stood around for a while – then
immediately on the appearance of bridal party from a private
room – they stood up like four cedar posts – The minister Mr Gil-
luvy officiating – gave them a free lecture first in which he made
out that woman was made but to make life more enjoyable to
man – forsooth! After the lecture – he said. do you [Joe?] Duff
take her whom you hold by the hand to be yours ect and faith he
got no answer at all but merely a stiff inclination of the head –
ditto from her after a repetition of former and all was over the
knot tied for life – I call it a slim tie too. If ever I get the business
done it will have more style about it than that and will be more
binding I trow – but what queer forms people do get into – we
then partook of 'dejeuner' – first the brides cake & wine – no
presents – no style at all at all – rec letters from Maud Dan & Jim
Dunn today & had a jolly good laugh over them too.

Oct 14

Letters from home & Edith today. I can scarce contain myself
now until I have been home. Sat walked up to Speyside & gave
music lessons – such a glorious day – more beautiful than words
can tell – balmy air, bright sunshine clear, blue heavens – beautiful scenery – beautiful road or pathway – and all the trees
covered with such a varied beautiful robe – and my heart could

not but feel happy & light – I could not but be thankful to the
Giver of all good for the blessings I enjoy tho' some would see
small cause for content if in my present situation. Sunday was at
church – lovely day a good congregation and a prosy sermon –
Sunday School in the forenoon and a very large attendance – I do
indeed try to do good in talking to my Bible class. If they would
take to heart what they hear with their outward ears I should do
good. I have hopes of doing some any way through the means of
His blessing. ...

Oct 22

Back again. Yes I've been and gone and done it. Thursday went
to school *hoping* it would not rain but the sky looking like it –
about midday it began & still I hoped on – & end in dispair –
gave a lesson at noon and came home through the rain and mud
in hope still – Mr Moore drove me all the way to Milton through
mud & rain. As I went jogging along in a one horse vehicle over
a dreary country road trying to be jolly and pleasant to the old
gentleman who went to so much trouble for me, I thought that
life was but a scale which went up and down at will – so much
pleasure so much pain. Sat an hour in Milton station – dreary –
dreary – no one that I knew so I had but the pleasure o the rain
beating on the window and observations on a few species of
humanity – one a commercial traveller, a perfect ass – whose
actions served to keep me from utter loneliness. After all it is
good fun to be among strangers, to observe the different types of
civilization – here one, who has risen from utter obscurity to
'golden mediocrity' – can not control his elation or greenness –
and trying to appears of some consequence utterly fails to be
thought anything – one buys a paper and elevates his feet to an
angle of 35% and wants the casual observer to think him a literary swell – a man quite blasé with travelling – when all the
time he is watching with lynx like eyes to see if he is thus appreciated – There one who thinks he would appear penurious or
unitiated if he did not buy some of the eatables presented to his

observing eyes. He buys a box of figs – looks closely at it to see if
there's anything alive in it and the getting out his knife proceeds
to dissect them one by one and masticates by eights – etsotera
etsotera – the literary – the greedy – the rich indifferent – the rich
proud – the poor content the poor ambitious – the would be
famous – the merchant wrapt in his own thoughts of loss &
gain – the bankers & his % the politician and his speech all kinds
and conditions mingling – rushing – pushing on to the end –
eternity – to take up the thread of my narrative – I finally found
my self aboard the night train for Hamilton – still raining,
arrived about eight to see under the gaslight Gertie Alice &
Mother – so glad so glad. All weariness – all loneliness vanishes
then – chatted with them for a time and went home through the
darkness now light to me for I was free from care or anything
else. ...

Nov 3rd

Well time flies and how quickly – how rapidly we run our
race – how fast the days go by and yet & yet it is a long road that
has no turning – always temptations & trials to be met with pleasure to be taken in doing duty as well as we are able and to take
other enjoyment as it comes as 'gratis' as something more than
our deserts but how many are able to do this – how many – oh
weak humanity where is thy boasted prowess & where thy superiority when of ourselves we can do nothing of good when all
tends to pull us back from the ways of pleasantness and peace
because 'Narrow is the way & strait the gate & few that find it.'
Soon it will be Xmas & then another rest for me another
reunion – perhaps only perhaps. Mine is a very humdrum life at
present – except for my letters I should be lost. They are the sea-
soning to potatoes, for as such common materials does my life
seem at present – Wrote Speyside Jottings last wk for the [Acton]
Free Press and behold it comes out under the head of 'From our
own correspondent' quite ridiculous – put it in too to the exclu-
sion of part of the New York letter, fun too for the folks wonder

who in the world put it in and of course their surmises are quite absurd. Teaching is hard work anyway and quite plenty of brain & body work for one person – That is to do it as they ought to. It's a long dreary task, day after day the same regime of lessons to be explained – simplified – order to be kept and when there is even one who has not the usual amt of brains it is very trying to the temper to keep order and temper: but I have so far succeeded as the have a good school – in fact quite a superior one if I do say it.

...

Nov. 17th

Ah well Ah well the days do pass quickly after all. It is all so strange this thing called time – it so swift so sure – and yet slow – our span of existence so short as compared with eternity and so long as we live it day by day – it would seem so little for us to 'fight the good fight of faith' – for our brief life – and we can not be of very great intellect not to – when so much is at stake so easy gained – so easily lost – indeed' we *are* such stuff as dreams are made of and our little life is rounded with a – sleep' and yet our temptations & trials are on a par with our capabilities – we are burdened no more than we can bear. How hard it may seem to us – never tried beyond our strength – however weak we may feel to meet the future yet in the self same hour we are given strength to bear. Never have I found the text of 'think not of tomorrow, sufficient unto the day is the evil' than so much exemplified in my life, as lately – When I looked forward to the weeks work the 'dull monotonous round' I felt like giving up the struggle – discouraged, heartsick at the prospect ... but by mental struggle & help from Heaven – I resolved to look no more to the future but to live each as a day apart from all other days & by 'opposing end the doubt & trouble of thoughts of tomorrow' and I *have* lived, *today* – I have tried. I have watched & prayed – and yet I have so often gone wrong – so often erred – when I

could, should have done better but it is so hard situated as I
am – when it is necessary to talk so much – not to let the tongue
unbridled 'slip.' Oh that unruly member, the tongue how often
does it bring us to shame how often do we wish something
unsaid. ... Well I am drearily plodding on – I am endeavoring to
insinuate learning into the minds of my scholars – to make it as
pleasant for them as I can and yet learn them more than any
other teacher in like circumstances would – I do not doubt but
they all like me, and respect me, as they have every reason to –
for have I not toiled incessantly for them – loved them for themselves alone – uncouth as some of them are, unkempt –
untaught – for the souls which have been given them for the
rough but kindly natures with which they are endowed, I have
tried to be a civilizing influence to them. I have tried by precept
& example to teach them cleanliness is next to Godliness that
politeness is great but costs little – to glory in doing good – and to
be truthful and honest – for truths sake and to learn them much
with the best means, to be kind & strict – plain and concise – I
have tried by getting up an examination to let the parents see
and aid me in my endeavors I have tried in so much as and by a
kindly influence to do them good & not evil & then the Sunday
School have I not tried to the best of my ability to so teach them,
that not only in their words but in their lives they should live a
Christian life – have I not with all my might by every means in
my power to promote the welfare of the Sunday School and the
section generally – and now does not every spare moment go to
work for the Xmas tree which I purpose giving them? And why
do I do it? What is my motive? I wonder what people ascribe as
my motive. *I* hope it is what I try to do all for – to use those
abilities which God has given me as I should for the ends of
good. I have the words 'to whom much is given much is required
and to whom little is given little *is* required' and whether I have
much or little I am trying to *do* to the extent of my abilities in
this Sphere of Life – trying to be one of the faithful in a few
things – for His sake who died for us. Wed night I was at Dunns
giving Lizzie a music lesson and not to affront so many, as three
came for us I went much against my own inclination to a party

at Speyside. ... I remained for 2 or three hrs and danced a few times. Some phases of it were very amusing – for instance two very tall specimens of mankind when swinging took their partners entirely off their feet – the great powerful monstrosities. Yesterday as I had strong invitation to go – I went over to see the raising of a building at Turners and the adjoining farm to this – About 40 or 50 men collected from the surrounding country and the timbers being ready for putting together – they – 'two men' choose sides and then a strife ensues to see which shall complete their side of the building first – Toward the latter part of it they excited beyond telling and such fearful yells as rend the air is quite appaling. Each one to a man – thinks the others will hasten & hear to his command and so each & every shout scream yell and tear ground like so many lunatic Indians. When all was up they make one grand dash for the fort – awh – house – with one rush each pushing shoving crowding, they get seated at table – as many as can – in this instance 25 and then they are fed to their hearts content – and depart for their respective homes – awk.

...

Dec 11th

Dear me what makes me feel so heartsick – I am weary let me rest. To look for the physical cause – my mind would instantly fly to the subject – sleep which from an extra taxation of duties impelled from what source of conscience I know not. Why I work so incessantly for the good of others without any aim but for the doing – is more than I can tell. Why I tax my powers of endurance so near the culminating point – without a semblance of gratitude or encouragement – among those who wilfully – perhaps misunderstood me is far more than I can tell, unless it is the lot of all in the time of youth to be so filled with youthful enthusiasm – so filled with a desire of praise – so filled with the idea of excelling others & of obtaining popularity ... Yes physically my despondence must be owing to the want of sleep for a number of nights – for weeks I have retired very late – trying through continued diligence in the way of manufacturing bric-a-brac to save in the matter of funds for the Xmas tree. There is no propelling power which leads me to do this when I would for my own pleasure & profit be reading books to hand. There seems to be a power which withholds and makes it my fatality to *do* for others If I seek for the cause of my depression of spirits mentally I need go back but a few hours to the receipt of the mail – Two or three letters have been late in coming & were beginning to make me feel qualmish at heart. When *one* of them coming this morning I am all misery from its tenor. I must, I will shake off this inordinate love of deep true lasting love from all my friends & be content with some few – and look for summer friends among my circle as well as that of others. I cannot tell the causa originam[?] of the partial – only estrangement – I *had* thought that she might have construed some hurt from my last letter but I do not now. Then I fear me it is in some manner owing to my jealous temperment as Ma has repeatedly told me – that I expect too much – Yes for all that precedes – they have in some manner spoiled me during my residence here, by making much of (in some cases only) my least act or word of such ovation of different kinds that I have become blasè with flattery of a common kind and unless it is very extravagant I am not satisfied. Perhaps if she had with great enthusiasm hailed my projected return to Hamilton – but then I am at sea whether she knows of it as yet – but then – hence darksome doubt – but – yes *but* how often do we see one sided friendships where one gives *all love, trust,* confidence and the other permits the giving – and that I cannot bear – I am so wickedly proud that I would live with a friend rather than such – so proud – I will not be the less let who will be the little – I must have all or none – where confidence of mine is given I must have implicit trust in its full return – else – it is not true friendship – I must look more to the end – to what I aim for – Heaven first – ambition next & *all* mankind last, not one. Put not your trust in Princes or in any child of Mars – not *one* but *all* Yet friendship is a holy thing – sweet & good.

3

Hamilton, Ontario
January to July 1879

At the beginning of 1879 Elizabeth leaves her Speyside school with mixed emotions to return to the Model School at Hamilton Collegiate Institute for the upgrading of her teaching qualifications. Soon an active contributor to the Literary Society and its *Quarterly*, she renews old friendships with Maud and Alice and reveals the same capacity for flirtation which keeps Jim Dunn of Speyside an active suitor. Not for the ambitious Elizabeth, however, marriage to a Catholic or life in a small town. Challenged by her own high-minded ambitions and encouraged by support from the medical pioneer, Dr Jennie Trout, she sits, for a second time, the entrance exams to medical school. Her anticipated shift from teaching to medicine was to be a road well travelled by Canada's women doctors.

Jan. 12th [1879]

To begin where I left off. I worked diligently at diverse things for that Xmas tree – nightly. That with music lessons – business – visitors and visiting kept my time fully employed. One Saturday – Mrs Moore went with me to Georgetown where I received the books & Chinese lanterns from Toronto and expended the money on the different things for the Christmas tree. ... Monday the usual daily routine – a music lesson at night and then work-

ing at Xmas presents – Tuesday night – a number of persons
in ... played hideous games and I could hardly walk – so tired &
sleepy & they actually did not go till near four o'clock & then
without much coaxing to stay. Must have been magnetism that
held them. Next day all work decorating the school & no play
made sad havoc with my sleeping time. Thursday I gave a holiday in order to have time to fix the tree. About eleven – I had
things ready to start and such a time. Mr Moore was to take Mrs
Moore & myself & presents over – & he took the cutter and such
a time. Mrs Moore with an armful – me with the large doll
wrapped in my shawl about the size of 12 mo baby – the doll, not
myself – baskets, boxes packed around so high we could not see
over & then where he was to sit – well he hung fast by some
manner of means & we reached there in safty to find the tree
lying outside whereas we expected to have it all ready – Well Mr
Moore went for a carpenter at Mr Hampshires & together they
got it up. ... About dark Mr and Mrs Moore & I went home – hurried our tea got our dresses changed – & off again in one large
sleighload ... I cannot tell my chagrin & surprise when on our
arrival we found a large crowd had already collected. Mrs
Moore, Mr Hampshire & I proceeded to light up the tree & then
we had to let in the impatient crowd & it had begun. I had Mr
Hampshire to take things off the tree and present them which he
did very well – only the oft repeated 'here's a nice present for
you Johnnie and remember your teacher.' ... Many many flattering things were said in my favor but the heaviest of all was when
they gave Mr Elliott a broad shouldered sixfooter the pleasure (!)
of presenting the album to me & the tears rolling down his face it
was earnest applaud for my labors in that place. He said many
pleasant speeches to my ears at least – of my superior (?) talents
of them not expecting to get another similarly blessed. We proceeded with the distributing until it was nearly done & then the
doll – a very handsome one – about 2 1/2 ft high which as yet
was at the top of the tree, was voted for. We had three polls – at
five cts per vote – & it brought it up to $14.45. This with many
more pretty speeches they divided equally between me & a dic-
tionary – I made my maiden speech in return for this & for the

album too. I said some few words in return. ... Next morning as I
was taking a late breakfast about 10 Oclock who should come in
but Lou & Dan to take me back with them – As I was not in [in a
state] to go just then they went to Ashgrove and returned for me
about four & then I went with them to Milton through the storm
of snow and with a severe cold – but I enjoyed it immensely as I
seemed to have escaped from all care for the time. ... Monday
morning Dan drove me back to the scene of my labors – as that
was examination day but as the snow was very deep – fortunately for me there were not many that came. I was so tired &
that feeling of only – compunction to do – so strong after having
for a time flung care to winds that it seemed if I could not pick
up the thread of my narrative where I left it. I murdered through
the day in some style or other & then came the partings with the
children whom I had grown to love as much as tho' they were
sons & daughters of aunts or uncles I will never forget the group
that I saw. The whole no. of girls standing in a corner with faces
very much distorted crying crying, crying, & I could not but cry
for sympathy. I had so crept into their young heart's that boys &
girls everyone thought me supreme of human flesh & blood. ...
On Saturday after New Years Cecil Gertie & I returned to Hamilton & here we are going to school. Yes actually I am at Hamilton
again going once more to the Coll. Inst. Sat Gertie & I went down
town & *etsotera*. Sunday we went up to All Saints – which was
beautifully decorated, in the morning – heard an excellent sermon – saw Minnie Drope. In the evening went up to Ascension
Church & heard another excellent sermon. Monday morning I
went up to the Collegiate – Saw Mr Ballard, Armstrong Sheppard
& McInnes who were very cordial in welcoming me back to
school. As nothing was doing I came home again. Went up again
next day & after arranging some classes they again dismissed us
for the day. Came home, went down town shopping – Wednesday after school Jennie Wood came home with me, had a good
talk etsotera, Thursday very common I received a letter from
Maud in excuse for not calling sooner telling me of her coming
on the morrow. Friday school as usual. ...

Jan. 18th

'Life's pathway seems full of promise.
And bright seems the coming year'

Yes the future is always bright to the eyes of youth. The coming
years can have trials & all kinds of trouble and yet they must
have some glory of happiness in store – some pleasant sunsets
tho' the days are dark. I often think whether I am morally constituted like anyone else or am I a distinct type of humanity. If
there is such another in all world then I would like to know that
one intimately and then, *that* is an impossibility – for of some
parts of our nature we would not speak, and other than intimate
we would not be known of one another. The ways of this world
are so dark so mysterious – we go *groping* about – 'we see as
through a glass darkly' but sometime it will all clear, all open as
the day & we shall 'See face' [?] to face. 'Know thyself' if a wise
axiom but [what a?] difficult task. It is a difficult task for me,
how I try to see myself as others see me, and I cannot. Some-
things I underrate, some overvalue and then I am in distress
worse than before. How I try to control myself to be a perfect Job
in temper and then how often I lose my self command & failure
is so ignominous and yet if I were at all times successful I become
too egotistic and that is not to be desired. Alls for the best all
must be if we cannot see clearly we can trust & there is where so
many go astray. ... When I was among strangers, in the country – where I had only hearts to win, where I became first in the
place, where I was the leader, above common criticism it was
very easy to feel – dress and station but empty words which
should be scorned as mere weakness, wickedness in fact – but it
comes to living once more among friends in city life it is vastly
different. I crave, not equality – not to be merely respectably
dressed but to excel – excel – excel – is the cry – is all – It makes
me feel almost bitter not to be foremost – not to be superior to
all – to excel in every branch – wit, music, dancing – talent study
and the thousand and one different ways of it all beside being

foremost in dress. And here it ends [where?] it began – Pride ...
Pride and ambition, but is not the last sometimes miscalled for
the former. ... Much need for self reformation, much charity
begins at home, and if we could be but missionarys to ourselves
we would do well. Another week of school has passed away, at
the Coll. Inst. [Things?] seem about the same as they were two
years ago ... the same scholars remain ...

Jan 24th

'The days go by and day and night are the same as one.' How
little we know of what a day may bring forth, our minds presage
us little of coming events. Tho' we may for a time continue in the
same grouve of daily business and our calculations for the morrow seem not far fetched dreams but realities. Tho we may go on
for a time in this routine we are startled suddenly by something – perhaps trivial in itself – but still startling us into thinking that we know *not* what a day may bring forth and therefore
as a direct result not to set our minds on anything earthly but
rather to live that each tomorrow finds us nearer a happy end. I
have been looking in my album at the faces that come to me now
as footlights of a bygone scene. What tho' at the time the acting
was all to real, all to great and endurance now it has become a
thing of the past – a has been – but so recently a vivid a trying
present. There are the children I taught, the children whom I
grew to love – and who are beginning their race toward the
destined goal. Oh mothers, teachers do you think do you know
the great the fearful responsibility that rests with you to make or
to mar this shroud of sentient clay as it best may be.

'The hand that rocks the cradle
        Rules the world'

What a great duty – a pleasant tho' onerous task – for where can
there be greater pleasure than that of a mother at the success of

her handiwork in thus moulding a nature, naturally evil into
something pure – honest & good as man may be. Ambition, true
ambition aims at something high, something beyond the most
common effort. Ambition would not hold that object attained at
a trivial price – as an achievement in which to glory – So
although it is hard to bring up a child, to instruct it without
detriment to innocence and nobility of character – yet when that
result has been attained, how satisfactory – how noble to thus
have achieved a great & a good undertaking. ... Where is the
influence of our ministers, of the many good works of great
thinkers – alas they are wafted o'er their heads and fall wide alas
so wide of the mark. When the young men of the age can so far
forget themselves as to jest – criticise, abuse correspond, in Gods
house on His day when His minister is holding forth the promise of redemption to one & all when they can so far forget all
that is good and worthy of respect as to swear at the scholars
committed to their charge, then what are we to think. We are
prone to look back to the beginning and think who instilled
these principles or rather left a void to be filled with. What of
evil came in his way? Who was his mother, who was his
teacher? But there are some exceptions else the world would
become a Pandomonium & chaos reign. There are still God-
fearing men & women who try to act up to a standard of
right – who educate their children to think, to feel, the truths
of nature, of religion & right. A scourge seems resting on our
land on our earth and so shall things be until the end is. For
among the good grain there are the tares also. And well might
Milton say:

'O shame to men! devil with devil damn'd
Firm concord holds: men only disagree
Of creatures rational, though under hope
Of heavenly grace and God proclaiming peace
Yet live in hatred, enmity, and strife
Among themselves, and levy cruel wars,
Wasting the earth, each other to destroy

As if (which might induce us to accord)
That day and night for his destruction wait'

Jan 27th

Last Monday when I came home to dinner who should I see but
Mrs Moore – the lady with whom I boarded at Speyside and who
was so very kind to me, kind as a mother and whom I will never
forget for that same kindness ... When I came home at night,
Maggie De Witt was here also – and Uncle Jonathan – Maggie is
just first class to converse with after her travels in Europe &
sightseeing at the Paris Exposition. How much she has seen, how
much she has enjoyed – I would so much like to travel and learn
what is in the world from very eyeknowledge – not all the books
printed can alone give perfect knowledge – without the sightseeing to make it substantial. I think when one is able to travel and
to see the world in all its phases while comparatively young –
enjoy it doubly as much as those who wait for maturer years. All
the zest has left their minds, at least of many things – the youthful spirit of enthusiasm and all the comparative superiority that
pleasure has over the trouble connected. But more than this there
would be the double pleasure – First at the time and through all
the future years of life – and altho' it is useless to long for it
now – I do so wish for that as well as other things which sometime God willing I intend to have even if I only have the single
pleasure of having it when old. The week went by much the
same as other weeks. The usual routine of study – the week ending with the meeting of the society on Friday night as usual. I
played an accompanyment for a song for Lizzie Rioch a very
sickly sentimental kind of a one – about on a par with nine
twelfths of the hackneyed songs that are sung by the modern
bells of society. We had a good debate on whether novel reading
was more profitable than unprofitable. One very able speaker Mr
Bowerman spoke as aforesaid with some eloquence – indeed with
great fluency & reason & I mean to keep my eye on him & hear
more of his debates. ...

Feb 9th

Well really it is amazing where time slips away to. I had calculated to have written at least once a week & when the end of the
week came I was so tired & it grew so late that I preferred to
postpone it till Monday – & Monday & all the week passed away
and here it is Sunday – I had also intended to have given up
writing on Sunday – So there are two good resolutions broken
and what excuse have I? Only this & nothing more a rush of
brain work. During this last week I have had to endure an
examination and I worked hard too, for I wanted to do well and I
was somewhat rusty from my long rest from study. How one's
mind can change. Why a year ago I had been quite indignant if
anyone had proposed my coming back to my old path of School
at the H.C.I. & then how easily I fell into the old tricks after I
once made up my mind to do it.

More than this how very much changed some opinions
become in the short space of two years. One thing for instance.
Then I had thought the world void and all mankind – false and
fickle if I had doubted the faith & friendship of Maud and *Now* I
could see her pass out from my life without a passing regret. If
she cares to keep up the farce with me well & good I can also
take my part without difficulty – I like to have friends oh yes,
indeed I do, but they have ceased to be the first essential in my
life. Alice is *my* friend whose ever I may be – By her my last faith
in friendship stands or falls. I believe in the love & faith of the
family but out of the home circle – There is only one who has my
entire confidence & faith & that is Alice. Others may say I am
singularly blest with friends, warm friends, but it is a difficult
thing for friendship to continue and an unfounded report, a
hearsay – a gentleman will soon dissapate the friendship we had
thought could not be broken. No Ambition is my first essential,
yes abused, untrampled ambition – for the achievement of which
is my first endeavor – What enjoyments come with it will be
enjoyed – But this first others second. Friday night I played
'Regret & Hope' at the Literary – the debate was whether Fear or
Hope exerted the greater influence. I am appointed as editor of

the Poetry department for the next issue of the Quarterly. Ma is home for a week while they are having their theatricals. ...

Feb. 23, 1879

How could I so neglect writing as to let two wks pass and in all that time not make an entry here. The days go rapidly by leaving only a casual remembrance to distinguish one from another. Life is a troubled dream of pleasure with some unpleasant realities – Five days of school of study day and night with the usual amount of fun and nonsense said and done – one hour in great glee another perhaps in thoughtful regret or disapointment. Five days of similarity and then Friday night the Literary Society and home again – to study – Then Saturday more study – music and the day is gone and then the peaceful sabbath crowns the week with a golden day of rest and of good words. On St Valentines day I received a nice one from J.P.D. [Jim Dunn] Oh where will all this end – is he actually past recovery without an explosion. Somehow I dread the next meeting but yet the weak fascination holds me to keep up a correspondence. I like him very much but like one other better [Dick?] – or rather could like someone better if that one wanted me to. Yes I have a story too – I could if I would a tale unfold but that its narration would be bitter to me.

I received an ugly valentine also – addressed to the poet of the Quarterly as I hold that onerous position. I opened it in the class and had a good time over it and left it pinned to the door – and never saw it again –

I was elected poetical editor ahead of Maggie White and M. Stewart & J. McIntyre the gaining it from the first was victory no. one for me – tho' a small one, it was quite satisfactory to me on acc't of persons – the first at least now. ...

'Men are only boys grown tall
Hearts don't change much after all'

Mar 4th.

Monday nothing unusual occurred but doubtless if I had then
written something here I would have found sufficient to say, and
so it is the small things of everyday make up the aggregate of
years long years as we live them but when we look back over
them they seem to have suddenly grown short – Tuesday at four
we were all on 'que vive' about our projected sleighride ect. Till
came over soon after four and after singing ect. & Jennie Wood
having arrived we set out – called for Frank Lawson and thus the
six of us set off for Stoney Creek where we were to have so much
fun. There was quite a no. already congregated – Gertie Frank &
Jennie – marched in defile across the room to the dressing room
and Tibb and I brought up the rear. But when we had arrived in
the dressing room there we beheld all manner of articles for public and private tableau. Tibb seizing a plughat & cane with distorted face begins pacing the room in the style of an old old man
much to our amusement for he naturally has a very old looking
mouth. Having divested ourselves of our outward apparel we
were conducted into Mr Whitcombs rooms to warm – There I
met Edith, Ursula, Mrs W. Robena and a no. of others after due
time had elapsed and much fun digested the programme was
started – and seemed much enjoyed – I played five accompany-
ments – sang once, & gave recitation and took part in a tableau – Altogether I had a capital time as everybody was ready to
pet and flatter me and make as happy as a queen. ... I have bar-
gained to write an essay for the Quarterly on Education of
women and so that is one more straw to the load that is on my
mind. Today – Sunday – Gertie and I were up at Ascension
Church and heard the Rev CarMichael preach an eloquent sermon – He spoke so pointedly and brought home such a feeling of
unworthiness to us that we were convicted in our sins and felt as
he described it as though we could sink down into the dust and
cry 'unclean! unclean!' He told us each one to go home and read
the commandments and our hearts and justly judge that not one
of us could say 'All these have I kept from my youth up.' The

sermon was based on the story of the 'young ruler who asked
Jesus what he should do to inherit eternal life.' He also said that
not one of those could look at each commandment and I have
kept that – & that & that I felt as he said it, that I should be
thankful that I was still young with my life before me to try with
help from above to do better in future – for how sad must have
been the outlook to those who had grown old – with their sins
and could not undo them – Then how much it behooves us who
know that life is to be lived but once and then the end decides for
eternity our destiny – Why is it How is it that this does not
weigh heavier on our minds. I want to do good to be good and
make many good resolves but seldom do I succeed – I know we
cannot be perfect – but to be the best we can be is so hard when
we are in lifes busy whirl.

> Through the deep caves of thought
> I hear a voice that sings;
> Build thee more stately mansions
> Oh my soul!

Mar 9th

Sunday has come again and another week has died – Oh the
compass of a week – what may it not contain of joy and sorrow.
Now tonight when there has been such a tempest swept over my
very soul – A tempest long and loud and deep – that has shattered my egotism my selfrighteousness if you will. Can I ever
forget it and all from so trivial a thing as a taffy party – because I
showed myself in a false light by singing two silly songs – I was
all remorse and I think no greater scourge can go over a human
life than that of deep – heartfelt remorse – Now it seems to me
that all I have in life is to show them I am not the trivial spirited
being my songs denoted – one of simple mirth the other what in
the expressive language of the day would be called spoony – If I
had written last night I would have said some bitter things but
now, the peace of the sabbath has in some case modified my
wrath. ...

'God bless thee then!
I'll see thy face no more
Like water spilled upon the plain
Not to be gathered up again
Is the old love I bore.'

March 22nd

So are many many acts and words which when done or said we
cannot undo – never undo – never, never. I wonder if there is
one in all the world who can say I have nothing to regret – I
would live the same if I lived again – I do not think so and yet I
believe it is best to not fret about the past which is beyond
retrieving – but to believe that is working together for our
good – And to look to the future as the subject for thought – to
improve on the experience of the past – 'to act in the living present heart within and God o'erhead.' Let the day be commenced
with never so bright a dawn there are sure to be clouds in the
calm surface of our life before the day is done. And we need all
the purpose of right; all strength of mind, all our heart & soul to
win the day against temptation to find when night lets her ample
curtain down, to find we have some things to regret – something
that in our human sight would have far better otherwise. Each
day as it passes over my existence each day is fraught with something that leaves its impress upon me – it must be so – each one
of us have an influence, more or less for good or evil on others –
and in my daily rounds of school I must needs be influenced to a
certain extent. Lessons, not of books are taught me day by day
observation is an open book that he who runs may read – it is a
pleasant task in some cases perhaps – to read it – but where one
sees oneself mirrored there, then it becomes vastly important
vastly interesting – and useful if we can but put aside egotism
and reflect on the picture there. Next to observation and sister to
it is experience that stern but thorough master which stamps
indelibly its lessons on our very souls – What is more pitiable
than to see – confiding youth – in either sex but especially in girls
commence life with a sublime trust in the truthfulness – of
everybodys friendship – and then to have that friendship wither

or shattered in the bud by some conniving wordly minded person who only seemed a friend while that seeming was beneficial to them – Much have they to answer for ... Friday night I gave a recitation 'Molly Meade' which was quite enthusiastically received – if they knew how sweet their praise was perhaps they would be more chary of it – I wonder if there is the same love of praise in the breasts of others as in mine. It makes me either on the mountain top or in the valley – according as I receive or do not receive it – It has been always so with me – always – I remember when first I could think so far it was manna for me to receive praise from father or mother – Perhaps the meagre supplies I received heightened the value – who shall say –? Yesterday I studied all day – a very few hours excepted from eight in the morning till half past eleven at night twelve pages of French – three hundred lines of Latin – eleven propositions and twenty six questions in algebra. ...

Mar 30th

The last week was another busy period of time that has passed away into the dreary past. Friday night was the quarterly meeting of the Literary Society – It was agreed on by the girls that Miss Wood & Miss Hager should be the ladies elected what was then my amazement when Mr Duncan got up and proposed me – as 2nd vice president after there had been some five already gentleman already nominated for that position – The gentlemen were very gallant and withdrew in my favor except one, but then Miss Mills got up & spoke for Jennie & said as she was one of the oldest girls of the society she thought her worthy of the position. We were ballotted for – the girls doing all they could for Jennie – not out of any malice they had for – as they all explained – but because they thought Jennie deserving of more honor than she received – so owing to the girls efforts Jennie came in a few votes ahead. Such a queer thing for Jennie & I to be opponents for anything – but this was not satisfactory – Hunter got up and nominated me for 3rd vice president and there were several nice things said – then Ratcliff according to instructions from the girls got up & said his word for Miss Hagar – so often a gent had been proposed – we were ballotted for & I came out ahead – I was glad of this as I did not relish in the least being put up for office & then being run out. I was as much elated by the kind of nominees I had as by anything else tho' I found that night that I had more gentlemen friends than I knew of. ... I may say I wish for many many things – There always seem something ahead that I want, nothing much that I have & yet there is too – if I had not what I have I w'd want them more than anything else – I guess I never will feel settled in life, that is can look ahead to succeeding years with a pretty fair certainty of where I shall be & what doing unless I should chance to marry & that is more doubtful than the abiding places of coming years ...

April 5th

This has been a very quiet week – the going to school makes up the greatest part of my life. Yes whatever the coming years may have in store for me I have had a long youth a long time at school. How discontented everyone is. All wishing for something they have not & then not satisfied when they do get it ... Friday night we had a very good programme at the Literary. Mr Dickson gave an essay – long & clever about the 'effects a man's surroundings had on himself.' Jennie Wood & I played a duet and *not* to my satisfaction – however they gave us an encore and there again I regret – for we went back too readily – but pshaw! Whats the use of so much sham – when they wait so long to respond to an encore theres always more or less sham & generally more. ...

'O'er all to throw a memorial hue
A glorious ideal the real never knew
For memory shifts from the past its pain
And suffers the glory alone to remain'

80 Hamilton, Ontario

April 13th

It was so in the long ago – before I came to know the shallowness of humanity – After years of the usual crosses and joys of the common school life – the troubles faded from sight and all the past seemed to have been bright. Even now I see where in the pattern of my life I might have woven brighter colors, but I would not wish to live again the twenty years of my life oh no – not if *all* would be lived over again. If in the space of twenty somewhat monotonous years I have much to regret what must be the feelings of those who have a dreary waste of eighty or fifty years to look back to. Especially if it has been an eventful past. There was only school on the first three days of the wk as the Inspector gave us Thursday ...

April 22nd

I am not in a mood to write all I would like to. My head seems quite befogged and altogether dizzy – but I must needs write before I forget. How much can be crowded into a week. I seemed to have lived long months since last Sabbath – feelings have changed likes & dislikes have paled before stronger thoughts & aims & resolutions have strengthened beyond belief in such a short time – and things that held some importance in my eyes before have sickened to my mental vision – lingered – died. I shall try to give a resume of the last week – Monday morning bright & beautiful spring morning. I arose betimes & after equipping myself I started for the morning train Cecil & Gertie going with me – saw Mrs Lawson at her door with wish for my success on which the smiling morn seemed to cast a happy augury. The rest & peace of the solitude, rather the tinking within self as we dashed o'er 'highways, hedges, gullys, ditches' across the beach with the blue waves on either side seemed chanting a reveille to all nature which seems slow this spring to come forth from the charnel house of winter. The conductor was very kind especially at the Junction at Georgetown which by the way is a miserable

affair and causes uneasiness to the minds of travellers. How
diverting it is to observe humanity in the varied phases which
one beholds while travelling. I had almost an hour of this diversion at Georgetown, first a lady – well dressed – trying entangle a
gentleman in the meshes of her talk – and then a mother with a
family of three on her way to Manitoba with all the care on her
face that must be in her heart – two old cronies of women talking
of smart sayings of smart children ect. Went on to Toronto
with[out] meeting any acquaintance but yet enjoying the diff.
specimens in the coach – arrived at To— about eleven and found
no one there to meet me – another mistake – always seems a
fatality for me to make such mistakes – to miss folks at the station – may be their faults too. I wandered up town – (as I missed
the st car from waiting at Station) and went into a confectionary
shop to inquire the way to W— St and a lady who was there
purchasing cake undertook to show me as she was going in that
direction – She was a queer speciman of the free souled American for she took me into confidence without so much as by your
leave – called me deary told me she had just come from the
Womans C[hristian] Association told me of her servants, of their
fidelity ect – mentioned things of herself, daughters, ect & even
told me her name but I did not distinctly catch it. Without further trouble except heat & fatigue I reached the domicile I sought
and took them by surprise as they did not expect me till the one
o clock train for which Dan was preparing to meet me at that
hour. ... Dan and I went for a walk up the the Normal [School]
but when we arrived there and found the door locked we recol-
lected that it was a holiday (Easter Monday) so we had the pleasure of walking back again. Dan is just a royal good fellow I can
talk to him & not for and instant feel that he considers our conversation otherwise than rationally cousinly – He never dreams
of what the beau monde would call flirting – pah! I only wish I
knew more – & I will know more – but not so much as I could
wish – For I get adrift on some subjects and am only secondary
in a deep argument with the learned – We spent quite a pleasant
evening and next morning Dan escorted me up to the Coll Inst
where the exam. was to be held and Mr McMurchy having put

in an appearance, Dan left me to his tender mercies. He told me I might hang my cloak & hat in his private room – I was settling my plumage – preparatory to my descent among the soon-to-be-featherless tribe below – when Mr McMurchy lead into my presence a nice sweetlooking red lipped & bright faced – rather delicate looking girl who also began to uncloak – Thinking her to be the Miss Johnson of whom I had heard intended to take this examination I addressed her, asking her if that was her name – then the ice being broken we were almost estatic in our self congratulations that we were not alone – she was quite nervous apparently but in her heart there was no quaking – There is much truth in the words of Byron that 'a kindred feeling makes us wondrous kind' for Miss Parmenter & I could then & there have sworn friendship as we were about to launch out in the same kind of a barque on the same sea of trouble. She seemed resolute to prosecute her medical studies there at the Medical school in the very teeth of her would be oppressors she said 'what did not hurt Mrs Jennie Trout[1] would not hurt us.' I was delighted to find one so sweet & girlish looking enternally have such an iron will – I fancy from all said & observed that it is blind necessity that keeps her there as they are not able to send her away to prosecute her studies & she is indeed to be admired for her courage to win her way against all disagreeables & difficulties. As McMurchy said there was not the least necessity for taking those subjects I passed in before I took my departure for the forenoon and as I was left to my own devises I called on Dr Trout who received me very kindly in her magnificent parlors. She sat on an easy chair before me on the sofa – I can see her now in fancy – her large kindly eyes, her hair which seemed coated with gray and lay back from her forehead high & white. I asked her what course would be advisable in my medical pursuits. She said She would very much like me to have a Canadian degree but would never advise me to go through the fiery ordeal she had subjected herself to in going to the Toronto School of

---

1 first woman licensed to practice medicine in Canada; a graduate of the Women's Medical College of Philadelphia

Medicine. She narrated circumstances to me appalling astounding & as she said, if the wives & mothers of our land knew the half of the depravity into which the students of medicine plunge – they would shrink from them as though they were leprous and would cry out in one great clamor for women doctors. Boys who before entering there were – moral – upright steady worthy sons of worthy parents – in a word religious and they came forth from that same place mured to the worst of vices and nearly in every participating in them – Because they had fallen into bad company because their professors encouraged & led them on. She had been before commencing her studies an invalid between the sofa & bed for six long dreary years – During this illness she determined to take up the study of medicine & she faithfully held to that thru' sickness – & discouragement – almost going up alone time when her health seemed to completely fail but by the earnest entreaty of her now partner Miss Left she was induced to try the Electro Theroputics which cured her and she was enabled to finish her studies & obtain her degree at Smiths College, Philadelphia – without experiencing anything that was repugnant to her womanhood – nothing but was fascinating & exalting to anyone – But as she was determined to hold a Canadian degree – she came to Toronto & with Mrs. Stowe[2] attended lectures for one year at Toronto. Then she encountered all the seathing blighting shamless villiany of those sons of Belial – which should make Canadians blush. Through the kindness (? !) of one of the Prof – they had been allowed to attend on promise that whatever occurred they would make no complaint and through all that long trying time they held to their word. Through a hole in a wall between the lecture room & an anteroom they kept the vigils over their seats in the lecture room & if the students had played any tricks such as laying parts of a body in their chairs they then would send to the janitor to have them removed – They would write naseous stuff on the desks & draw

---

2 second woman licensed to practice medicine in Canada; a graduate of the New York Medical College for Women; founder and first president of the Toronto Women's Literary Club, later the Toronto Woman Suffrage Club

caricatures on the walls – which had to be whitewashed four times during that session – And worse than this the Profs themselves with two honorable exceptions Drs Barrett[3] & Richardson – encouraged the demon in the hearts of the students infuriated them with sickening stories quite irrevalent to the subject and one went so far as to insult them more than they could bear & she told him if he ever dared to tell such smutty stories in her hearing she would go straight to his wife – And he a professing Christian an apparent gentleman took her advice & refrained from such wickedness, that neither his feelings nor the sense of decency had debared him from. On the whole she strongly advised me to go to Ann Arbor as it was quite equal to N.Y. or Phil. Colleges – She was at present engaged in a correspondence with a friend at Ann Arbor who had also attended at Phil & N.Y. & by all odds gave the premium to Ann Arbor. She said she thought if a number of girls say eight or twelve could be collected for the same study they would have separate courses for them. She saw me out and asked me there to tea in the evening – I strolled home to dinner ... After dinner Dan went up with me & deposited me safely in the Coll. Inst. where not having the first subject I had the pleasure of rem. in McMurchys room & reading English history or anything else I liked. Soon a boy appeared to usher me down ... to the lower regions of the building and then 'in medio conspectu turbatus mermis constito' I actually had the temerity to move along before the eyes not of the Phrygian band but of a masculine troup of male men and take my seat deliberately promiscously and to all intents & purposes maliciously in a not overly commodious seat with the flipperty flop of a desk before it. I sat next Miss Parmenter (Emma) and I was not such abashed by the more than 100 eyes turned upon me but moved with deliberation & during recess moved my chair up to Miss P's here had the felicity of one of those delicious smiles of Sangsters as he passed me & also recognitions from Hodson – Also saw little Richardson from Milton there – &

---

3 Dr Michael Barrett, professor of physiology at the Toronto School of Medicine; in 1883 a champion of the Toronto Women's Medical College

was very much stared at & kindly treated & felt altogether as tho' I had the best of it for however much they gazed at me I had a greater variety of them to look at & I did & enjoyed it too. The Latin paper was very much harder than last year & I pity those poor fellows from here who I am almost sure did not pass even if I did or do. I came forth from that felicitous abode home again & stayed for a while & then went up to Mrs Trouts – a girl afterward introduced as a niece of Dr Trouts admitted me & went for the Dr. She came to me in her brilliant parlors & conducted me thence up stairs through splendidly furnished apartments – to an exquisite bedroom to lay aside my wraps – thence back to the parlors. I had quite a chat with her niece Daisy who is a fragile thing who seems to have been intended by her aunt to have become a Dr – but health forbade – Soon the great bell rang and Miss Margeret Johnson – a would be aspirant to the degree of M D seemed to have tacitly become my chaperon. She conducted me through many halls & passages until at length we arrived at the large dining room where I found three large tables pretty well surrounded & well laded. I was introduced to numerous persons but whose names I did not catch. After a hearty tea which had been served with good taste and better [for] waiting I was led in a different direction tho halls – down passages – up stairs until we reached another parlor very large & well furnished where I found the other persons who had been at tea had assembled – Hymnbooks were distributed – & Miss Left officiating at the organ we all joined in singing a hymn, then, a patient Rev Mr Rand read from the Bible & prayed – then being left to our own inclination – Miss Parmenter soon left to study & Miss Johnson undertook to pilot me over the premises which she did quite satisfactorily – enlightening me very much on the subject of their importance. She said they generally had about 60 patients staying in the Inst[4] for treatment and that they were all very busy treated about 40 patients daily – The rooms where they performed this part were very small & warm & contained apparatus which I did not understand and bath tubs ect with little corners

4 Therapeutic and Electrical Institute

curtained off for the patients to robe & disrobe in. We finally
reached Miss Parmenters room where seeming very welcome we
stopped for a time & Parm & I read French together – Johnson
lying on the bed listening – I on a chair – Parmenter leaning
toward me from the side of the bed. A scene which will probably
never fade from sight. After spending sometime in this manner I
thought that I had stayed long enough and bid Miss P goodnight
& Miss Johnson & I filed our way back to the starting place viz
Mrs T elegant parlor & herself. We had another talk she showed
me her office – husband & parrot ect & after much more talking – myself – Ma – profession & humanity in general I left her
much elated in spirit much encouraged in mind & if possible a
lower estimate of a certain class of men, left her resolved to go
through my profession and do in what measure I may be able the
work that she has done. But never will I be able to do the great
good that she as a pioneer has done. She is a dear noble woman
and God only can estimate her work as it deserves. Miss Johnson
& Richardson came home with me & I met Dan just at the gate
coming for me. We went in and had quite a pleasant evening ...
Next morning I spent studying & in desultory conversation. Dan
went up with me at noon – The French paper was a vast sight
harder then before – and I was short on time but n'importe I
guess I'm through – The examiner from Kingston Mr Knight was
extremely kind – He examined us in Latin & French – in the oral
part too – He is a capital man & was very kind – said the Kingston College would admit ladies & he thought would have a
separate course if there could be a number of ladies join together
for that purpose – He made kind inquiries about where I
intended to pursue my studies – said he would do what he
could – was a believer in lady doctors and sent his regards to Mr
Dickson by me – I was well pleased to hear him say this as so few
men are quite willing to see ladies assume privileges which they
have by right. I went down town & purchased some toys for the
children & when I arrived home I found William had returned &
was ill – also that the 5 Oclock train would not connect at
Georgetown & I would have to remain over till next morning – a
card had been left me on the table – J.P.D. & said that he would

call again, which he immediately did. I entered the door dressed
à la mode in my black with array of buttons and he a perfect
Beau Brummel in attire arose with eager outstretched hand to
meet me – a hearty handclasp & I took my seat with back to window. Then the tirade began – reminiscences of last year at the
Spey with much fun at recollections & words a glimpse at both
our societys – at our various literary productions and then he
began the great plea of the time – that I would have my 'profile
took' as an accessory to this that I would stay till the 3 train next
afternoon – He would do anything from telegraphing them to
blowing up the track if I would only only stay little beauty – But
refused again & again – he besieging me with flattery – wit –
persuasion of sense & nonsense – 'Tho his tongue dropt manna
he could make the worse appear the better reason.' He pleaded
hard but I thought I saw what I ought to do & I was firm in my
resolution to go at 7 Oclock. Often I think myself too easily led
and then when I make up my mind to do something and stick to
it – I am quite proud of it and it may in some cases amt to stub-
borness – Jim said it did anyway – we were both standing & I
thought he had been convinced & was about taking his departure when he turned once more and said Now won't you – I'll
call at ten tomorrow anyway – for the last time won't you I said
quite firmly & looking straight at him for the last time no! Then
he said he thought I was stubborn & I told him I believed him –
He took his departure much crest fallen for he saw more in that
refusal than the mere not getting a photo n'importe it was a good
thing ... Reached Scotch Block quite unexpectedly & no one to
meet me – waddled along toward 'Moores' & on my way met Mr
Colin Campbell II who was quite delighted to see me – Well!
Well! Well! What next and pressed me to come & spend that
evening with Miss Fletcher & Grant at his house. I went on to
Moores and quite took away their breath with surprise – When
Mrs Moore opened the door & saw me standing there she
seemed to turn to eyes & then to arms for she grasped me with
some strength. Then after due salutations questions ect & duly
domesticated the little girl Mina was dispatched for the old
gentleman – Who came in to see what was the matter & behold

the great (!!) arrival – After dinner Mrs Moore & I went over to visit the school. As no one knew that I had arrived I thought we would manage to surprise them – but unfortunately one of the youngsters being outside espied me at quite a distance and went in & spread the news so that was no surprise at all – I and I am quite sure every chick of them agonized for about an hour until recess then such a time – they were so delighted & yet they did not know how to express it. I ran off with the girls to see their play houses & then came back to see the boys play ball – and had something to say to all of them – the dear little children. On our way back we call at Hampshires where I saw what one would usually see there – work misery and youngones – 'A woman a dog & a walnut tree the more you beat them the better they be' seems to be the motto of that man and he pretends to hold up his head as a Christian member of society and one to meet & converse with him see's only a pleasant witty man – Went on home & in the evening went over to Mr Campbells to spend the evening. Had a very quiet time and much talk and went weary to bed only to talk till the wee sma' hours with Miss Fletcher. We had a good talk – and she very much amused me by telling me that there had been a report current that I was soon to be Mrs Campbell. – That at a party at his house a girl 'Gilles' had the audacity to say before the assembly Mr C where is Miss S. tonight. He turned it off by saying they had not notified him soon enough to send me word (a surprise party) & they say that Jack Hume congratulated him sefl to someone that 'Miss S. being absent his sister would have a chance' – If I had know this I would not have run my head in the trap of going over there today. Next morning the Turners were there bright & early to hear me sing & then I went across the fields with them as far as McNaughtons where I called. ... I went on up the Speyside road and soon before me I saw the Beau Brummel form of Jim coming toward me. ... Between us is a great gulf set which never can be budged unless he changes his religious faith. There is something so entirely repelling in it that I can not abide it – I always feel it in my inmost bones it seems ever staring me in the face when with them – everpresent – ever repulsive – We went on up to Speyside.

The Miss Metires shaking their wise heads (!) one saying 'It looks suspicious', the other 'Must have been understood' ect and I suppose all Speyside had their nods, speeches, scrapes & guesses – although nothing animated was to be seen save a forlorn dog. Nevertheless their ambuscades behind windows & window screens were not for naught. Met with a very hearty welcome at Dunns – Mrs Moore thinks they are ambitious of having me in the family (Ugh!) Had a comical time always do if Jim is near & lots of music. My ci devant pupil Lizzie is doing well, very well in her music & is the pride of the family. Jim showed me his photo & some pretty girls opposite in a double frame & on my expressions of admiration he looked quite downfallen & said plaintively he had only put that there temporarly that he had been anxiously waiting for another for a long long time to put there – Showed me some appropriate poetry & sung me some ah! some luny songs but all for nothing the impression failed on me & he was off. ...

Do noble deeds not dream them all day long
And so make life death & that vast forever
One grand sweet song –

April 26th [back in Hamilton]

I know when I finished reading it [*St. Elmo*] [5] I was resolved with a stronger resolve not to let trifles come between me & my object in life – to overcome obstacles to rebound higher if aught seemed to pull me down. Monday seemed dull enough to go back to school drudgery – although I received a warm welcome back – warm enough to assure me that I was of some consequence at any rate, but I do not feel much affected by homage either – I am grateful I wish to be influential & yet when I receive it, it palls on my taste – & I only take it as I would my dinner as a matter of necessity. Today Friday has been very warm – sultry – exam this

5 a novel by Mrs Augusta Jane Evans Wilson

afternoon – hard paper in Eng Grammar. ... Came back to literary – We had quite a time to night – got quite befogged in their
movements & amendments – and that poor creature the president was completely lost amid 'not nineteenth century English' – We also had election of officers for Quarterly & I was put
on for one of principal editors by acclamation – quite gratified
Ahem! ...

May 11th

Beautiful May and beautiful life – I am happy these days – at least
nearly so – I am indeed *very very* thankful for the pleasant life I
lead but will it last. I am only doubting what will appear to mar
its beauties. The awakening of nature reawakens all dormant
energies – and puts a new impulse in our veins – that propels us
forward with lighter hearts. Jim alas for Jim – all the romance
connected with that friendship is dead – It grew rapidly and died
shortly. Just one year of life and now I am so wearied of it that I
cut the chord without a feeling of regret – new scenes, new
friends & new society have only served to make the ending, to
me – one of relief – It was all well for a time all well in so far as
friendship was concerned & that is all I every meant it to be with
him and he I hope that his words belie him & that he too will
not feel bitterly I do – I do – If he should feel revengeful I should
be in despair – but then, he should have gathered from everything that – that – a wide gulf was between us & that I would
never go down in my own estimation by turning renegade to
myself or my religion – All this tho' did not hinder me from
admiring his cleverness or from liking him as a friend but that
one act of his when I saw him at Speyside when he showed me a
paragraph which I doubt he wrote, in a paper of Toronto, I
forever cancelled his claims to my friendship – I hope I shall
never see him again – never again – but I doubt I shall hear.

...

'The sun comes up & the sun goes down
And what is all when all is done.'

May 18th

So are the weeks – they pass much the same and then at the end
'what of it.' What is done. We have our Boat Club now and have
been out several times. The bay has been very very smooth last
week & I hope I shall never be in such a hardened state of feelings as not to appreciate such wonderful beauty & calm in
nature as last Friday on the bay – oh it was glorious. The air *very*
clear & the sky so blue the bay calm and a May Sunshine over all
beautiful beautiful everywhere these days. ... Ma was up & Pa
went home – lots of letters from home but no news from Kingston. Today is beautiful day I am going up to Mrs L[awson]'s &
then down to Alices & back with them to church.

May 30th

I cannot cannot tell all that happen here I have not time – I have
not energy enough to do so. I was home for Queens Birthday had
a rest & saw home in peace. Ernest drove me up Tuesday morning just in time for school – & since then it has been hurry scurry
all the time – from morning until nights. The picnic has weighed
heavy on my hands & then we have but got over the examinations of Magill [McGill] Wednesday night were at Lawsons & I
enjoyed myself very much ... Wed's night 28 May 1879 a paragraph read thusly – 'Three ladies presented themselves before the
Council of Physicians & Surgeons for matriculation exam – two
of them Misses Augusta Stowe & Elizabeth Smith were successful but the third was "plucked"' – I cannot understand because
there certainly was but one lady beside myself there & that was
Miss Parmenter its a mystery to me but I think I will solve
it – Tonight we had a very tiresome meeting of the Literary – an
extemporanious debate of ten speakers on each side – whether

city or country life was the more conducive to happiness – & was decided for the country and yet we know better away down in our hearts we know at least some of us that this city life is the most exciting at any rate & thought of by the mass more enjoyable – I like both alternated – city life while strength & undying ambition animates the body – but when worn & tired with lifes troubles the quiet country then.

June 1st

Well I shall endeavor to describe my doings yesterday – Early in the morning I tried to do some studying but only did some Arithmetic. I went for my music lesson at ten & got back about half past eleven – fixed sundry small articles for wear & entertained Sutherland for a few min had dinner – donned my white basque & hat & started with my bundle of provisions for Maggie Ramsay – called for her – put my cakes in her basket – & after having a glass of cider took my departure for James St. called at Edwards & at another place for gloves – then for Mary Varey & then for Jennie Wood but as I was late they had both gone. Maggie & I tugging that baskets along under a blazing sun were so fatigued that when we reached James st we took a st car & were conveyed to Steamer Eclipse where I was hailed with numerous salutations and some business – Got through with that & seated myself – near Jennie & Ina while they disputed to which I belonged – Tried to read Molly Lawn but was assailed on all sides with reproof for wishing to be so unsociable – Reached Oaklands, Sutherland carrying our basket up the hill – to the tables on the grounds – There the crowd that had somewhat divided into twos mixed up again & I deputed Suth to go for the croquet & then Maggie McCoy & I got sixteen started at that – & went off & sat down by ourselves with Molly Baron but not long to be alone – first came McInnis tramping to us to have a talk & gradually seats tables – around was a crowd around us talking fishing arguing – Mcl. kept up a desultary confab for a time & then asked me to go out on the Lake for the afternoon – get on a

steamer & go back & forth for the sake of the fresh air. I agreed &
we hurried down to the piers only to see the steamer leave without us – We stood on the piers for a long long time – He told me
of his trip on the Lakes last summer ect & was very nice – we at
length sauntered back where I was saluted with 'we want you' so
we started to get supper ready ... lots of repartee & fun – then
Maggie & I sauntered off whilst they should set the tables. I read
some of Molly to her but was soon interrupted & then we got up
& being soon surrounded we talked hard – I especially at Code –
& pinned some leaves ect – for him & more nonsense – but supper being called, Sutherland came up & of course I had the felicity of taking my lemonade next to him because Code had been
ruthlessly called away to wait on the table – Ina sat at my right
hand & I had a real jolly time talking at everybody. Code in particular as he seemed to wait more at my table then anywhere
else – told or started to tell my fortune but I rudely cut him short
at the first mention of a young man in the scene said he w'd
come round to tea & would finish it then. I looked exceedingly
amazed & he quite abashed – laughed & said I should not mind
all he said ahem! During this time Suth was sitting meekly at my
elbow & a word in every five minutes was enough to keep him
in good humor ... We all waddled off to the boat & Mr Armstrong again secured a seat by me until we arrived in Hamilton
when Suthe. had the cheek to want to see me home – We went
up in the street car as far as Caroline & just reached the corner
by the collegiate when it began to pour. Miss Hagar, Martin,
Suthe. & I all took refuge in the Coll Inst. & although somewhat
damp we struck up a programme – lightened the gas and had
some fun music reading speaking reciting ect – till about nine
when the rain having abated somewhat – we again started for
home – when it again began to rain & I could not but in mercy to
his new coat ask him to come in when in he seemed dubious
about going out again & did not till about half after eleven – I
then retired – tired – glad & sleepy – footsore & tongue tired –
until about eleven this morning – I have slept nearly all day
intending to go to church tonight but as is so rainy I staid at
home – & am now going to bed again.

June 3rd

In broad daylight that I should sit down & write in this is
strange passing strange – Yesterday – Monday the morning went
much the same as usual with the exception of much talk about
the picnic – who did this & who that who got wet & who did
not. At noon for we had our lunch there – Ina & I were sitting
together alone when C.Coventry came up sat down before me
and began in a solemn voice to tell me that G.E.F. our mutual
acquaintance & friend was at the point of death from hemor-
rhagge. Now he is Ina's declared lover & I knowing the height of
bliss in which those two last met & the unparalleled worth in
which he was held by – trembled for the consequence – when in
a horrified tone Cora began to tale the pitiful tale – Ina could not
contain her tears nor shocked feelings & Miss C – all astonished
kindly left her to me. I got her down to the yard where poor sensitive darling cried & sobbed on my shoulder – She shook like
one in the ague & I seeing her sufferings – counciled her to go
home & I went with her despite my sore foot. I stayed for a time
& tried to comfort her – & then I left her alone with her grief.
Came back to school till four & then Alice & I according to
agreement came up Caroline & met W. Snow – our quandum
schoolfriend of two years ago – We came up home here & he
showed me how to doctor Alice's eyes which had been troubling
her but which she did not want her parents to know. He is very
much the same as formerly – talks incessantly – rather interesting
and has got through two years of his medical course. He spoke of
sending me several books, one of which I received this morning –
I don't know whether to think ill or well of him – I have a sound
distrust for all boys who have attended medical lectures for it
seems to have a very baneful effect on them – more so than it
would on girls ... tonight had scarce let her sombre curtains
down when Ina came for me to go & stay all night with her & I
went knowing how desolate she was – We spent a sadly quiet
evening & not much study – she could not & I could not for love
of her – She showed me his letter, where if ever I doubted the
ecstasy of lovers I was confirmed – happy Ina – whether he lives

or dies – to know that one manly heart beat truely responsive to thine – I hold it true what e'er befall – I own it when I sorrow most tis better to have loved & lost than never to have loved at all – There seems to be a gloom over their future – in fact ill forboding incline me to think that he will die – & then poor Ina sweet little pure hearted Ina ...

June 22nd

About this time every year I seem to be very happy. I will not go back over the days not recorded here for I should but imperfectly describe them and that would be an immense pity – old time is still a flying – Shall not recount the diff. answers I have received about medical & other matters – from Parmenter, Carson, Lavelle, Sanderson – but will pass by the wk. but to say that Wednesday night when we had our last committee meeting we had a splendid time – talked for about two hrs and talked not the greatest nonsense but about religion & politics principally & such a time I was sorry after I spoke so bitterly & generally about the Methodists – I was amazed to find Mr Hambly to be a Methodist – I was very sorry for I like him very much – Saturday was *the* day of the session. The boys picnic – One Oclock Simcoe St. wharf. I called for Mary Lavelle & we for Mary Varey & so on till there were quite a crowd of us before we reached the boat. We found Miss Coventry there monarch of all she surveyed – We disposed ourselves here & there waiting for the male men to put in an appearance which they did very slowly – we started with about twice as many females on board as there were gentlemen. When we got to Oaklands – Jennie Wood & I took the lead & sprang away to the well to get a drink & so on around the hotel to the seats at the other side. We were followed by the others marching two & two as solemn as a funeral procession & as orderly as a troop – girls together – boys ditto Presently there were arrayed some eight of us on a bench but no male man put in an appearance. Miss Coventry comes to me with 'For H— sake lets go & find a man' & so we started off Jennie & Navie bringing

up the rear. We went to the other side & reposed us in a
swing – soon Mary Varey & Lavelle & Ada Grover came up &
began a desultory talk & Ada stayed with us. Soon we were
joined by Ratcliff & Coutts & then soon we went from there,
Miss C with Ratcliff & I & Miss L. with Coutts just for a little
way & then I met a no. of others Ballard, Armstrong ect. Then I
don't remember except that Ratcliff, Jennie & I went for a stroll
around to the bank through the wood & reposed us with some
half dozen others under the trees on the bank. I had but settled
myself when the Commercial Master Sutherland came up &
wished me to go back to the grounds & play a game of croquet. I
went & soon had the three gents. – Lawson, Kapelle & Suth.
playing with me & having fun. ... After supper I went off ... to the
wharf & then as I had escaped everybody & was walking peacefully down the wharf with Miss McDonald, the other Sutherland
came up & asked if he might have the felicity & all that sort of
thing & see me to my paternal roof – I assented & when I had
reached the boat & got seated up comes the other Suth. that I had
left in the lurch & makes room beside me to explain what I had
against him, & we had lots of fun – Kappelle hovered around the
outskirts of the circle till he got tired & gave it up & delivered
over my parasol that he had taken such good care of all day.
When we arrived at this side – H. Suth stepped up to me &
walked off with me according to agreement. Oh for a painters
brush to depict the look on Suth no 2's face – He had nothing to
do but turn & ask Mary Lavelle to go with her & so we came up
st. & then down King to get some soda water ect & there Suth. 2.
hurls at Suth 1's head that he credits him to a good deal of
malice for taking Miss S. away from him – Well Suth 1 came up
& really acted as if he did not know when to go away. ... Sunday
afternoon according to agreement I went down to Alice's &
whatever evil destiny so ruled my star at that time I cannot tell.
Suffice to tell I met Suth. 2 down Main & he must turn about &
go down with me to Alices & the great soft booby actually came
in & bored us till five o'clock if he knew the inward anathema's
he received perhaps he would not have stayed so long. Maud
was there & Minnie Morrison too & I received a grand teas-

ing – to add to all. ... School again today – One could see there
had be something up by the diff. manners in which one would
address the other – comical. Tonight we had another editors
meeting & lots of fun. Kapelle keeps me in hysterics almost. Such
twinkling eyes & hearty laughs – Such a merry was & witty
speech if he were some 6 or eight years older I might be in
danger of losing my heart – but if he were that old I would not
like him so well. Perhaps I may never see him & the others again.
Alas! helas –

Sigh no more girls sigh no more
Men are deceivers ever
One foot on sea & one on shore
To one thing constant never

July 1st

Just one year ago today I was in Speyside vicinity visiting on that
broiling day at a farm house, so slow – so terribly slow – today I
am in my study, and studying hard, at Mrs Lawsons. ... Sat.
Myrtie went home & Ma came up. I went to church on Sunday
morning thinking to get a good sleep at night but who should
come in about 8 Oclock but H. Sutherland & bother me to
weariness – excuse got a letter for me at school – if he only knew
when to go home it would not be so bad. Monday went to school
in the morning & finding there would be no school till Thursday
morning after the forenoon – In the afternoon we moved. Ernest
& Cecil taking the things home & Ma & I coming here, what a
relief to my feelings no one knows here. Ma staid till today &
visited Mrs L. & I have been studying. Maud called yesterday &
wants me to go & stay a week with her after school closes. I
think I will for a while. This removes a barrier between Maud &
I for whether she knew it or not I would never have been quite
so much a friend unless she had. What shall I do with pride?
Why is dust & ashes proud?

July 6th

Wednesday night I had a call from H. Suther – a lengthy one –
and it was so comical. I waited till half past eight to make sure of
no one coming in & then I put on my wrapper & had not so
ensconced myself five, nay 2 mins before a ring at the door & the
appearance of Suth caught me – I went down & endured the
infliction in my wrapper – en dishabile with a vengeance. He
asked me to go for a row on Saturday & I assented – but the next day
repenting & the next more so I sent him Sat morning a note saying
that untoward events prevented me – ect but lo at noon – I was
called to the drawing again to meet his egotistic phy[siognomy] –
& I told him I would not go & also refused to go the the beach
& to church with him. Well I ate my dinner in a risable frame of
mind – as we had some fun over it & then after dinner before I
had dressed for calls I was again summoned to the drawing room
to meet Suth No 2 horrors, horrors. How shall I be able to write
what followed. In short I acted a part & successfully & I have as
often before I have found it polite to meet deceit with the same
tools & I put on the face of indignant innocence about the information he gave me with reference to the other Sutherland how
they had both tried @ the picnic to cut one another out. And the
gossip of school which he said coupled our names indeed over
this. There was no sham indignation – because there was no
grounds for such a report as I had never gone with him anywhere & he had only escorted me home a few times. But he was
so proud of what he had done that I honestly believe he has
boasted of it to the boys – miserable miseres cor. Well I quizzed
him & was agreeable for the mere love of wickedness I believe as
I do not like him in the least. He went away at last. After wonderfully astonishing me by offering to kiss me but I made my
way out of his reach in a hurry & told him if he dared to offer
such a thing I would strike him. Little do they know me here,
little indeed, does he if he fancies me that me to be that kind.
After he went away the reaction set in & I laughted till I cried –
almost hysterical @ the deceptive part I had played. Mrs. L. joining in the fun – Sunday afternoon Alex & John were in I cannot

forget Alex – he seems to try against caring for me & as he expresses it his greatest bump is caution, poor fellow. He is ambitious & good & yet circumstances are unkind to him, and he is thin & depressed in mind. Well as to the latter I do not wonder as he gives some of his wages I do not know how much to his people as his father is not employed – a shame a heartless shame. A boy kept on supporting his people when rather the father should have helped him – Went to church with the rest of them & when we returned we found Suth. No 2 @ the door & that great donkey came in & stayed till after ten Oclock much to my chagrin. He certainly is obtuse @ taking a hint for I gave him very broad ones to go. Friday night I was at Dalleys & enjoyed myself very much a great deal of fun & nonsense. ...

4

Nelson Township, Ontario
August to December 1879

Nelson Township provides Elizabeth with her second stint of rather more uncongenial teaching. Unruly students and home-sickness crowd the pages together with the delights of new friends and flirtations. Her unvarnished account of rural teaching with its difficulties as well as its opportunities for the single woman suggests why the turnover rate in the profession was so great. On October 7th Charlie Roberts first appears. Soon he will supplant the two Jims and Dick in her affections. Future developments are also anticipated by the arrival of her satisfactory Model School grades. These, like her successful attempt at the medical entrance exams, allow her hopes to range beyond that limited stage offered by rural schools.

> Time wasted is existence: used tis life
> How blessings brighten as they take their flight

July 27th

That week after my last entry was the week of the intermediate exams ... I think I got through of that more anon but Mary Varey failed. My exam. lasted till Sat. noon then in the afternoon I went to Services & stayed there till Thursday. ... Since that Thursday I have been home fixing up my correspondence and business gen-

erally. I have felt not at all energetic since the last wk of school –
too little sleep. Alice has not only passed the matriculation exam.
but got the scholarship in Modern Languages. hurrah for
Goldie – Our Allie. ...

Aug. 19th

I am here in Nelson township going to teach I guess tomorrow –
but first I will record what I clearly remember of the intervening
time between this & when I wrote last. ... Thursday I drove down
in the covered buggy for Maud as I expected her. Standing at the
station who should my eyes rest on first on the approaching
train but Dick – and soon Maud alighted to my great delight.
Then we proceeded to the buggy & ensconced ourselves. Now
can any one picture a more ludicrous scene than three trying to
sit in a buggy made for two. Well Dick had the centre seat & he
unknown to us was actually sitting on space by bracing himself.
We talked quite desultory tis true, owing to the different states of
mind in which we were. Maud had a peculiar dislike of Dick and
was annoyed that he had come at the same time as herself – and
Dick was enduring a species of agony better imagined than
described. While I was divided between delight at their arrival –
the comicality of the whole thing & a wish to keep up a friendly
peace and make things go of smoothly & sociably – per se to keep
up the conversation.
    Well we at last arrived the happy isle and made another fiasco
in alighting. I hopped out before Dick could reach the buggy
from the gate ... Dick got out helped me out & was about to assist
Maud who stood on the step of the carriage when the horse
started on & poor Dick wavering between a desire to help Maud
& to stop the horse was allowed to do the former when the horse
was stopped. ... Next day passed quietly with reading talking,
music croquet ect. ... & such a night, beautiful night shall I ever
forget. The purest harvest moon – a lovely breeze – and I was
happy – yes so lighthearted – such buoyant spirits that as Betsy
Bobbets would say 'exhilarated.' I was in the wildest spirits – I

made game of Frank, fought battles of repartee with Dick, laughed with Maud and I could have 'chattered chattered and gone on forever.' I wished it would never end at last it was necessary to retire – & we did so with a challenge which would be up first. After we had withdrawn I gave the girls theatrical performances in the most *hilarious* manner & made them laugh so long & so loud that it was to much for them. Next morning we breakfasted at ten (?) and after eating a good many apples & reading some we went for ferns & a walk to the mountain – and we missed our path & had to go through brush untold. The sun broiling down on us & burs innumerable – at last we reached the mountain and had comfortably settled ourselves with our books when the rolling of thunder & a few drops warned us of an approaching storm & hastily collecting things we started on our homeward way – We had almost reached home when it began to rain so Vi went to the house & brought umbrellas to us & we proceeded. Dick tormented me more than I can write by pretending to drive me before him and I was such a tempest that according to my temper I would not be driven and so we had quite – a fiasco – in fact – it was so ridiculous that I can not forget it – he was such a tease & I told him some plain truths too – and we got home without being very wet tis true but quite a drooping appearance for all. We kept it up pretty well all day – quarreling till towards evening when he was going away & I gave him cake & wine for a peace offering & he said G— bless you & threw a kiss to me when going. Ernie took him away to the station & we consoled ourselves by playing croquet – & singing & games. Next day Sunday we wandered about each on his own destruction bent; I read Evangeline to Maud & in the evening went to Stoney Creek to church – a good sermon & a lovely drive. Monday & Tuesday were only ordinary days except that there was a great deal of company. ... Sunday I dreamt away, went to church & then over the place & about the house. The next week was very quiet as Myrtie was away. ... [Sunday] We went on to H[amilton] & I went to see my dear dear friend Alice – my *best & truest*. She met me at the door and then we went to the parlor. I nearly broke down for I had been grievously disappointed that she had

not been to stay with me on the holidays as agreed, and then my
nerves were somewhat unstrung from going away. She told me
she thought to come to me on her way back from the Port but
had got a letter from home calling back immediately She had just
posted a letter for me, I felt more than I could say for I love Alice,
more perhaps than I ought, but then she is indeed a friend. A
friend. I went over to Arlands & waited for Ma. Then after doing
some shopping we drove to the G.W. Station where Ma left me &
my baggage. I went to the waiting room – observed human
nature in many different styles for a time, got my ticket & check
& then as the car was in I ensconced myself therein to wait till it
should leave for B— [Brantford] having during this time a good
observing place from the window of the car, to see the man of
business – the idler – fox, the philosopher & the flirt. We were
soon on the way to B— all right – found no one there to meet
me – a blessing in disguise as the sequel proves. I took up my
quarters in the waiting room @ B— & sang ... for my own
entertainment & waited for about half an hour ... then a man
disturbing my desolation by coming in for a drink. I questioned
him about the mails for Lowville & so by questioning, he found
out where I desired to go & said he was going within a mile of
there & would take me if I would ride in a lumber waggon
which I had for once the sense to do & so straightway behold
me, the conceited originator of ladies medical school ... the
haughty editor of the Quarterly – perched up so high above
terra firma that me feet could only reach the top of the lumber ... by dint of much exertion. ... About half way up he asked
me my name & declared his was that same ubiquitous cognomen. I laughed heartily, it seemed so absurd at the time. When
he had reached the corner where he was to have landed me – I
had so evidently made an impression that he insisted on taking
me all the way to Mr Wilson's, one of the Trustees but not the
one that was to meet me at the station. How fortunate, how very
fortunate! after events proved. I asked if Mr A Wilson a trustee
lived there & by that they knew who I was – & received me
cordially – one of the girls (Mary) took me off to the sitting
room where her father came and chatted. To my delight I found

them educated and modernised. The girls of which there were three Mary Janet & Ellen have each been to Brantford College[1] & have gold watches & chains ect – & its not every farmer who has done so much for his daughters. They are nice sensible girls with no glaring faults that I at least have observed. Their eldest brother is a B.A. M.A. & L.L.D went to the Collegiate @ the same time Ernie did. Their next brother Jim is also nice – funny and reminds me of the late Jim of Spey. and they have a nice little brother George about 13 who his father remarked was to attend the other school as they had more advanced scholars and he wanted him to get on fast. We shall see what we shall see. ... After I had partaken of a hearty dinner Mrs Davidson & Clara called & I was duly introduced & made friends. Mary & I then came up to the schoolhouse & over to Thomases, the trustees and I found they were Methodists – lived in a large stone house & nice flowers about but also plenty of mother inside the house as well as outside. They had evidently to me made up their minds that I was to board there but I also made up my mind that I would n't when I saw the condition of things. So on my way home we called @ Davidsons. There are two young ladies in the family one is now ill – convalescent – the other has been in Waterdown where she knew Mary Smith very well. They have a very nice place & nicely furnished – a piano ect – nice family. Got pretty well acquainted that night. Next afternoon we drove up to Freemans, school, & Spences. I found that Freemans were first class too, saw Willie Tallman there. At School was introduced to a good number and we arranged to call a meeting for Friday night to get up an entertainment to raise funds for school furnishings. And at Spences I found that I could get board after while & I was very glad for it is the only place beside Thomases that I know that I could. It will be the better for me too as I will not have so many incentives to idle away time & enjoy myself only. Next day school began such a school – 40 young ones that had – at least some of them, never been to school before – very

1 Brantford Young Ladies' College, founded in 1874 under the auspices of the Presbyterian Church

laughable and very tiresome one boy standing by me waiting for his slate hears another of the same grade trying to struggle through his lessons, turns to me & says 'he does'nt know it very well does he?' Another informs me that his pa got 'this book & one for John and Mary Jane a nice dress at the store today.' Well I survived the day. Mrs thomas called in the afternoon & seemed very desirous of having me there sometime at least – but I was proof against the 'witchcraft' or 'curious art' & hastened away home – found lots of company at the house. ... Friday evening we had a [school] meeting. They were present Mrs Inglehart, Freeman Spence & Thomas, Mary Davidson Mary Wilson & myself. I was modest at first & gave them a chance to have it their own way but I soon saw that that would be a very strange way if it was any way at all & so I went forward & said how it should be & thus it is. Went back & found more company there & spent a very sociable evening – Mr & Miss Wilson cousins of theirs were there we had lots of croquet & next day Saturday I sewed most of the forenoon & wrote most of the afternoon, had a couple games of croquet with Rev Wilson had a very nice chat ect. & then Mary Davidson having put in an appearance for rehearsal we betook ourselves to that & had a jolly time. Mary Davidson told me I had passed my examinations. Nobody on earth could tell or know how glad I was. I have not said much about it but thought all the same. So many plans were either to be grounded on that success or overthrown by failure. Oh I am & was so glad. I clapped my two hands at sides of her face & kissed her for her good news. I am sorry too for the girls for I only saw the no's of Lucy Bowes & myself among our girls & Rickark & Code among the boys. I am more delighted perhaps because of the long anxious but silent waiting & then too I got such a start of some of those conceited ones but yet I am truly sorry for them all, especially some. ... Hugh McCoy & George W took their pockets full of pears to church & kept us eating going & coming. Took a sleep in the afternoon & read McCauly essay on Milton. We the young folks Hugh Jim & George Mary Ellen & I went down to B. in the evening to hear the Rev. W. Wilson preach. Such a lovely drive – incomparable almost, lovely – & such fun if it was Sunday

but the most fun came in coming back. When we started we
wanted Ellen to sit in the back seat with Hugh – but no she
would not & created quite a bit of fun – a fiasco in short –
enough to get Hugh a little riled. When we started back Jim
wanted her to sit between him & Hugh but no she wouldn't
have anything to do with him & it was such fun to tease them.
So Jim just faced about and sat facing us & between him & me
we had most of the repartee – I like him firstrate and hope he
will be as obedient as the last Jim. We had a great deal of jesting
& consequently of laughing – it was a beautiful moonlight
night – by the time we reached home Hugh was almost in a
white heat with rage, so comical! ... Next morning – Tuesday I
rec. note from home & Kingston letters from Parmenter Service
& Cummings. Jolly & interesting. In the afternoon we had
another womens meeting here at school. Just before school was
out Mrs Freeman, Thomas & Inglehart came in & after the two
Mrs Spence Mrs Coulson & Mrs Davidson Mr Freeman, & Mr
Inglehart. We had a better meeting than before & most everything was arranged to our satisfaction. We kept it up pretty long
as women generally have so much to say & then extend it over
the greatest possible limit of time. ... Mary & I drove over to
Wilsons about 7 o'clock and we spent a very pleasant evening
rehearsing & Rev as critic tho' he never criticises me nemo lae-
cessit me impune & he has found that out. About 9 or ten Rev
Mr Henderson arrived to stay an indefinite time. He is a very
odd genius – very – quite eccentric & quite folly he's a married
man but seems not the least like a clergyman. Next morning he
told that as he was driving near Princton he met a friend whom
he recognised but who did not know him but said 'I think I
ought to know your face' 'Yes' he replies 'You ought to know the
bishop of Hyde Park.' He said this would have been so rich if the
companion of his friend had been an Episcopalian. I looked up &
quietly observed 'Probably if he had been an Episcopalian he
would not have believed you.' This took splendid as there was a
general laugh @ his expense. Well we were up late that night & I
felt anything but quick witted next day. However, I managed to

get through the days proceedings & crawl home @ night. ... At
table Henderson asked me about the no. of my scholars & on my
reply being 'Something over forty' – Wilson says with his usual
dignity 'You have a good chance to teach the young idea how to
shoot' – (& I said) peas – which brought in the laugh against him
& he said I see classics are no use here or something like that.
Well Friday afternoon I had no school – went up with Mr Engle-
hart for dinner & came back with them, cut some cake & engi-
neered the arrangements in the schoolhouse – saw the platform
made the carpet down lamps up etsotera (!) And as Rev Wilson
was waiting for us we took our departure, had a nice drive
home – then it was all bustle till all were away again up to the
school. Came up here & found Mr Dean waiting for us. We came
in had some fun & a little rehearsing. Soon the people began to
come & among them a great many infants which more than kept
up their reputation as terrible. I was almost satiated with praise
– a perfect ovation & I was introduced to the Audience as 'Our
much respected teacher' amid great applause which fairly over-
came all bounds when I had finished reciting. The Chairman seeing some going out offered as inducements to them to remain
'that I was to appear again' and when I recited Mary Queen of
Scots I had the best the most rapt attention. I carried their feelings with the piece & fairly took away their breath. It was flattering to say the least & I was the first one nominated for the cake
& got by far the most to vote for me & the first pool was a long
way in the majority but a girls brother being angry that his sister
should be outdone put down a four dollar bill & she carried off
the cake by a small majority. Everyone who knows of the $4
thinks very little of her success – all right tho'. It was a perfect
ovation for me. Rev. W. says it was a pity I had not had my
photos for sale that night & I might have made quite a heavy
sum. The cakes ran up to near $18 & the boquets were auctioned
off for 38 cents. So that the net proceeds will come somewhere
near $50. It was quite late when it was over & Jack McCoy & the
two Miss Chesnuts went over & stayed for a couple hours so that
it was near two oclock before we retired that night. Next morn-

ing Nellie & I came up with George to help wash dishes but found the most of the things cleared away. Went home & put in a jolly kind of a day – lazy rather. ...

Sep 2nd

Last night went up to Mrs Freemans found Janet & Nellie there before me & Rev W. came soon after. Had lots of peaches & spent a very pleasant evening, – played Lotto. They went away early and I stayed all night. Went to bed early & had a good sleep which is a great relief and, a variation, to the usual order of things. They are very nice sociable folks and are *very* kind to me as everyone else is here. I have more fruit stored here in my desk that I can manufacture before spoiling, peaches, plums & a host of apples. A year ago Jim used to arrive about 4 Oclock & I divided with him but the present Jim is too busy. Little Tom Stewart brought me some peaches this morning – said his father sent them from Saltfleet. I was very much flattered & accepted them in toto. Well I do think peaches and cream is the 'sumum bonum' of civilized 'grub' whatever the ambrosia of the gods may have been. Received a letter from home just now with lots of home news in it – dear old home and dearer inmates. Who can be like them. They can forgive faults till seventy times seven. If seems to me I always show the worst side of my character at home and the best abroad.

>'Often in the course
>Of lifes few fleeting years
>A single pleasure costs
>The soul a thousand tears'

Sep 4th

Yes it is too true – not that I know of any at present but we all by dear experience gain that pleasure ever bought with pain ... Last night was very quiet very. I read some from Sarah Tytlers 'Papers for thoughtful girls' and like it very much. I have enough to do and might do more if time would appear for the doing of them. Here am I at my desk in the schoolhouse with some industrious youngsters studying waiting with me. The children on the whole are pretty good. What should I do if they were not. I suppose I should then have to rule by fear as I do now over *some at least* by love. Now that would be capital to tell for there is one *ganache* who is nearly my own age as he is soon 19 and it seems so ridiculous to look up to a pupil – a great brawny man of a fellow but thank fortune a well disposed one. One feature of the pupils likes is manifest in that they bring one fruit in abundance – from tomatoes to peaches – until I think I shall have to give up in despair & let the fruit rot – *drefful* nuf sed (Oh for the touch of a vanished [hand])

Pass through this life as best we may
'Tis full of anxious care

Sept 5th

That's so and whether tis as teacher, doctor, student or farmers daughter anywhere everwhere there's the bitter with the sweet making life pleasant enough to wish us to live even tho' we have trouble in the main. It seems to me that I have left all philosophy behind or before me and am actually living in the present. Oh I sometimes think I am I must be made of queer material, for it was but so late and I was in all the effervescence of 'Loves young dream' and now contrary to all I thought possible I think not care not about him. I doubt then I could be content to live with one man for life – oh dear what an idea. Yes I'm a queer case – now theres another flirtation simmering with another, in fact, James VII. What a confession, but how can I help it. I like gentlemen friends and they like me and there's an end 'out to me at least. Well & I like to get ahead of the other girls – thats a confession. Here I am in my sanctum – the schoolhouse with the

trustees – they are having a confab about diverse things & I am
writing & listening – a beautiful beautiful day. ...

Honor & shame from no condition rise!
Act well thy part; in that the glory lies

Sept 8th

Monday noon – a right clear, cold atmosphere just such a day as
makes the heart feel light & the frame buoyant – and what is like
unto that. Friday night things went off quietly I practised & J[im
Wilson] read by the same light while the girls were in the sitting
room. Saturday a nice sort of a day had several games of croquet
with Jim & won every time. Yesterday we all went to church in
the morning had a nice drive a rather pedantic sermon – so
abstract in idea that the closest attention was necessary to imbibe
any good. I honestly try to listen & understand the gist in fact
the whole preamble as I hear it in that pulpit portrayed by Rev
Mr McMichan but he gives such uninstigated confusion of verbosity that it is exceedingly execrable and delivers it in such a
hackneyed man[ner] with closed eyes & almost a stammering
speech. In the afternoon I left arguing with J on religious matters
to go take a sleep with Mary. Had a good short one & then got
ready for Church again. We drove again to Waterdown & heard
the same conglomeration of words. Some parts of his sermon
was good & some I did not like. One allusion to our church of
the turncoats from it to Rome whilst they had none. Another
when speaking of Marquis of Lorne[2] said 'we as Presby. have a
great claim of respect for him on account of the Martyr blood'
Forgot likely that the endeavors of Lornes ancestors to stamp
them out would or should counterbalance that.

2   Sir John Douglas Sutherland Campbell, Marquess of Lorne, Governor-
General of Canada 1878–83

Sept 9th

Why is it that we live so culpably, why so lightly when the
things of earth are gravissimus as weighed in the balance
whether our future will be bright or not. Last night I received a
letter, the receipt of which was something of a marvel and yet
something of a relief. If ever I flirted alas that I should say it it
was with J.P.D. [Jim Dunn] oh dear why will men deceive themselves. When we used to meet so often – oh just one year ago –
and these days bring it back vividly to remembrance. Those days
of jollity, walks, music & fruit, those days when the beauty of
earth & the lightheartedness of youth and the attendance of
handsome witty J.P.D. They were golden if they are regretted, oh
that was one of those instances where 'a single pleasure costs the
soul a thousand tears.' I have regretted & yet what have I to
regret – only this he will not cease from keeping himself remembered by letters & music. Alas poor Jim what shall I do shall I
answer or not thats the question whether 'tis nobler in the mind
to suffer the slings & arrows of not answering his letter or to
take up my pen & put an end to his trouble. Aye there's the rub
for in that correspondence what speeches may be made that may
not lessen the difficulty. He also sent with the letter 'The Blue
Alsahan Mountains' ...

It was as if remembering they had wept
And knowing they should some day weep again

Sept 15th

Monday it is – Monday the renowned in the annals of Hamilton
ah – why am I absent from the city of my adoption when the
Princess Louise & the Marquis of Lorne are to be on exhibition
in Wentworths ambitious city. Helas! – helas. But to go back to
the thread of my narrative ... Went to church in the evening
[Sunday] to Waterdown & heard Rev Mr Fraser preach a firstrate

sermon. 'Out of the depths have I called to Thee' a very good sermon one that leaves an impress. He said that in prayer there should be an earnest cry for some particular thing that we needed not to pray for everything in general. For if we prayed forgive us our sins how would we answer the question 'what sins?' if addressed to us & gave the example of blind Bartimus who forgot everything else in the desire that he might receive his sight. He also said that many did good deeds not through love of pleasing the Heavenly Father but in hope of being rewarded by gaining heaven or equally culpable those who did so for fear of going to hell & said as much as tho' we should set forth our religion not only with our lips but in our lives. and that is my creed 'may I live up to it.' This morning broke bright & clear & I was very glad of that for it makes the irksome duties lighter if nature is in a good humor. ...

'The boast of heraldry the pomp of power
And all that beauty all that wealth e'er gave
Await alike the inevitable hour
The path of glory leads but to the grave'

Sept 16th

Everything went off so well in Hamilton yesterday. How I should like to have been there. ... This morning came up to school very early ... James came in with me took a survey of the school and an apple. Chatted & went on. Thank fortune they are digging a well in the yard. I presume by Xmas they will probably have the school furnished. It will be nice for the next teacher but what a tiresome time for me. ... I do get so thoroughly disgusted with teaching to stay all day away from civilization & try to instil knowledge of the most primary description into such infantile minds – oh dear. I thank my fate that it was nor will be my portion tho' it is for so short a time, but I've no doubt but that it is good discipline for me. I know that it is – therefore why

do I murmur when my sky is wholly bright to view   Kismet –
Kismet – Oh fy

Sept 18th

Oh dear this is a dreadful task. So many quarrels & bickering
among the young ones & then I have to settle them, be judge
jury, & lawyers. Well lately have not had much time to write at
noons & neither is this, but after the opera is over & the children
for the night are dismissed. ... Thursday & Friday went I suppose
as usual, I had not time to comfortably write so let it go. Gave
Clara her music lessons & went through the usual drudgery of
the week. Oh dear I am so tired of this – how shall I ever live
through it till Xmas. Such a long dreary dreary time ahead but it
must pass away. God give me strength of mind & body to do my
duty without flinching to do my duty to the children & to all
men. It *is* hard to do right & it is harder yet to know the right to
be sure we are in the straight & narrow path but I am going
home on Thursday wk if alls well & then I shall be better
minded. I wish I had Jennie Wood to talk to just now. She is the
one I was wont to go to unbosom myself when aggravated or
depressed. Dear Jennie, I do wish I had you with me ...

  'To make our idols & to find them clay
   And then bewail their worship'

Sept 25

How often in life do we do this. We place a high appreciation on
someone and then find that 'too much familiarity breeds con-
tempt' Thank fortune that I *have* friends that I'll never bewail –
but saddest sharpest of all these idols would be like the one in
the original 'Rispahs Idols' where in young girlhood she had
loved passionately entirely as only deep natures can and then

when she had reached womanhood & the end of her education
to find him so far different from her – that wanting respect for
him, love, vanished with it. Ah me – ah me we are all heroes or
heroines in our own particular dramas. ... Today is *the day* @
home – The Bazaar. I wish I were there & if wishes were horses I
would. Really it almost seems too bad. I have not been home this
season in so long a time – but I fancy – things will not alter much
in a week except the bazaar which I shall inevitably miss. Oh
dear what is there to make me like this part of my novel – so
dull, so slow so slow – – –

Sept 29th

'We know not what a day or an hour may bring forth.' How
little I thought when I last wrote here that I should be home so
soon. Friday night when I went back to Wilsons the old folks
were away & Jim was going to Josiahs & wanted me to go I had
the strength of will enough to resist all his coaxing & his sisters
persuasions & stay at home. Soon George came in with letter
from Maud & a card from Mater summoning me home the next
day. As they were going to take James to the station next morning I saw my way clear for that part of it. Went in by the G.W.R.
early train with Jim to H— up to Mrs Lawsons & found that Ma
had been there but was down at the station. Went down town
found Myrtie, had walk & talk. In afternoon visited Alice &
stayed to tea. Alice just looked 'chic' in her silk dress & cap. ...
Reached home about ten as we had to wait a long time for Ernest
who was away, up at Walkerton & around there. Found my
receipt of 10 $ waiting me for books on Duncan & Stewarts, also
a very satisfactory letter from Dr Lavalle.[3] It was indeed *very*
satisfactory – all that I could wish. I am just delighted about the
University – everything goes on so well. I have small cause to
complain or look melancholy – all my days I may be sure I have
had all that was good for me. ... Sunday I was over the farm in

3 of the Royal Medical School at Queen's University, Kingston

the vineyard over the house. The place looks so well & all the
farm looks thriving – looks like the 19th century. Came away
about 4 on Monday morning – Ma brought Cecil to H— to commence again at the Coll Inst. I was just in time for the train got
aboard & reached Burlington at 7 Oclock, waited for more than a
halfhour & Mr Wilson came for me drove up & got to school a
few minutes after nine. ... I think I will go to Spences on Saturday
if I can get my traps taken. Then I will at last be settled down &
have time to write & read & study. A delightful calm before the
storm a rest before commencing the arduous rounds of a university course. I hope I shall be able to get into the Normal [School].
I must make my application right away. I received a letter from
dear Jen Wood last night dear faithful Jennie. how I used to
abuse her good nature by telling her all my trivial crosses

Oct 7th

Yes the days go slowly surely by and each day is a small aperture
in the curtain of the future. I wish how I wish that I were a better Christian there is a constant worrying knowledge within that
tells me I am too much of earth. That I do not think enough of
the Hereafter ah Hereafter. 'A whip to keep a coward to his
track'? No! No! no that were an atheistic speech – terrible. I wish
I knew could always know but one way one narrow sure way
wherein to tread but sometimes I cannot see which to choose
how to act. Is it the true & the right way to abstain from *all*
things but religion in the heart & mind on Sundays? Is it the
right way to keep a painfully solemn face on that day more than
others? I cannot believe the last at any rate I cannot think God
would delight in such worship. '*they* disfigure their faces and
make long prayers' is that to be good? I do not think so I am not
the only one so troubled. Charlie Roberts said the other day that
he was almost an heathen – 'that he had queer thoughts.' I hope
he will think better of it all and go back to the church it has been
the Methodists that have disgusted him I am afraid I like Charlie
first rate never had such a good talk with him before

Oct 8th

Well a day we shall [see] what change of place will do for you old diary. I have shifted your quarters from school to my room and here goes for a 'retrospect' Last Thursday I went in with Wilsons to the Central Fair in H. ... Went from there over to the Coll Inst to see Cecil. On approaching the West Entrance who should I see but Sutherland No 2 coming to greet me and he reminded me as usual of 'Peter Dick' with his guffaw & self assertion. He offered to hunt up Cecil & did so I only had chance to see Cecil for a few minutes & so Suth. walked down to King St. with us & told me some of the Hamilton news. We went on up to the grounds – saw several friends from the country and presently caught sight of Ernest & Gertie made up to them introduced Helen & almost at the instant Mr J. Shaw & Young. Carruthers came up had a regular pitch battle of words with Carruthers – like him I'm afraid my mischievous or some would say flirting propensities stood out in *base* relief; for Carruthers, yes Shaw too roused me to veni vidi vici. Went on for awhile – met several friends Mary Smith, Senior among them – picked up Charlie Roberts in the fruit department and had a real good walk & talk with him. Soon after I parted with him I fell in with our crowd Joe & wife – John & wife William & wife & soon up came Dan & George. I was real glad to see Dan. I think a great deal of Dan and maybe they thought too much for a mere cousin but I see in Dan a possible *beau ideal* cousin – A cousin next to a brother – a friend & adviser of the other sex & that I like let them think what they will. Had a good talk with Dan Gertie & Ernie bade us goodbye as the[y] had to go by that train & so Helen & I wandered off & fell in with Mr Wilson the bachelor, who is a rich confirmed old bachelor. He manifested a desire to fall in rank & asked if he might we graciously gave our permission and we continued our march – Met Mr McInnis & he asked me not caring for those about if I were free to walk round with him. I was constrained to say no where I had much rather have said 'Yes' & so I was compelled to continue our round. ... On again till we made the circuit and then fell in with Jack McCoy & wife a

little banter & then behold Sutherland making his bow to us. He
sauntered up to me & conversed madly for a while, told me he
was doing duty to a female cousin that afternoon and that she
was 'awful quiet' could n't get her to talk except in monosyl-
lables – 'how distrait.' He lingered till common politeness bade
him go. He actually had the audacity to ask for my photo & there
before Wilsons very eyes & ears, how absurd! ... George & Dan
again appeared but Helen & I were forced to go. The brightest
the most beautiful skies do not last. I tore myself from them ... Mr
Wilson followed & walked down to the Hotel with us where we
found Mary & James VI quite delighted & all that sort o' thing.
Had a long lovely drive home by moonlight and all that delightful day was done. The next day Friday was but the dregs of the
cup of pleasure – A dull listless working day with the same tale
told that so many days tell, of lessons, tried temper, exhausted
patience delight at success regret at failure, impatience of stupidity of case where I was defendents & plaintiffs lawyer and judge
of all squabbles. Saturday came away from Wilsons. In the morning went round by Zimmermans to see about music lessons up to
Davidsons to give Clara hers. Met Rev Mr Straith there a fat fair
fish for which some of the girls seem to be angling. Well it was
really comical to see the household at Zimmermans. The boys
popped corn for me the old lady brought honey the girl nuts &
peaches till I was fairly gorged with eating. The Wilsons were
very kind Mrs W. especially. The girls came with me to the
woods where we had a quiet ramble so that I did not get here till
about sundown. Spent a quiet evening. Went to church on Sunday afternoon at the St. heard Mr Belt preach a good sermon but
it was very warm. ...

Oct 13th

How one gets accustomed to most anything. I am getting quite
happy & content with this Bohemian sort of a life. 'Vagabondia'
forever. Probably it is because I think of a speedy release from –
perhaps because I can ride – & study & think – here – where I can

keep my own room – But @ Wilsons I was in perpetual trouble because if I kept my room I was afraid they would think me unsociable and so I must needs keep about the house talking & dawdling when I would much rather have been in my room. I have studied a little, read a little & several other things a little altogether keeping me quite busy – quite. Here it is Monday morning again – the weeks speeding by till Xmas will soon be here – good. How much less one feels time drag when one is busy – I am quite – so, so now. Sat I was out again for a ride, three times last week & I had a lovely canter. I enjoy it indeed. What a jolly useful life I can lead if I try not if I try, but if I succeed – because I will try. I think tho' that teaching makes one selfish. Always thinking of *what* I shall do, when & how and of results, of plans for the future & altogether I do not get time to get everything thought about. I am shamefully neglecting writing – especially on business. I must do that now right away. Everyone is kind to me to my face at least N'importe – I don't much care.

Oct 16th

What a very pleasant existence mine has been so far, thank God for it. Yes I will say this time what I mean for how often do we say 'thank fortune' when we mean a higher power by far than that. And yet if we should say out bluntly what we did mean it would smack of blasphemy and would rather frighten – hurt the hearer rather than make a good impression. Todays programme has been the same as a great many others. In the morning rise at dawn – don my wrapper & hasten down to breakfast & prayers. Then back to my room – tidy it up – dress myself and then sew or study or write till – half past eight. Then off to school. Perform the duties of the three hours forenoon – then noon & I eat my dinner with the children on tables they have erected at the back of the schoolhouse in the girls yard. At this time and others, I teach the children to love me rather than fear me – to like to be with me rather than shun me. The noon soon passes & then three hours more of even harder duty – and then release & hurry home – equip myself for the ride get my horse & self ready & off. Willie with me & that ride compensates for the days labor almost. Teaching may be irksome, it is sometimes, but yet it has its brighter side. I have everywhere met kindness. Whatever they say – I think theres no reason for a girl sitting down & bewailing her incapability to make her way in the world. Why even that year I taught just on a third & yet I saved up 250 and paid my own board. Now if I only continued in *that* way for 5 years I would have enough to keep me on the interest and free to marry or not as I chose without any impelling motive to make my fortunes sure by marrying. Come back again when darkness falls – cheered tired & ready for other work – go to my room read study or sew till supper then descend for a chat & a hearty meal & back again to my room for work. I like study this kind of study – the human frame really I like it. Whatever the world says what do I care – I am free to work out my own salvation without regard to what man thinks provided I do all things to the glory of the Father. Can we *not* do so – we *can*. I can foresee that in the future course which I have planned I must only think as one possessing brains – must forget that I am a woman, forget there is a trait called sensibility and only think there is a great Creator, over all, who has fashioned us & called the work – good – think only of it all as a wonderful study – a study worthy of all the powers of the greatest mind & therefore less than all mine would be unworthy the subject I pursue. Go forward I must and will in this. Yes distasteful as it may be in some phases to that ingrained false modesty which recoils at the study of what we are and how constituted. Oh Society! Society! Why do you weaken while endeavoring to purify mankind! why do the barriers first raised become covered with the slime and moss of falsity & prejudice, until those barriers of or rather from evil become walls to shut out good – Why are most peoples so strongly conservative in its true sense? Why so apt to cry shame to any new code. The Reform comes at last by someone. Someone of your caged and trammeled creatures break those barriers and in the breaking suffer much wounds suffer and bear all, sacrificing self – for the

hope that they may bear the brunt whilst others may follow
scatheless – scatheless of what? The 'on dits' of the public. Why
should that daunt or hurt? Ah we are only mortal after all & we
like our fellows good opinion. We like to be great in the eyes of
the present man. We that is the majority are not content like
Burns, Milton Shakespeare to be slighted in life, to be remembered for aye in the future no – no. let us have sufficient courage
to throw off that trammling – unworthy bondage – pampering to
public opinion – which is fickle as the wind.

...

Oct 28th

Last Friday night Mary Davidson called at the School to see me
& if I would not go out to Waterdown to the Literary Society
with her. I thought I would & hurried home dressed & off.
Reached there about dark waited awhile and then we – Mary
George & I started off in the buggy. Were not quite in time for
the beginning but soon enough to see plenty. About the biggest
sham of a debate I ever saw. It was 'Resolved that the Negro has
suffered more from the hands of the white man than the Indian.'
There were some five speakers. The first arose & with some difficulty reached the Reading Desk looked around – blinking like a
weak-eyed man in sun & snow. Made a grimace – said a word
made another grimace laughed covered his face with his hand –
broke entirely down covered his face with both hands. Made
another start & grimace said we all knew that the Indian had
suffered more from the White man than the Indian & as he had
another chance of speaking in the reply he would take his seat
which he did to our infinite amusement & delight. The next
speaker said the first had brought forward no arguments and as
it was self evident fact – that the Negro had suffered more from
the hands of the White man than the Indian – he would take his
seat which he did amid somthered groans. The others copied

their leaders with little variation and so the debate was closed
and the unlucky chairman was called on to decide. ... On Thursday night John Thomas ... big old & ignorant thought himself
justified in ringing the bell & this was against orders as he knew
altho' I had never said in so many words that it should not be
rung. So next morning I spoke to him about it & he was imper-
tient so summoning all my dignity & straightening my spinal
column I said 'if I say the bell shall not be rung it *shall not* be
rung' & went on with my lessons. The children being quite terri-
fied by my tones as I think I never spoke to them so before. So
that night he took it upon himself to ring it again & hasten away.
So Monday morning I told him he was to write me an apology
before I would hear him any lessons for his disobedience. He was
very bold & said he would do no such thing & would come there
to school as long as he liked. I told him he might take his books
& go home & said he would not – I told him it did not matter he
might sit there but *I* should never hear him another lesson until
he wrote the apology. He sat there till noon & then went home to
his dinner & when he came back he found the door locked on
him. Then the run began – he tried the door but found it
impregnable. Then he mounted the window ledge outside &
yelled frantically at me all manner of absurd speeches such as 'I
command you to go & open that door – I'll let you know you're
not boss around here' ect. I paid no attention to him more than
some scraps of his oration came floating in to me & made me
quite hilarious with laughter & the children too. This made him
angrier still & he could think of no better plan than going down
to the window next the boys & trying to induce them to go
unfasten the door but they only laughed & turned away & this
made us merrier still for he screamed 'I don't see what you are
laughing at.' He then went to the door & barricaded it from the
outside then shouting that if he did not get them open today he
would soon   he stalked off. ...

'A heart at leisure from itself
To soothe & sympathise'

Nov. 7th

I must continue the thread of my narrative where I left off to do
so has been a mountain to write up the whole but by putting it
off it has now become so great that the writing is unsatisfactory.
Wednesday I thought the best thing would be to have the trustees all in and have it settled so I sent a boy to Mr Wilson & one
to Mr Inglehart & notice to Mr Thomas & waited to see results.
They came at noon Mr W & I & Mrs Wilson long before Thomas
& I told them the story. They both thought I had done well had
acted best under the circumstances. Then Mr Thomas came in
and if I could only remember what all he said it would fill a
goodly number of pages and such Billingsgate such a monster of
ingovernable temper as he showed himself he has completely
astonished his neighbors & disgusted them too. He was in just
such a mood as you would expect an Indian mad with drink to
be & he very resembled a native at that time. Mr Wilson kept his
temper well or there might have been I know not what. Thomas
would hear nothing but would insult & storm at us & the other
trustees expelled John T think of that ... He went away in high
dudgeon after having successfully made a fool & laughing stock
of himself. That evening according to invitation Mr & Mrs
Spence & I went to Tassies. They bear marks of good society
Paters brother is Principal of Coll Inst Galt & one of his sons a
B.A. was a teacher there too & happened to be home that evening.
We had a very singular talk – very & I wish I could see him again
for I was so miserable that I was but a listener & assented to
more than I would if I had been well. They live in good style &
are well educated. I like them very well. They as well as every
one else think Mr Thomas – noncomposmentis especially in his
treatment of me. I was very tired and busy last week for I gave
the music pupils their two lessons apiece during the week that I
might have Saturday to go to Hamilton. I thought I would
crochet a pair of cuffs for Cecil so sat up till midnight in order to
finish them & was up before daylight to go to town it was bitter
cold but I arrived safely about eight oclock in the fair City. Went

up to Mrs Lawsons to see if Ma had been there & found Cecil keeping house & getting his lessons. He almost demolished me with his bear hugs & I was real glad to see him he's a very affectionate boy and of a strange enough temperament to be interesting & very clever is he. Had a good talk with him & Frank coming in I chatted awhile with him & then Cecil & I went down town to do some shopping & meet Ma. ...

'As I have seen a boat go down
In quiet waters suddenly
When not a wave was on the sea
Nor in the sky a frown'

Nov. 10th

Saturday was a very busy day with me even as all my days are. In the morning I rode down to give Clara her music lesson & back again to do my washing then gave two music lessons and did sundry other things that kept me late & then I read till near two oclock. Sunday morning bright & balmy like a spring morning. I busied myself helping Mrs Spence as her girl had left her the night before. We got ready for church & just before going Miss Jennie Panton came in & then just as we were off Mr Culloden drove up & so we stayed at home. I was seated in the sitting room chatting with Miss Panton of Milton news & folks in general when she told me of Ella Sanderson's death. Dear dear Ella dead & forever parted from me on earth. I cannot tell how I felt grieved shocked, stunned. I can fancy how people faint at such blows. I bore up for awhile & then I made my escape to my room & had a good hearty cry – a cry such as I have not had in a long time. I can scarcely realize it. To think that she is only dust & ashes now – what would I give for her photograph? Oh it is a sad solemn warning to be ready at all times for 'we know not the day nor the hour when the Son of Man cometh'

Nov 11th

Monday morning the first thing wrote a letter to Mrs Harrison
for information about Ella – dust & ashes. Who's got thy bonny
arm? dust & worms – how well I remember her telling that ghost
story to Wes McCollom & the driving out of Milton one Autumn
night just two years back from her death. Mors janua vitae. ...
This morning began to rain – dark dismal & constant rain, paddled up to school, thirty scholars went through the first part of
day much as usual and about two Oclock Mr Little came in. He
is indeed a strange man – a noticable character – one to make a
book popular a Daniel Deronda[4] – an iceberg – an automaton.
The second class made 96.26 in spelling which was very good
indeed. I do not admire his inspection for its justice but I do in
some things for its thoroughness. Kept me there till dark. I sent
for Mr Wilson too as he wished one of the trustees & he was
there also – It was thoroughly dark when we did get home. Gave
Johnnie Spence his lesson & ect & now write tired so tired.

Nov. 15th

Already that date; how glad I am to see the golden moments go.
It is getting nearer Christmas nearer nearer and I am nearer
Home, 'and it may be I am nearer home – nearer now than I
think' I have been so unnaturally tired these last few days. Not
myself at all. ... The people here are more than satisfied with my
teaching & desire me to stay but no I'm off for pastures new. I
like to instil knowledge but oh the worry and bother and dirty
faces that one has to encounter – bah – not for me ... I hope I shall
have strength & skill enough to fight the good fight so that I
shall not be one of the foolish virgins when the Bridegroom
cometh. Aye God give me strength & skill.

---

4 title of George Eliot's last novel (1876). Perhaps Elizabeth is thinking of the
   cold and mechanical Henleigh Grandcourt rather than of Daniel Deronda
   himself.

Nov 21st

This week has gone by very quickly & very quietly. The trivial
round the common task has furnished all I need to ask, Music
lesson beside the other round of school work keeps me busy
indeed. Today Mary Wilson was here to see me. This morning
down to Davidsons to give Clara her lesson back then dinner &
then Johnie & then Mary came & stayed till dark. She says her
brother is to be married on Xmas day to St Mary's for a wk &
then home for a week & perhaps they will come to see me the
second week of the New Year. I wonder now if they are afraid of
my wiles are they afraid that I'm ambitious to carry off James
and live on the old place. All families I believe have a fancy that
their own are the ones that every one is endeavoring to capture.
Pah – it takes some folks a long time to find out one's opinions. If
they they knew how I well not exactly despise but consider
utterly out of the question it would be for me to have any of
these or any other common person they would perhaps not think
so. I believe in marriage and would fain marry sometime but
where will I find the 'beau ideal' of my fancy where – echo
answer – where – I wonder sometimes how & my life will go
on – here the loitering length is – dull and slow indeed –

Sic transit gloria mundi

A marvel seems the universe
A miracle our life and death
A mystery which I cannot solve
Around above beneath

Nov 29th

Yes indeed it is all of that, is beyond our depth. So little brings us
near death, so little. I have by some means or other secured a
most severe cold indeed it is congestion of the lungs. I was very

much frightened when on awaking this morning about five
Oclock I was very near strangling – so hard to get my breath.
This last week has been much the same as usual. ...

Dec 5th

Monday night two music lessons & very tired. Yesterday night
about exhausted & Matilda Shyman, Mrs Spence's sister came a
sweet gentle invalid confined to her chair with rheumatism –
how thankful might I to be that I have life & limb & so many
blessings. Wed night down to Davidsons gave Clara her lesson &
stayed all night. He (Mr D) brought us up next morning – The
roads have been and are in a frightful condition here & I think
that helps to increase my cold. Thursday night – two music lessons and as tired or more than usual. Tonight a regular feast of
reading the papers & a letter from Alice & one from Myrtie. I see
so much news in the papers – among other things mention of the
Separate Lectures at Queens and another piece bearing on that
subject. Today like all days has been very tiresome at school. I do
indeed like the majority of my pupils – and I do not like to
punish them. ...

Dec 9th.

Yes I am so tired of teaching here. So tired of battling with overgrown boys – and boyish impertinence. And yet I suspect all
lives have their troubles. Into each life some rain must fall. Some
days be dark and dreary. Saturday was a very busy day. In the
morning went down on 'Polly' to give Clara her lesson & when I
got back found Agnes waiting for her music lesson. Gave John &
Bella theirs too and found the day only to long & the rest at
night so sweet. Today Tuesday has been very much the same as
usual only Charlie Thomas refusing to do as I told him a great
over grown booby – but yet I punished him. I would not like to
be in circumstances that compelled me to be country school

teacher all my days or marry – ah no. I have written a long letter
to Maud a special one. In it I give some reasons for not believing
in foreordination to 'Work out your own salvation with fear &
trembling' ...

> One thing must still remain in dark
> The reason why they do it
> And just as lamely can ye mark
> How far perhaps they rue it

Dec 11th

Oh it is getting so near going home time so near & I am sae
glad – sae glad. I have had such a time here. The other day I saw
Charlie Thomas whispering and told him to stand – he's a great
booby of a boy & is taller than myself – he refused to do so. I told
him to remain @ recesses for the week & when it came recess
time he said he would not stay in. I told him to stay out & he
took his books & went home. So I was duly notified that there
would be a meeting of the trustees on Friday night & I was
requested to attend. Well Friday night came & with it trouble,
trouble. I never doubting that he would attempt to prove a lie
detained no one for witness but Thomas brought up his sons &
John Draker a boy very much resembling swine and tho' a half
grown boy in the first book & had them to say what they had
been tutored to say – and then by blarney they got Mr Inglehart
to waver & go halves & support the motion that Charlie should
come back if he were obedient. Mr Wilson stood out bravely &
spoke well & warmly. I shall never forget him for it he stood my
friend & a gentleman. I may say the only one present. He called
to condole rather to comfort me on Sat but I was out & did not
see him. I bore up bravely while that shameless affair was going
on but cried silently all the way home, & when I got here I
nearly had hysterics. I do n't know that I have had a cry like that
for years – ever. ... Sat morning when I awoke I felt one of the
dreariest of mortals to be sure. I had the future to look forward

too but ah the intervening days how could I go forward through all their dreariness and blank ingratitude, and the days work before me. Well the only way was to ask God's help & I did & found strength to go cheerfully through my duties ... thankful that the morrow was the sabbath – had a short peaceful day, got ready to go to church but the storm came on & we did not go. Today has been a struggle & God has helped me this I know – or I had never got through it, so I have the sympathy of the community.

5

Ottawa, Ontario
January to March 1880

In her few months of attendance at the Ottawa Normal School Elizabeth explores not only the attractions of the capital, especially its sermons, but discovers a strong affection for Charlie Roberts or Carlos as she nicknames him. Although good times are very much a part of her life with the other 'Normalites,' the aspiring medical student also hardens her resolve not to imitate her more frivolous companions. A typical nineteenth-century feminist, she argues that women have a special moral purpose. In much the same way as ministers, they should remind men of their higher nature. Her preoccupation with moral reform, again quite typical of the age, leaves her largely indifferent to the injustices of the economic system. This outlook is evident in her description of the E.B. Eddy match factory where she ignores the working conditions to voice a liberal's delight in the technical ingenuity it reveals.

'Then looking back upon thy life
  Thy one regret shall be
  That thou hast done no more for Him
  Who did so much for thee'

Jan 1st [1880]

Yaas weally – it is New Years evening and I am here under the home roof glad to be there ay – so glad. That last week over there at Nelson was very busy. The Wednesday after what I last wrote we Mary & George Davidson & I went over to Wm. Wilson's. Spent a very pleasant evening I got back about one. Friday night Jim Wilson took Mary & I to Waterdown to an entertainment & the distribution of prizes. It was very good especially the farce at the end. 'Popping the Question' They all did their parts well – very well! We got back about one Oclock – I liked Jim firstrate & he returned it. If he was better educated & had seen more of the world I might like him very well but never mind there's more fish in the sea. ... Next day I bade them a tearful tender adieu & Mr Spence drove me to Hamilton where I found Myrtie & Ernie at Lawsons a warm welcome truly, Myrtie & I went shopping and did not get through till about nine when we set sail for home, tired & drabbled for the streets were in a very bad condition. When we reached home & had had our first chat over, Myrtie & I went to work to make Xmas presents & did not get through till two Oclock Christmas day Ma & Pa were at Uncle Ransom's & Cecil was spending a week in Buffalo. He had carried off 1st proficiency prize & first French at school, & now we hear Myrtie has secured the ten dollar prize at St. Catherines as she come's out head of the girls. We went to Church in the morning & heard Mr Craig. The church was splendidly decorated. Next day Cecil came home – the dear boy – having had a very good time. Saturday Frank Lawson came down and in the evening Kennedy & Roberts were here and we spent a very pleasant evening very – Roberts stayed till next day. I like him very much, very much, because I respect his genius he's so *clever*. Monday night the Lavalle girls – Hannah & Will Corman, Kennedy, George & Lizzie, Joel, & Walter Thomas were here & we had a capital time just capital. ...

Jan 7th   Ottawa

'Man's inhumanity to man
Makes countless thousands mourn'

So I said at the beginning of Model School. So say I now. The great inhumanity to me just now is that I cannot talk with Charlie [Roberts] or Shields. oh dear you may laugh if you please but no one but one placed in a strange city with two friends from home and then debarred from seeing them, can tell how hard it goes. I suppose I may as well begin where I left off and give a synopsis of my doings down to the present time. Saturday a number of callers. Sunday peaceful as it was a stormy day we did not go to church. Monday morning started at dawn for the station – Pa & Cecil going with me. Waited at the station for a good while. J[im] W. Wilson came in – was going up on the same train. Took charge of me up to Hamilton & saw me off on the Toronto train. I arrived in Toronto about half past ten went up town did some shopping then went to Wm. Smiths, somewhat surprising them. Stayed there to dinner & tea & came down on the St car about half past five to G[rand] T[runk] Station. The baggage man had had my luggage transferred from G[reat] W[estern] Station to G.T. Station. About seven we were aboard for Ottawa. When I had almost given them up I saw Charlie's tall form looming in the door of the car & glad was I. They had been detained & had at the last moment to get their baggage removed from the G.W. Station to the G.T. Charlies friend Shield came with him. We settled ourselves for the night & a jolly good time we had. Charlie & I in one seat & Shields facing us. We kept up a pretty lively chat among us most of the night. When we would get tired we would tacitly agree to a rest or perhaps a short sleep tho' I did not sleep till about 5 Oclock in the morning & then only for a few minutes – for who could sleep with their head bobbing around like a footballs. Its almost a wonder how babies do sleep when they are being bounced around in a cradle. We changed cars at Prescott about 4 Oclock. When we had reached Ottawa it was still dark. Charlie wanted to hire a fine sleigh & Shields wanted to take the 'bus for some hotel. We jumped in the Windsor 'bus & went to the Windsor House – a fine hotel on Metcalf St. We straightened ourselves up waited till eight, had a little visit in the meanwhile went down to breakfast & soon after set out for the Normal. We entered the main hall & the boys were told to go one way and I another to the rooms for each. I chatted with some other unfortunates while we waited our turns to go upstairs. Saw a girl there I had seen at the hotel & so we went together – & when we had had our names enrolled & given a list of boarding houses, Miss Linton & I set out to find one. We were recommended to come to Mr Brown's third house from Normal on Nepean St. We came but he said 3.00 per week & so we thought we could do better & set out again to try. We were discouraged of the idea however when we called @ the poorest looking place of all & she asked three so as it was storming we came back & said we would stay for a week & went to the Normal to see Charlie – he said he would have my trunk brought up. So we went back to the Windsor House & Miss Linton hired a hack & we came up with her trunks, had dinner, & then sat drearily waiting for my trunk or Charlie. They both came & I was so glad. Charlie & Shields both thought we were paying too high as they had very good places for two fifty. After they went away we started out to make a tour of the boarding houses & by way of competition & talk secured a place @ Mrs Roys for 2.50 on Albert St. I liked her looks & I think it will be more of a home there. We came back told Mr Brown had tea & wrote letters home & soon after retired to rest after 36 hours of waking weariness, got up in time to school next morning. We were given some instructions & again dismissed till afternoon. Saw the boys again & they said they were going to Parliament Buildings. I saw a girl coming through the hall with a paper in hand of boarding houses & I told her of Mrs Roy's. She came down with us till we got ready & then we took the express to take her trunks to her boarding house & then went up to the Parliament Buildings. We three girls entered the main entrance of the east building. The man at the door gave us in charge of another man to pilot us about. He did so. (The Parliament Buildings are in three separate edifices – immense stone structures with heavy magnificent towers. The main building forms the centre flanked on either side with similar smaller ones.) In this building were the private chambers of business for the members. As we passed along the corridors – two very long ones – we could read the names of the

members on the doors, among others he called our attention
to His Excellency's room. He showed us the way over to the
main building in which the chief attractions are the Senate
Chamber – Library and House of Commons Chamber. At the
first hall on entering I asked for some one to guide us over the
place – a gentleman (Mr Wheeler) belonging to the buildings
offered his services. First he showed us the Senate Chamber –
Not such an extensive room in regard to size as you would perhaps expect to see – but gaudy almost in its adornments. The
length of the apartment is about too thirds greater than its width.
At the upper end of the room is a dais – reached by three
steps – semi circular almost in shape at the back of which is a
canopy gorgeous with crimson cloth fringe, overhanging the
vice-regal throne on which are placed two heavy crimson
chairs – large – massive oak wood – one a little larger than the
other in which His Excellency sits. The other – the smaller one
the Princess Louise sits in, you see e'en tho' royal blood flows in
her veins she takes an inferior place to her husband on account
of his appointment. The floor is carpeted with crimson. The arm-
chairs for the members the same, each chair has a crimson
covered desk before it with ink & pen. Around the apartment is a
gallery very nice. The room itself is lighted from the gallery by
windows of stained glass – three arches forming one arched
shape window. Over the throne is inscribed 'Dieu et mon droit'
In that apartment your voice sounds unnatural because of the
closeness of it, sounded as though you were in a big drum or
your head under the bedclothes. We passed from this to the
library – The most gorgeous room I ever saw. I have come to
such a degree of satiety that tho' I do say it myself it takes something pretty nice – out of the common to astonish me, to exceed
my anticipation – but this was almost a marvel. Words will fail to
do it justice ... it was a circular apartment with a very lofty ceiling in the shape of a dome – with frescoed ceilings arched &
groined. Then the wall for about twenty five feet high around
the building was covered with books. It is reckoned @ about
90,000 volumes. We have the privilege of going there to read any
thing we like but can not take any away without a card from Mr

Alpheus Todd, Librarian & the thing is to get introduced to him.
This is the case out of session but when Parliament sits it is
closed. There were several men there engaged at their desks
either in the centre of the room – in enclosures or at the sides. ...
In the middle ... a good statue of 'Our good Queen Victoria', the
statue is like her pictures & I suppose like her. There's a crown
on her head, & a wreath in her hand. This is saying little of a
sight that is truly brilliant. We went from this – with almost
reluctant steps through other corridors. On the walls of several
of them were large oil paintings of great men who have been
connected in some way with progress – the House or we may say
remarkable for their intellect – speakers, statesmen, literati &
many of the originals are now defunct. Among others I noticed
Cauchon – a Frenchman in dress as well as in nationality. The
lace on his bosom & sleeves costing £50 in Paris – all vanity for it
is not even customary for men of his position in this country to
wear it, beautiful to be sure but think of the hungry fellow creatures it would have fed – ay! truly it is easier for a camel to go
through the eye of a needle than for a rich man to enter the kingdom of heaven. McGill too – the founder of the Montreal College
of that name – a stout figure a rather intelligent but noble face &
somewhat sensual mouth but still a noticably clever man. Anglin
the last Speaker of the House – a decided look to his face, thin
firm lips a face indicative of thought. We went next to the House
of Commons department similar to the Senate Chamber in size &
shape but different in two noticable points – 1st the members
here set two together & the dais is at the side of the room instead
of the end, thus changing the position of the seats ect. This did
not present a striking appearance because it is now undergoing
repairs as it caught fire recently. The ceiling of the room is glass
set in heavy mouldings of wood – seemingly walnut & the light
is transmitted from the room above or windows in the tower.
The plumbers have often to repair the room above & one day
while examining leaks they carelessly left a hot iron lying there
which set fire to the place – but the water used in extinguishing
the fire did the damage. Our pilot asked us to enroll our names &
said we had seen everything of interest on that building except

climbing the tower & he directed a man to show us the way – & bade us adieu after having promised to use his influence to secure cards of admittance to parliament when in session for me. So you see I did not use my powers of pleasing in vain. He found out that I was attending the Normal ect. Mr Wheeler is a middle aged man looks as tho he was part of the institution & was shrivelled up with the heat for it was *very warm* in there. He was very very nice & obliging everyway. We then commenced the ascent of the tower & such a long long way up – innumerable steps – & how tired we were to be sure when we reached to top & looked down on the capital so airy – so fair – so grand. There we stood far above the city with our soul in our eyes – seeing – extended in succession gay broad fields – mountains – rivers & directly below the well built city of Ottawa with its domes ... It was cold and icy up there – countless names inscribed there. On our descent I met Charlie & Shields & had a little chat – then followed on after the girls – lamenting bitterly that in a few hours McCabe[1] would proclaim that for ten weeks we were to be as strangers to each other – oh dear.

Jan 13th

Oh dear I don't know where to begin do you? Well then last Friday night we had Adah Grahame & Topsy Hall here to tea – wild, jolly – Normal girls ... Sat morning we wrote letters & went down & posted them. Back again & I read Davies Higher Education of Women – a capital book – & by a woman – Emily Davies[2] – capital. Roberts sent me some Canada Educational Monthlies to read & in them there are some capital pieces among others – Agnodice's letters to Clyte setting forth the why & the wherefore of lady physicians. They are indeed good – April May June July August 1879. In the afternoon Adah & I went for a walk a long

1 Principal of the Ottawa Normal School
2 a very influential English pioneer in the cause of higher education for women; principal of Girton College, Cambridge University in the 1870s

one too – a very long one & I came home tired enough – Sunday
morning Adah called for me & we went to the Dominion Methodist. Charlie & Shields were there I believe I'm becoming
infatuated. I'd smile at them in the furnace I believe. ... Monday
just about the same old programme. I like Miss Mosher our
teacher of elocution very much indeed – I like all the teachers
pretty well if I could only talk to Roberts & Shields when I
like – bah what an Eastern rule to be sure as tho' we were in a —
well I wont say it. Mr McCabe Herr Principal is a R. Catholic so
Dr Baptie our science master – prays in the morning. Mr McCabe
is a clever man – stern, clear & somewhat kind. Dr Baptie
reminds me sometimes of Dr Spenser and is such a fussy fidgty
fellow – never knows where to put a thing or where he left it and
creates in me a hearty desire to laugh. Mr or perhaps I should
say Prof Workman is a singular looking man – forehead slants
right back & has some queer bumps I'll be bound ... Mr Swal-
low – a nice fellow decidedly embonpoint – Mr Cope – drill
master & librarian – tiptop lively – I tell you. ... I am seriously in
doubt sometimes whether or no I shall keep the rules – that is if I
had a good chance to break them. I went for a walk with Adah
tonight after school. She's nice but a little too fact [?] – for my
notion & much as she objects to Miss Linton she is not half the
girl she is.

Jan 17th

Well life is a very strange thing, even in my wonted humdrum
existence of a year past – there has been so many unforeseen
occurrences – much of change – much pleasure – some pain and
take it all in all much reason to thank God truly.
    Oh I am weary tha' night – ill in fact. I have been lying down
since tea & now am almost stupid from sleep. I am enjoying life
now. I am not one to wear a long face continually & can adapt
myself to circumstances and the only particular reason why I
should not be happy is that I cannot talks to Roberts & Shields or

as Miss Linton has facetiously named them David & Jonathan. It is a strong temptation to meet them face to face & then content oneself with smiles – well I can practise the language of smiles with a diligence for that is all the satisfaction I am likely to get in that quarter. Another week has passed of the Normal Session and next Wednesday we are to begin to teach. Here I think a difficulty will present itself in this wise – If we should see a teacher call up a class in a slovenly manner & when it came our turn to do so & we should wish to change the way of doing it (1st what benefit would possibly acrue from the diff. methods – to the class 2nd If we did do as we thought we ought, the teacher observing what we evidently think an improvement in his way would he or she not be liable to mark us ill rather than well? 3rd If we passed over this & look up the class as they we would be doing an injustice to ourselves and leaving a chance for the Normal teachers to mark us – low).

In the Educational Monthly April – May & June – July & August 1879 there are letters from 'Agnodice' a fictitious name after an ancient female hero of medicine. The subject of the letters is that a girl with no especial claim – young strong & vigorous should have some aim in life rather than the shameless one of husband-hunting. Why should a girl condense her energies into the few small so called accomplishments necessary for entree into society. Why should she spend the best part of her life for 'Society' when Society has done nothing as yet for her. The first objection that so called strongminded women dress so peculiarly and assume such unladylike airs & such fanatical phraseology 'as the painless extinction of man'. True there are a few such who do a great deal of harm to the majority of women thinkers who wish 'to use the reason God has given them to form a just opinion'. Women should not be condemned on account of the few as all clergymen should not be deemed fanatics because John Knox in the zeal of Reform defaced altars mutilated carvings ect. Next comes the plea – womens' modesty as tho' a woman fighting her way in the world could not remain unsullied – are charwomen, seamstresses teachers any the less modest & virtuous on account of their public duties. Is our

innate modesty so small a thing of so frail a material that it will
bear no contact with externals. 'If it is then she has neither virtue
or honor for good & holy men have lived & worked in the public
field & still remained good & holy.' We want to fit ourselves for
any office whether we shall be called upon to fill them as
another thing. 'The first thing to be done for women is to raise
their standard of education. These women who feigning humility
desert women thinkers thinking thereby to win admiration &
affection, forgetting the intense selfishness of their motto of live
& let live.' Then again speaking of nerve she says if girls were
brought up as boys are – with a knowledge of animals she would
not be afraid of a beetle ect. If girls were not expected to scream
@ sight of a beetle or the firing of a pistol they would learn to
control their nerves. Her sarcasms on indifferent musical performers and painters & of the smattering of the Modern Languages which girls get at school is both true and amusing. A
'Women's Mission' The express thing a person is sent to do, the
actual end of their living & being. She then describes a picture so
named which seemed 'to take' pretty *well* in Paris – It was in
three parts signifying – daughter wife – mother. In the first – She
is picking up a handkerchief for a very infirm decayed old man
& both looking very pleased (a fact which tells against the
daughter for if this were common it would not so much surprise
the old gentleman.) Next she is leaning on the arm of a frowning
man and apparently soothing his ruffled temper. Next she is
learning a child how to walk. Now she says 'will you admit that
any creature with a God given soul with reasonable & imaginative faculties can make it her mission, the end & aim of her existence to pick up any no. of pocket handkerchiefs for fathers – to
coax husbands when they are ruffled or to act the part of a walking chair to an infant' She says she does not wish to underate
these but that this should not be all. Things will improve & in
future times they will wonder at us even as we have wondered at
the dark ages. Prof Agassiz says Whenever a new & startling fact
is brought to light in science people just say 'it is not true;' then
that 'it is contrary to religion;' that everybody knew it before
And it is just the same in social reform.

She mentions another picture – that struck her as ridiculous a namby pamby sort of woman leaning against a horse with some hounds gazing up at her. Not but what she likes to see women have pet animals but the title 'My Wife – my horse my dogs' was what shocked her & she if the young wife had had sufficient spirit she would have insisted on a companion picture of My husband My bonnet, My boots. She then laments that there are so few men on our side – but I do not so much feel with her there – for I think the best educated the best thinkers *are* on our side & why should we care for the great unwashed. She characerizes those men who stand out boldly for us as 'men whose souls are larger than their bodies – who can lose a little creature worship with equanimity' & moreover asserts that such men will gain more than an equivalent in the respect they will gain. Then she expresses how much happier will be the union of two similarly educated minds – both for contemplation formed – & she will still be able to soothe him with her finer fancy – touch him with her lighter thought. Then she mentions the insipid way in which commonplace men insult us with their commonplaces their hackneyed expressions & attempts to make the whole thing appear ridiculous. That the majority of men if you speak of a reading thinking woman immediately construe it into a neglect of household duties – always making a Mrs Jellyby[3] in their imagination as that is their beau ideal of a literary woman. We are told that we alone must overturn all this accumulated mass of prejudices & selfishness & when we begin to feel ourselves capable – when we get accustomed to harness we may even tho' those who have brought these things to pass look on in scorn & indifference. Then she goes on with an oration about John Stuart Mill as one who wrote for us spoke for us – who strove for liberty for all liberty in its truest & purest sense – No one can stand still either must go forward or backward & to go back one can only read Kingsley's 'Water Babies' – Where a people prefered to go into the land of readymade rather than hardwork &

3 a character in Charles Dickens' *Bleak House* (1852–3) who sacrifices her family to her philanthropic interests

degenerated into a Troglodytes – & could only climb a tree & sob
out boohoo boohoo when what it meant to say was 'I am a man
& a brother'. The old story of One must sow & another will reap.
She expresses a hope that in another generation women will not
be ashamed to own they have aspirations & desires beyond the
'daily round of their common task.' Then the argument is sometimes advanced that women are too frivolous – too much given
to detail too diffuse – & wordy to attend to anything serious.
They fritter away their talent & are too fond of the precept 'here
a little & there a little.' The answer to that is 'try us.' When we
are allowed something to interest us of a higher order of things
than new bonnets or lawn tennis the old charge of idleness &
levity will be exploded. Fuller says: The study of physic giveth
wealth; the study of law giveth honors. When high birth &
beauty are compelled to go on foot. To prevent such foot travelling it is good to be mounted on a gainful vocation to carry
one out of the mire on all occasions.

Jan 19th

Yesterday I was twenty one – ah think thou well upon it 'twenty
one and what have I accomplished?' In all that twenty one years
what a comparatively happy time I have had. If as the minister in
the Baptist church said last night we are all punished more or
less for our misdemeanors here on earth then I may expect more
suffering – & less of pleasure in the years to come – I suppose
that minister believes – 'That the mills of God grind slowly but
they grind excedding small tho' with patience He stands waiting
with exactness grinds He all' He also said that as we did not all
sin alike here – some would receive their due of punishment in
this world while those whose sins were deeper would inherit
everlasting punishment. He said that it was an impossibility with
Him to let us escape punishment, that we would be sure to
receive it sometime, somehow. I wonder whether I shall live to
be twice twenty one or three times twenty one or mayhap four
times twenty one – a dried up swiveled up old woman with one

foot in the grave. Will I at forty two be a matronly mother of children. I hope I shall – I should not think my destiny fulfiled if I lived to be an old old maid. ...

'One by one the sands are flowing
One by one the moments fall;
Some are coming some are going;
Do not strive to grasp them all'

Jan 22nd

Yes it is. How fast the days go by – and am I doing my part in the world's great drama well? I wish I could – I wish I could use the talents committed to my keeping – so that when the end comes I will neither have wasted them nor have hidden them. The life I lead, from an outsiders' view might seem blameless – That is I commit no very flagrant sins and yet it seems frivolous – for want of proper depth. I am too happy – and tho' the girls would laugh to see these words I write them in a different sense than heretofore 'There is e'en a happiness that makes the heart afraid.' Yes I am afraid when I look around me and see so many worse conditioned than myself – and think how lighthearted & happy *I* am that surely. I shall suffer for it sometime that I ought not to be happy & gay – but ought to be engaged in alleviating the sorrows of mankind. Then arises the question 'how?' Now take today for instance. I arose soon after Miss Linton with a quilt around me – hauled off the bed & put on my boots while she was meandering about & then threw it on the pile – (I might have placed it somewhere else to be handy for her) – Dressed & was ready to go down with her waited awhile for breakfast. After that we went up to school. I was a little inclined to moodiness & kept watch out of the window for 'David & Jonathan' saw them go by & then turned to talk to the girls. Now I just take it for granted that they are like me & I get along very well with them – but there is a constant desire & temptation to criticize the girls now I suppose it is very unkind – and why do we do it – just I suppose to make ourselves believe we are better than our fellow students – now that seems resolved into pure and unmitigated egoism. – Ay poor me there's a sad fault I must strive against. I think too there is another reason why I say these unkind personals, that is to make the girls laugh and to show *my* clearness of insight & tact in discernment, another rotten prop which I must pull away. Of course if I see defects – I see them, but I can at least be silent when I can do no good by speaking – now thats a good resolution – to quit that wicked way and turn over a new leaf. ... Education notes always first thing in the morning from Mr McCabe ... And as I go to my seat or Charlie goes to his we always exchange smiles & that is a cause of satisfaction where that can be all. Next hour we had reading with Miss Mosher. I read for her for the first time, she gave me some praise a great thing for her for she said she only had time to find fault & make corrections. She cuts up some of them bad. Next hour over to George Ward School & Miss Grahame & Brown taught this morning. They did not do very well & Mr McCabe was there & took notes on them. Now again when I saw Adah make a failure of her teaching and when she was suffering nervous qualms on account of her felt failings before Mr McCabe – And when she came back to my side hoping and wanting some praise to solace conscience how hard was it to keep to the truth. To tell her faults seemed like adding Scylla to Charybdis & to praise her was not truth. Every day there is a serious conflict in mind over things like this – for more especially if they have praise me – it seems but what they expect to praise them back. A not very elegant comparison & proverb truly but nevertheless trite 'You scratch my back & I'll scratch yours' ...

Jan. 28th

How very true that 'procrastination is the thief of time' as well as of other things. Now last Sunday night I had a whole budget to write but got interested in reading this & so left it till Monday and Monday has resolved itself into Wednesday – and here we are. Last Saturday morning 'Mine host' Mr Brown came to us and unfolded not his tail but a tale. Previously to this we had noticed many strange things & had made merry over all mysteries (to us). The week before – silently without word or warning there was installed in the front parlor & hall a real live man or rather boy – a green silent animal that took his meals after the family had finished. Silently he came – silently he moved – silently he invaded the lower regions for his meals – silently he lived a week thus silently on Saturday he stole away and thus next morn we missed him from his place no more he came & we were left to wonder. Next unfathomable mystery – We came home to dinner one day – and found the stair carpet up & all the steps & floor covered with plaster & commotion generally – on ascending we found the cause to be the cutting of a door between that & next house at the head of the stair – query – why? No word of explanation. Again we began to miss the ornaments on mantel & tables till the mantel was left – bare – & yet no explanation but lo! on the eventful day Monsieur Brown came to build a fire for us and he did what he intended us to think – explained. We at least gathered this that there was to be a sale there on the following Tuesday & they were going to move away – & thf. we took the hint by the forelock & went to find another boarding place. We securing one here at Mrs Bradens – went down town and I bought stuff for an apron which I actually made that afternoon. ... Monday night a cabby took our trunks down to Bradens and we remained till next day – altho' – sundry hints would have led us to infer that our absence that night would not have been lamented. We did not take them however as we intended to finish our week. Next day for dinner we were here – and we are not sorry for we are well put up & well fed – & have a very comfortable room so therewith let us be content ... Last night I was out with Evvy Mac & meeting David & Jonathan they said goodevening – against the rules tonight – Jonathan lifted his hat, against the rules again & meeting him again he *said* 'here we are again' & said yes but really this must not go on – or there will be danger – – – oh I wish not.

'One by one in the infinite meadows of heaven
Blossomed the lovely stars the forget-me-nots of the angels.'

'Night let her sable curtain down
And pinned it with a star'

Jan 30th

Yes so the nights are – cold, crisp & starlight as it was *that night*
travelling down to the Capital. Is this me or not me? am I
awake? – So many things seem dreamlike – & I cannot get in my
cranium all I would like. For instance today in religious instruction there was a storm brewing so that it was almost twilight.
We – six girls & four boys sat facing Rev Mr Pollard as he dis-
coursed about the history of the Church to us. It did indeed seem
a dream – I was in one of those deadened moods when our
minds are away & our bodies are present. Again & again I tried
to rivet my attention on his remarks & as often I found myself
away. I was in a soil of stupor & doubtless he thought he had an
attentive listener – but I must confess much of it fell short of my
brain.

   In Hygiene Adah said 'Jonathan threw me a note' – well I
could not find it & so wrote – 'did not get your note – try again &
I'll reply.' ... Adah gave this in Rel[igious] Instruction to Jonathan & he wrote back to her 'did not send any but no matter. I
see you do not think Mr McCabe finds out everything 24 hrs
after neither do I. What is your address also acquaint me with
Miss Smith' Adah brought this to me & when I read & showed to
her oh but was n't it rich? We had a good laugh. Well I came on
down with Miss Linton & before we got near home I saw Davids
head appear round the door looking for us. So when we got as
far as there – there were four of them standing outside & as we
turned in our door I looked back & saw Jonathan bareheaded in
the door waving something at me & I shook the note at him (he
knew it for it was blue) & laughing went on in. Now is n't that
good original too. What ever he shook at me I do n't know –
something like a letter & something like a book – I got 71 marks

in Education today, the highest was 74 – Miss Conlon – I rec
honorable mention now for the second time I'm glad – ahead of
David & Jonathan both.

Feb 1st

Oh sweet are stolen sweets. I am in such a dilemma – have
been – am still. Yesterday as Adah said she wished I would
explain – we were for a walk down to the Library so when night
came I wrote a note to 'Jonathan' telling him how it was & sent it
in the magazines I had of his. Miss B took them to the door & I
went with her but stood behind the outer door. She nearly broke
down for 'David' came to the door – however we got the door
shut & left. When we came in after being down town there was a
book & in it a letter for me. He wanted to know several things &
asked if I would violate any of the rules for instance Sunday
ev'ngs & said if I would be at the Dominion Methodist it would
be 'all right' ect. Well no one can imagine the lacerated state of
my feelings during the last forty-eight hours – to go or not to go
that was the question. Well after a great deal of thinking I concluded to go & run the risk. This morning I went according to
agreement with Adah but as it was so very cold we did not go to
St. Albyns but stopped at the Dom Meth. I was fairly electrified
coming out to see 'Jonathan.' ... [Later] Well we came home had
supper & off again to the Dom Meth rather late but as we passed
to our seats we saw 'David & Jonathan' & I could scarce restrain
a smile which David did not. Well when the service was over – I
tied on a big veil & prepared to get my shawl around my neck. I
saw Jonathan waiting at the door but as some of the girls came
along he moved on to the outside. When I came out with the
girls I saw them both standing outside looking for me & I nearly
ran against them but I would not make a sign if they never
found me & so I passed on & the girls were going Sparks St. but I
wheeled them right about face & saw Jonathan rushing frantically to meet us. It was very laughable he scarcely knew me then.
So complete was my disguise. We had a hearty laugh over it. I

had Miss T's arm but when Jonathan stepped up she sped forward when he took my arm. We marched off & so did they. We had quite a talk coming home but not half enough. What shall I do – shall we go on running this risk or had we best stop. He seems to think we *might*. I do not know what to do. Whether to follow the bent of my inclination or to pause on account of the risk.

Feb 4th

Well Monday dawned as usual on the fair city Ottawa – and things went on in their usual jog trot fashion ... This morning I found a good long letter from Myrtie & a post card in my box. Now the last is a mystery to me – it runs so – 'May I have the pleasure of your company to the Mechanic's Hall tonight – will call @ 6:35' – signed We Us & Co. On the card is the Nelson stamp but there is no Ottawa stamp & yet it has been through Mr Copes hands. It is a mystery so far – for no one has called tonight. I am almost sure it is from C.R. but why did he not put in an appearance sometime tho' the card bears date Feb 2nd & Nelson Feb 3 & says call tonight – its evidently not the handiwork of an adept in deception. ... I wish I were strong-minded enough to overcome listlessness. Here I am just going on – drifting, I may say – All the studying I do amounts to little very little & what do I do beside. Oh I wish I could be true & strong enough to cultivate all that is good & train myself to entertain only noble & lofty thoughts – if I only could exclude the little soulless thoughts words & deeds that come to light every day. I wish I had some noble, honorable, highsouled cultured person to lean on as it were – mentally – someone that I could look up to & be led by – for no one knows more than I how much we are the creatures of circumstances. Those with whom we associate leave some impress on our lives they do, they will. We can not retain our individuality complete we are always being moulded anew – I am weary of waiting, so weary.

Feb 10th

... Friday night Charlie called & left a note or rather a letter for
me gave it into my own hand. I answered it next day. Sunday
night he faithfully put in an appearance at Christ Church with
Mr Case. It was such a fiasco coming out just as ridiculous as @
the Dom. Methodist. Charlie introduced Case to me. We Carlos &
I had a long walk & talk did not come directly home. He is very
kind nevertheless we are going to abstain from such digressions
of rules for awhile. ...

Feb 11th

Sent my letter home today. Today much like other days – with its
pleasures and duties and failures in acting the noble part & overcoming the weaknesses of poor fallen humanity. I know so many
faults I have & I want to correct them. How true that we cannot
touch pitch & not be defiled. The company one keeps leaves its
impress on us. I cannot well avoid the company of the girls &
what am I to do? Why to overcome my faults in the face of all
opposition & be the nobler for doing so in the face of temptation
to the contrary. I have been rereading Blackies *Self-Culture*[4] and
here are some notes from it – ... Difficult things in fact are the
only things worth doing & *they* are done by a determined will &
a strong hand. In a word Virtous Energy sums all up. In a noble
life one paltriness after another must disappear or you have lost
your chance. If you cannot always avoid the contagion of low
company you may @ all events ban yourself from voluntarilly
marching intact – moral contagion like physical is injurious
'There is nothing more proud or more paltry than Man' (Pliny)

Feb 13th

Yes the days go by so swiftly so swiftly & will soon land me @
home for awhile. Yesterday we had a half holiday. Got excused

4 John Stuart Blackie, *Self-Culture* (1874)

from the Normal [School] & straightened myself – went down to
Dr Leggs for Adah & Topsy – waited till they ate their dinner &
then Miss Robinson came & we all went down to the Parliament
Bdgs. Found several there before us among others Miss Linton,
Tomkins & Braden & soon other N[ormal] Students came &
many others too. Still they came – The Opening of Parliament is
momentuous affair. To see the madding crowd's ignoble strife –
to see them like dumbdriven cattle – for none could be heroic
with his arms pinned to his side unless heroism consisted in
using brute force for you could see 'one brawny arm was round
her friend & in one was clenched her ticket.' Charlie had secured
me a ticket & a gentleman of the House had also given me one.
We went down about 12 Oclock. We got pretty near the inner
pale – All were allowed an entrance to the first hall & then there
was a gate put up to prevent further progress till half past one. I
have felt & seen crowds before but never I solemnly avow did I
get in one like that before that gate – and they were women
too – with but few exceptions near me. Curiosity – thy name is
Woman! There were steps – broad ones – leading to this gate & a
landing directly before it. This was *all* filled, packed like her-
rings – with people possessed with a mania that more than one
body could occupy the same space. I had prepared in some sort
by leaving off all unnecessary garments & yet I never was more
nearly killed by over prespiration, bad air & jamming. I thought
of the changeling crowd as the common fool. They certainly did
not act like animals endowed with intellect. Topsy said I was to
take the few buttons & the scrap of fur – that would remain of
her & convey them to her father – after the ordeal would be over.
I thanked my lucky stars that I was tall & weighed 145 Avoir du
pois else all that had been left to my sorrowing relatives had
been my switch & a rubber or two. Fancy me packed in there in a
mass of humans – with my arms pinned to me like a straight-
jacket for about an hour & a half. It was truly characteristic of an
animal for two to try to stand in one place & to go through a
door wide enough for one & was enough to take all sentiment
out of even a Betsy Bobbet. At last they did open the door & then
such a grand rush – pel mel as hard as weary legs could carry

them – up the stairs through the hall into the Senate Chamber gallery. This whole room is elegant. Nearly the whole of the back wall of the side gallerys were a blaze of stained glass of different designs. The front at the top of the gallery are four grand arches held by massive marble pillars. The end gallery facing the throne was reserved for ladies in full dress – there were no windows at the back of this but two splendid oil paintings. The other end gallery had five smaller stained glass windows & similar arches & was open to holders of tickets. There are only three tiers of seats in the side galleries but these held quite a multitude. I sat in a very good place in the gallery & a gent accommodated me with a glass & I had a full view. Downstairs in the Senate Chamber proper were arm chairs on either side, two tiers of these & two tiers of other seats back of these. In the middle of the room was a large table around which six dignitaries sat. Then the Supreme Judges in their crimson gowns & ermine. The clergy were represented too. At the head of the room was the throne – on which were two chairs – the larger one for the Marquis & the other for the Princess. The arm chairs, the table, carpet, dais & canopy over the throne were all crimson cloth. The Usher of the black Rod was performing all his numerous offices. He was dressed in black with broad gold stripes down either leg with breast plate of gold – an ebony & gold wand about 3 1/2 feet long. You may be sure the galleries for spectators were soon filled & then we had only to wait & watch – very soon there was a rush of 'full dressed' save the mark ladies to the end galleries – very pretty some of them & very elegant & various costumes. I cannot describe them, many were non-pareil & seemed to have come from Norths & Stewart. Many middle aged ladies in full blast. I noticed that the majority of them all were decidedly fleshy. Of course the centre of attraction was the floor and the ladies in the gallery tho' a phalanx of beauty will remain unnoticed further here. The first lady to sweep across the room well if you could have seen her you would have felt an inclination to laugh outright at the weakness of humanity. I am speaking in a decidedly figurative sense because otherwise it would not be at all suitable to her – that she was fair fat & forty would only give a hint of the

last two. Something over 200 lbs I fancy & not much cloth to
hide her fairness above the waist. I blushed for my sex more than
once. Soon they came in two's & threes & such magnificent costumes. They only agreed in one thing & that was to leave their
dresses off the upper part of the body & let two or three yds
come creeping after them on the floor. In many cases the trains
exceeded the wearer in length. They did not speak much for the
intellect of the 19th century – so extreme they were absurd.
There are 206 members in the House. There were about 130
ladies below stairs in this kind of costume. Many elderly ladies
wore black velvet or satin but the majority wore diverse light
colored silks & satins with abundance of lace & exquisite 'lin-
gerie'. They were *all* so grand & various, that I cannot describe
them & do them justice. Lady MacDonald wore a canary colored
gros grain – low corsage – gold ornaments – yellow & cardinal
ostrich tip & cardinal fan. Not quite as becoming to her as it
might be to some. It was quite evident she did not powder for her
shoulders were a human red. She is just moderately good looking & her manners are perfection. She bore out the phrase to 'the
manor born'. She had the seat next the Premier the best next
royalty. Lady Tilley sat next in mulberry velvet trimmed richly
with Koniton lace & next her Lady Tupper in black velvet – the
three ladys that sat in the front row on that side. About a quarter
to 3 Oclock the form began by a clergyman reading some prayers
from the Ch of Eng Prayer Book. The Bishop (Lewis) was there
too in knee breeches, black silk stockings slippers & a purple
apron – a dress of the old school. The Mayor (McIntosh) with an
immense chain of gold around his neck. ... Soon a distant bustle
& noise was heard then louder & still more loud & the salute is
fired & all eyes are turned in expectancy on the door to see the
Governor[-General] enter. First came the Usher of the Black
Rod – & then the Marquis – after proceeding a few paces – the
usher bowed very low (I don't think he belongs to the class ver-
tabrate because he seemed quite boneless when he bowed.) This
he continued to do across the room till the throne was reached.
The clerks came after the Marquis & arrayed themselves on
either side of the throne. The Marquis wore a splendid uniform

with much gold trimmings (By the way Sir John A. Mc[5] was
dressed in an elaborate costume of black & gold. The Windsor
Costume – like those in the Eng Court) One of the finest things I
saw was a chat between Sir John & his wife – a tableau I shall not
soon forget. It was before the Marquis came. They were jesting
about something. He was evidently telling her some amusing
story or quizzing her & she took it so well & tapped him inter-
rogatively & playfully with her fan, the play on their features
was quite interesting. The Princess came in by another door at
the left of the throne – very regal very womanlike she looked.
One to pin one's faith to & live & die by the venture. She wore a
two shade grey satin gown & train trimmed with grey lace with
tiara & necklace of diamonds. They stood for a moment while a
man read them an address – then they sat down. The Marquis
wore his hat throughout the whole performance except to raise it
twice when reading his addresses. Both remained seated all the
time. A man in uniform stepped forward – bowed, handed the
Marquis a paper which he read aloud i.e. The Speech from the
Throne or vulgarly called The Bill of Fare – which the Opposition
have already critized. ... After the ceremony was over Charlie &
Shields came over to me. They had been sitting not far away with
a crowd of Normalites & wanted me to come too but I did not. So
he came up & talked for awhile in full view of anyone who
might look & then Shields came up & actually shook hands to
the amazement & envy of the other girls. We got out of the
gallery through the hall & down the stair all right but then as the
people were not allowed out till the Marquis passed out – there
was another jam @ the door after he did go out – just as bad as
the one coming in – terrible – two trying to get through a door
made for the exit of one & pushed on by the crowd. ...

If you to me be cold
Or I be false to you
The world will go on I think
Just as it used to do;

5 Sir John A. Macdonald, Prime Minister of Canada 1867–74, 1878–91

Feb 19th   (or 17th)

Yesterday morning the postman brought me a lovely valentine from James VII [Jim Wilson] – kind of him too after my long silence. Went up to school & Mr McCabe told us we would finish our term in March that means two weeks holidays for me – hurrah – hurrah – then Mr McCabe began reading out the marks and I could only blush with joy when above all my came out first & best. Mine the best out of seventy eight second class teachers – hurrah. I was glad – glad – he praised it too – said it was a '*very* excellent paper'. I have been second or among the leaders all the time & have had honorable mention every time but this was the climax to my delight. Roberts & Shields came out well this time too. Roberts – 2nd among the gents. ...

Feb 25th

Yes really it has got as far as 25th. I must really try & write more regularly in this. Sat afternoon I was for a walk with Davidson Mc & Fraser. Went down to French Cathedral & home Sunday morning. Evvy Mac & I went out to St. Albyns Church liked it very much indeed & purpose going next Sunday. ... Went to Dominion Methodist in the evening with Mr Newman – they came back with me & we talked long & nonsensically @ the door. He's very nice, as far as he goes – but is not a very deep personage – I fancy. ... Today Wednesday we – about 20 of the Normal girls went to the Parliamentary Pinafore – It was good. I went with Mrs Lelwyn & Mac & Evvy. It is one grand Political Satire. The characters represented were natural as life. In the first place the music was excellent, the orchestra better than that of Neilson [Theatre] I think. ... But what made me most enthusiastic was the last scene – where England is in the form of a robust handsome, full blown looking young woman – with Eng shield and other trappings red white & blue, characteristic of Eng with sceptre advanced is represented as talking with her daughter Canada – a youthful maiden – slim & graceful with blue dress &

garland of maple leaves who is wanting money of her mother to
build a railway – for how can she live parted from her children &
some of them in B. Columbia. She accuses her mother of thinking
more of her children Australia & Zealand than of her & then
England chides her for this telling her that had she not sent her
Lord Dufferin & his peerless wife & then her favorite princess &
her husband. Then Canada asks pardon & then introduces Sir
John to Eng. who says she is happy to see him – he looks like
some of her own people – that perhaps he is a little too fond of
party but that nothing can be said against his personal character.
Then Tilley is brought to notice & she says something about glad
to see him if he did not come too often – & then to Mackenzie
something about she was sorry she could not address him by the
same title as the others & he said brusquely he did na care for sic
baubles & she said something to the effect that 'haps it was this
same disrespect of her gifts that kept him from having it. Then
turning to Canada she says – I want to speak to you seriously
now about Coz Jonathan I hear you are flirting with him ect –
Canada denies the charge & says it must have been some gossip-
ing bystander who has told this false story – that she likes coz
Jonathan very well as a neighbor & nothing more – then all
acclaim their fidelity to Eng. & shout in enthusiastic song – their
patriotism. Tilley Sir John & McKenzie slide off the stage &
appear waving each a flag – the Union Jack, Red White Blue &
McKenzie the Stars & Stripes & stand at the rear of the troup
waving them while all the troup sing to the music of the orchestra 'Rule Britania' it was very good – exciting. That last scene
excited me most of all & therefore pleased me most. I think there
must be a goodly stream of patriotic blood in my composition for
that sort of thing always tickles my fancy.

Feb 28th

The shadows lift from my waked spirit
Airily & swift & I could write – on – & on ect. ...

Today Saturday has been a strangely quiet one for me & I have
had some time for thought & self examination. The morn broke
beautiful & bright like fairest spring but in the forenoon it
turned to one of those days of rain that bring to mind the old
home life and 'a feeling of sadness comes o'er me that is not akin
to pain but only resembles sorrow as mist resembles rain.' Adah
Grahame came in for a chat in the morning – oh that girl! I suppose I have no right to judge but oh the shameless wanton wickedness there is in that girl and yet she wears the mask of a caste
which infest the earth, who go about like doves & are serpents.
Not that she has broken the letter of the law, not that, but she
has no thought of principles – religion or maiden decorum. Alas
that I should be so. Alas! Alas! I see around me girls making
themselves cheap who act speak think things no true virtuous
sensible girl should. They are all agreed on one thing – to be bold
& hoydenish as concerns the opposite sex – to attract their
notice – no matter at what cost. – no matter that they make the
first advances – No matter that they sacrifice dignity & respect so
long as they gain the attention of even one milksop, they are not
unhappy. Oh the shamelessness of such conduct – oh the
unwomanliness that marks the generality of girls of the middle
class. If they only knew – if they would only think that they are
sowing tares for themselves – whirlwinds – & more than this –
they are in many instances – learning the boys to estimate *all*
girls cheaply by their knowledge of them – & how can we hope
to receive respect or consideration from them men of today when
they have flaunted before their eyes such manners – as are worn
by so many. That it should be so is a vast pity – and that it will
continue to be so is there a doubt so long as such become the
mothers of the land & in their turn allow their children to grow
up in the way they may rather than the way they should. People
might well wonder whether such girls ever had a home – or
mother – when they are lost to all principles of truth – when religion has become a thing of mirth & their speech is interlarded
with vulgarisms & even oaths – Alas! Many talk & with reason
of the fastness of the young men of the day – but when we come
to know of so much shallowness as is found in the young

women some at least – can the gentle moulder of finer fancies –
should be the help & stay of man – to lead to better things she is
in many cases the reverse. Although I have been ill today the above is not the result of
bile or dyspepsia but I'm sorry to say too true. I have been think-
ing about myself too – how weak & frail the mind is, how many
times I have said to myself 'judge not that ye be not judged' &
made an inward resolve not to say ill of my fellows – but where I
could say no good to say nothing at all – and always some noticable act or word would make me lose my self respect by breaking
that resolution – often I am lead on to this by others more often I
fear by a desire to create a laugh or to infer to make known that I
am not to be caught with chaff – that I am clever enough to see
through masks & paint the flaws I find – often was a desire to
have the hearer think that I know that it is wrong & that I am
made of better stuff than to be caught at such or too good to do
such things. Oh I am afraid that there is too much of the Pharisaical cry of 'I thank the Lord I am not as other men are' or too
much so.

Again the life I lead – it seems so shallow – so barren of good
works – I live & move & have my being and am to all appearances – happy – but there ever runs through all – & I feel it most
at retiring – that the day has been passed in fickle pleasure and
not in self culture – not in a strive for good – not in nobleness –
but has left me farther from the goal of a noble character &
achievements – strange I think of this as a queer lesson in my
life – strange persons – strange ways – and a strange – strange
world. When I look forward to the work before I pause for very
wonder. I who am drifting as it were now, who am gaining
strength as it were for the onset. I will soon be in the battle &
then where will my strength carry me – comforting words 'As
thy day is so shall my strength be' Heaven grant it may be so – I
want to be of some use in the world – not a mere statue to fill up
a corner – or a faithless steward – but to use faithfully the talents
committed to my keeping. When in my daily tasks – I find myself
displaying nervousness & the false timidity so inherent to girls of
today I must school myself to do away with nerves entirely and

be a woman – womanly in my strength – I received a letter from Mrs Hunter who says that she had money laid by to enter college with me but lost it all last fall & now as her husband is sick she has to support the family & she has to give up the long cherished scheme of years – the ambition of her life – I wish sincerely I had to means to pay her way – how thankful I should be that I am so happily situated. I am grateful I think – however frail & wicked I am – I thank God for the good things He sends me. It is past the midnight hour and I here in my cosy room in Ottawa – with all the hopes and ambitions – all the aspirations for good, and desire of future good to my world. I will close this diary not with filling up its last page with trivial tales of mistakes of giddy girls of A Lane or any part of that 'fiasco' which occurred last night on our return from the House. Nor will I say anything about Roberts or the progress he has made – of the thousand & one little things that go to make up the sum of a days doings but will say to my friends –

'Mizpah' – 'Mizpah'

March 3rd Ottawa

The days and the weeks go by and bring me nearer that day that has always loomed up in the great future – the day on which I shall begin my medical studies at College. All that has gone before and now is will be but as play to the real study that must then come. I feel it – know it – that that will be no mere pretence – no flimsey structure on a superficial foundation – I must throw off all fickleness of purpose – all trammels of shallow fun and be 'a woman with a purpose' must be and do what some are expecting of me. 'All I would do it all' rather than live the frivolous life of the majority of girls. I have seen a great deal of human nature here whatever else I may have seen. Such girls I never saw & never wish to again – but there I shall not begin this volume with a tirade against my sex –

March 4th

Has Spring really come or is this only a fore-taste. Is it possible that winter is done. It seems like a dream & the ending of this session will appear strange. It is strange how we accustom our-selves to a life – no matter how strange in the beginning – and get even weary of the monotony that was not monotony at the first. Today we have had the drear music of the rain on the roof – balmy air – but filthy streets. I may mention the three most pleasing points in todays events. 1st Miss Mosher our teacher in elocution gave me praise for my reading – said I read the best in the section. 2nd Mr Connell M.P. called but unfortunately I was out. However he said he would call again. 3rd. Charley called & we had a good talk – I enjoyed it very much. He wants me to get two other girls to go with us Shields & Cody & have our photos taken. I hope C. will continue to be the frank, nice fellow he is and not let the world spoil him ...

March 6th

The same old story yesterday. Friday and exam paper on Mental Arith & Hygiene & then Religious Instruction. It is so like a dream to sit there in the Laboratory – with the flowers around & Rev Pollard before us – teaching us or trying to – the history of the church. ... This morning Sat. we arose betimes & went out before breakfast – did our errands & came back to breakfast & then we four went exploring. We went out to the N. West of city around the lumber yard or rather through it. This is quite a sight – so many acres covered with piles of lumber from 20 to 60 ft square. There are canals made from the river to go through the yards & down these the rafts of lumber come from the river. Next we came to the Ottawa river & standing on the suspension bridge over the river we have a good view of Chaudiere Falls – very grand as all striking things in nature are. ... The greatest

thing that I saw today was the Match Factory (Eddy's) at Hull in
Quebec. When we received permission from the headoffice we
were guided along alleys & rooms past barrels of brimstone
ect. – we were shown from one foreman to another through the
buildings. To begin with – the blocks are made of similar sizes
– just twice the length of a match These blocks were made to
exactly fit an iron box that had a knife at its bottom – the blocks
were quickly transformed into slips of wood the thickness of a
match & passed to another part of the same machine where a
number of knives changed the slips of wood into a number of
sticks just twice the length of the match but otherwise complete
in shape. The matches were sent flying down an iron trough &
piled up of their own accord, a girl stood by lifting the piles out
as they collected. This was all done in a twinkling – quicker than
you could imagine possible. In another room there were numerous girls engaged at machinery in rolling the matches – in this
way. Fancy a hemp strap – like the girth of a saddle – only this
was only two inches wide & this strap wound on a pivot – one
layer overlapping the other – just as you would wind up a piece
of tape – & between each layer of the hemp strap there were
matches at regular distances apart about 1/8th inch. When a
goodly roll had been made – about same in circumference as the
top of a washbowl they were dipped in melted brimstone. There
was a long brick furnace in which of course there was fire about
3 1/2 ft. high at one end of this there was an iron trough in
which was a sea of melted brimstone these circular rolls of
matches, were placed on a carrier or pulley which went sailing
through the brimstone – just dipping the end sufficiently – they
were dipped at both ends – as they were yet of double length.
Next comes the phosphorus. There is a cylinder covered with
sheet iron & this passes through as it rotates – phosphorus
heated by steam – in a semi-cylindrical iron vessel. There were
gauges to prevent too much phosp. adhering. The rolls of
matches were just given a rub – on this by a man & was done
very quickly – The rolls of matches are next hung on pegs to
dry – and then are cut in two pieces. This is done in incredible
short time by a machine for the purpose. The belt of hemp is

fastened at the end & as it unwinds gives up the matches & a knife divides them in twain & the match is made. But the work is not yet complete. Hundreds I may say are still at work in making the boxes of paper & wood & putting the matches in the boxes & then those sent to the United States have a ct stamp for every hundred matches to be pasted on.

We were taken up stairs & then across the street through an avenue built over the st into the tub & pail manufactory. This was not so intricate – but very interesting. The staves are thrown in the dry houses from the roof – & lay there in immense heaps & are steamed from beneath by hot air. Then men & boys are engaged in placing in fitting, in making the hoops, that is cutting the strips of iron the proper length & fastening them by a pivot into a circle. There are then filled to the pail or tub – then they are painted a coat of white & then by a curious contrivance they are grained. They are pressed against a roller which as it revolves leaves an impress of its irregular surface in paint of the pail or tub – they are dryed & then the hoops are painted green or red. Then again – the bails or handles a man puts the wire through the piece of wood on the handle – another – twists it into shape over iron, another puts the curl on the end of the wire – others – fasten the handles on by ears as they are called of similar wire – jammed in by machinery. Then they are packed for transfer. One of the men said there were about 2000 persons in Mr Eddy's employ. In the match factory alone there are about 350 or 400. The machinery was beyound comprehension to an observer – so various so intricate & it did the work so speedily. On the home-ward way we visited the waterworks. I went to a gallery at the end of the room – sat down & lost myself in wonder at the inventions of man. Oh Man! So proud so paltry – when we view the grand inventions – the wondrous machinery and think that in thy brain originated so vast a scheme we may well talk of edu-cation & culture as mans highest earthly good. When man can be so paltry as we see in some instances & then see the results of mental training can we but lose ourselves in wonder at the wonder 'man' that God created and placed here for purposes known to himself.

March 13th

Oh me! It is thus the days pass away and our lives – & all seems but as yesterday. ... Sunday Lizzie called for me & we went to Christ Church in the evening. In the morning went to St. Albans with Evvy. Of course Roberts & Mac were there & the usual walk followed. We had a splendid talk – good for both of us I think. I was quite delighted & liked him better than ever. Monday the school life began again in all its sameness – of course there were unusual occurrences but now they are as tho they had not been. Tuesday night I went with the three girls Robertson Powell & Crepar to the Par. Bdgs to hear Cartwright ex. Finance Minister make the unslaught on the budget speech. He did so with much verbosity & his satelites thought exceedingly well. ... Today I think should be marked at least in black letters for we put on the climax – by getting our photos taken – the eight of us in a group. Shade of my ancestors to think that a descendant of Aimeke Jeans Bogardis – the descendant of a line of kings[6] should so far forget rules & the terror encumbent on broken ones – should so far forget everything as to go in open day & get 'her profile took' She did – alas. It was quite comical too – quite lots of fun. Well then this afternoon ... who should call but Connell M.P. I expected him – as he called before & sent me some tickets I wrote my thanks & 'that I would be in this afternoon.' He is a middle aged man, was very cordial in his greeting. I wonder if it is the custom in N. Brunswick to kiss cousins however far removed? I do not like him overmuch – in fact between myself & you, diary, I think he had had overmuch wine for desert. If he is a sample of the energetic (?) politician pity the country – pity us all. It was rather a strange interview we had take it all in all – he had an appointment at four to call on Lady MacDonald so he only stayed here for an hour. Said he would take me for a drive – secure me tickets for the Senators gallery ect – ect. I don't believe he would be very anxious for his wife to accompany him here for he calls

6 a family legend. The Smiths believed themselves to have a British king in their ancestry.

himself a *boy* & speaks playfully of me telling me he called on me
ect & that he is a bad boy.

Mar 14th

Ah well the end draws near and I am not studying very hard
either. Today we had two exams. Music & Elocution hard too. ...
In the evening the three girls Powell, Crepar & Robinson called
for me & we went to Christs Church. After church Roberts & I
had a magnificent walk & talk & I enjoyed it *so* much – a lovely
evening – talking confidentially on serious subjects. I felt more
than I can say when I came in. He spoke so openly of his inmost
thoughts & feelings & that woman like I was touched. Tonight
Mr Connell called – made me a present of a mass of stationary –
gold pens – cards, ect. He made quite a lengthy call. I do not
understand him perhaps will know him better after Wednesday
night. ...

March 18th

Tuesday was just an ordinary day with its troubles & pleasures.
Two examination papers. So tired when through them but the
feeling soon wore off when out in the air with the girls. Went for
a walk with Lizzie Robertson. She is a nice girl – I like – she is
one of the few modest reticent kind – faithful unselfish toward
friends – a motherly quiet sympathising girl. She is nice. Wednesday the same old story of school – came home early – studied
chemistry then dressed for the theatre. After tea C.R. [Charlie]
called – asked me if I was going to 'Hamlet' I had do intimated to
him – said he had just made up his mind to go & if I was not
going with Connell would I go with him. To tell the truth I
would much rather have gone with him for more reasons than
one – especially that he could understand & appreciate the play
better than Connell. He was under the necessity of shortening
his call. Soon after Connell came & we set out for the theatre. ...

Mar 25th

The end has come to the Normal session and so may it be. It will be the shortest way to write a resumé of the past few days. Sat. night Roberts & Shields called. I was so very tired after the days examinations, drill, chemistry ect that I did not appear very jovial I'm afraid. Next day Sunday I took advantage of the opportunity and remained quietly at home in the day went to the D.M.C. church [Dominion Methodist] according to agreement. Mr Stafford preached a very good sermon, one part where he expiated on the chapter in St. Paul where it speaks of wives obeying their husbands & husbands honoring their wives he spoke splendidly on. He did the subject justice & reconciled me to the precepts there held up more than I ever was before. R. thought he spoke well & so did I. We did not walk much that night as we knew next day was exam day. Next day came & a hard days work. I think I did fairly & do not dispair of getting through. In the evening there was quite a fiasco here. Miss Mosher had not left when in came Miss Mattice & Dunbar – Miss Mosher had but left when came Misses Kane & Mellville – they had but fairly seated themselves when in came Charley, Case & Thomson. Such breaking of the rules was something terrible. They soon all left but Charley & Case & presently Lizzie Robertson came in we spent a very pleasant evening. I noticed however that my head was not as clear as usual. Well I spent a most miserable night & found in the morning that I was indeed ill, with fever & rheumatism I was ill indeed – & as I did not have anything to do that day I managed to get along

March 28th

I will just continue where I left off. Wed. morning I was ill as ever but learned that I had to teach that day as I felt a little better I got up put on my wrapper & soon knew its value for Roberts came in to see how I was as did also several of the girls. I 'screwed my courage to the sticking point' and struggled up to

St. George's Ward & taught before the examiner Mr Glashan.
Everyone was kind to me Roberts & Lizzie each called for me to
see me over to the school but I had gone. I went after teaching &
spent the afternoon with Lizzie. She walked down with me &
read a story to me while I lay down. I had but dressed for the
evening & taken my supper when Connell called & shortly after
Roberts came in according to agreement to go with me up to the
Normal to our last 'Union' There Connell detained us for a little
& bade me goodbye When we reached the Normal we found
them assembled. They seemed waiting for us – they made a regular pow wow over me as tho' I had been through a whole gamut
of sickness. They seemed as tho' I was first in their affections &
yet I know I am not, but it was the social effect of the occasion. ... Next day we packed our trunks ... After tea Roberts
Shields, Lizzie & McLaughlin came in & spent the first part of
the evening. R. & Mc went for a cab & took Lizzie & I down to
the depot. It was a most glorious night & sleighride our last @
the capital. All was bustle & confusion @ the depot. The students still kept coming the trunks were still mounting higher. We
at least the boys got our baggage checked all right. Went on
board, secured seats vis a vis. I never saw Charley in such a
mood never. I told him he was playing a new role. Soon as all
were on they struck up some of their songs & such a rolicsome
time as we had. Charley left the seat once or twice & as soon as
he was out of it someone would sit down by me. He came back &
wanted his place – but left again afterward for a short time I suppose but I thought I would learn him better so I sat myself to
entertain those who came & was as vivacious as you please. I
soon had both seats & the aisle full. Just a regular crowd around
me – one sang for me – another a recitation – then a song then a
speech & I gave them Molly Meade which fairly set them wild.
All the students who were away wished they had been there. I
held high carnival. I could see Roberts face over the crowd to see
what was going on – but he did not get to me till Prescott and
then & after he knew to keep by me & I was glad he did. I liked
him better than ever. We had a good talk indeed. After leaving
Prescott & they had somewhat quieted down – we had a confi-

dential chat – as tho' alone. That journey I think I will ever remember – We all enjoyed it very much. The member for Hastings 'White' & his friend were with us & helped in a great measure to heighten the enjoyment. I played cards with him and White looked over my shoulder – they were very kind. After daylight came the hours went more slowly away and it was near noon before we reached Toronto & near three when at Hamilton. C. & I went up town in the st car. ... I slept so hard that night & so long for I was quite exhausted.

> Words but half reveal & half conceal
> The soul within –

Ma came early next morning & I started out to do some shopping but felt so miserable that after selecting the pattern I went to the hotel – about noon. Roberts came up soon after Shields & then Kennedy – they bade me goodbye & waited on. Again Charley came back as it commenced to rain & stayed till we left. We came home through a severe rain storm but did reach home. I slept most of Sunday. Yesterday according to promise R. came. I was very glad to see him. I am not made of wood or stone that having associated with a person like him for so long I can part without regret from him. Myrtie left last night. Cecil & Roberts this morning. I am nearly deranged today. What has come over me. I have written – written & yet I feel –

6

Winona and Kingston, Ontario
April to October 1880

As these entries reveal, Elizabeth's first term at Queen's Medical School was most heartening. Although critics were always present, their carping could be ignored in the company of the two other female students, Elizabeth Beatty and Alice McGillivray, and in the support all three won from the local community. This was just as well for the work was arduous; the dissecting and surgery in particular rather intimidating. Elizabeth's moods also reflect her maturing relationship with Charlie Roberts. She suffers the doubts and misunderstandings which are an inevitable part of a love affair so largely dependent on correspondence.

> 'Farewells if ever fondest prayer
> For other's weal availed on high
> Mine will not all be last in air
> But waft thy name beyond the sky'

April 2nd, 1880

Yes we seem to be such stuff as dreams are made of & our little life is rounded with a sleep. We meet – get acquainted – think the world of each other part and grieve o'er the parting for awhile and then enact the scene again perhaps with less feeling and of shorter duration the scene. I will not write here for fear it may meet other eyes and again who shall say there is not down deep in my heart a hope – a desire that all is not over between us. If he [Charlie] can go on in his career without casting more in the matter then he is not what I think him. I did indeed feel desolate the last time I wrote here & yet I would not tell or write half I did feel. I would not gain the exact sympathy I wished if I told indeed would not desire it & if I wrote it down – might be sorry. Such utter prostration of mind – void of all cheerfulness and shirking duty, feeling that earth held nothing of interest I must as usual attribute to ill health – if not dyspepsia. Then weariness – mental & physical fatigue. I have somewhat now recovered and have more stamina in me & yet I do not anticipate the work of my future but am drifting carelessly to it waiting demurely to take the plunge. Today Gertie has been sick & I have been doing housework, washing dishes – getting meals – making beds ect – now for me to go on doing this day after day – month after month – to years would be continual awful punishment to me I wonder what I would do – die of inanition or become mentally petrified & yet & yet when I hear Gertie saunter off – humming a ditty to milk I wonder whether the simple pleasures that always please is not best yet.

April 6th

Ah me I am so tired but I will write tonight. Sunday was a very quiet day, did not get to church as it was so muddy. Monday ... Had a good talk with Ernest. Where they are all so busy in the household one hardly gets a chance to have private & confidential but we had a good chance and we improved it. Ernest has his romance as well as I. I don't know why it is exactly but I can never speak freely of the subject nearest the heart. True confidence I think consists in confessing everything & when C.R. [Charlie] told me in his manly way of his first flame – I was gratified with his confidence – & trust. And so it was on that memorable night coming from Ottawa shall I ever forget. I think I never shall nor my companion either. I guess in that lay the

charm. Well I shall soon be away again from the home circle. It
does not seem 'comme il faut' now because Myrtie & Cecil are
away & have been. I had always seemed the truant bird but now
they too have flown perhaps forever from the rooftree. What a
queer sort of life we live at best & I am sure each life is a story
strange as fiction. Here am I for a brief season – living at home,
in which I have long since ceased to live long at a time, here am I
doing housework for a change. Gertie sick – ma sewing & I doing
the work. I can do it & that is some consolation tho to continue
in that line long would be for me as complete drudgery as desirable. I wish I had more real active energy that would not be
daunted, but would overcome all possible things. People deem
me energetic but they do not know ...

April 13th

As usual I begin where I left off and give a summary as near as
memory permits of the circumstances that have swept over my
resistless head. During the succeeding days until Thursday the
routine consisted in Ma sewing for me, I doing housework,
Gertie sick – those were busy days – busy. Thursday morning
early Ma Ernest & I drove into Hamilton who should but in
appearance right at the minute of arrival but the one I most
wished to see. I longed to see – had craved to see for more than a
week – poor fellow he was agitated – he has not learned the trick
of concealing his feelings and in some cases I am glad – that he
cares for me very much I have not a doubt, that he loves yea,
loves me even passionately I do not doubt he has let me learn so
much and yet he has not made an exact avowal I think him wise
in thus keeping his aim his success in the future before him. I
think I understand him fully & I know we implicitly trust each
other. He very reluctantly bade me goodbye as it was past
schooltime. Ma & I went shopping then I to the 'Spectator' office
where I read ma's recent article on medical Education of
Women – it was very good. I then after bidding Ma & Ernest
goodbye turned my steps toward Maud's. We had a good old

fashioned talk in the sewing room – dinner went & visited Mrs Lawson & Cecil. Went down town & home – just as we were finishing tea there was a call for me to the drawing room & there he was – my own friend Charley. We were both delighted to again have a private chat presently I called Maud to me & introduced her. She likes him – I promised to go out with him on the next evening & he slowly took his departure. Friday morning we read 'The Princess'[1] together Maud & I enjoyed it very much. In the afternoon went to see Alice – they are just moving into their new residence – we took her with us up to the Coll. Inst. to the L[iterary] S[ociety] ... According to promise Charley put in an appearance after tea & we went to hear Dr Peck lecture on Pluck vs Good Luck. ... The lecturer dealt creditably with the subject – sound sense and much wit interspersed with sentiment & narratives. We had rather a quiet uneventful walk home we both knew it was goodbye & we felt it & yet could not say plainly to each other that we grieved or fretted. It was hard for him to go that night & hard for me to say goodbye, but he said he would write & I am anxiously looking for it. Maud & I had a hearty human sympathetic talk that night after retiring. Next morn I was very quiet & felt my loss. I really think I did, very quiet & given to moping melancholy. The day dragged away & about four Maud & I went down to the G[reat] W[estern] depot here I found Cecil, Sutherland & White to see me off. Maud with me too. Suth got my check & we went on board – presently Maud bade me goodbye & Cecil going with her followed suit & White also took himself off like a silly boy & left Suth master of the situation. Then that great cream faced loon sat & gaped & talked at me until the train moved off & he had to leave. ... It was storming furiously when I reached Toronto – got the st car & arrived all right found William had gone down to both trains to meet me, was down then & came up in the next st car. They are so nice both of them. Sunday morning Mr Breckan her brother came me. We sang hymns till noon & then Miss Parmenter came in stayed

1 extended poem (1847) by Alfred Lord Tennyson, largely concerned with the higher education of women

to dinner I was sorry to hear she was unable to come [to medical school]. I think money is the great hindrance would help her if I could. ... Monday morning before seven found Wm & I at the G[rand] T[runk] station he bought Mail & Globe for me & I breathlessly perusing their columns for the Normal student's list saw my illustrious cognomen among the successful candidates. How often in my little life am I surprised at the great goodness of God to me who am so unworthy of even the smallest favor. Yes my name was there & those I held dearest of the Normal Students. I went on my way rejoicing. How amusing & interesting it is to travel. So many types of humanity – illustrious of many traits of character – & how many fine landscapes. Arrived in Kingston about two O'clock found the town rather city to be about a mile & a half from the station. Secured a cab & set off to the scene of trial – went to Anna Davidsons had my baggage deposited there & we set off to see Dr Fowler. He was very kind directed me to come to Mrs Days where Mrs McGillivray a medical student in embryo was. We next went to see Mr Knight who was also very kind, came here saw Mrs Day & settled to board here. Mrs McGillivray is a very young person – fair to see & good to talk to, has been married over a year and is not yet nineteen – determined – clever & girlish a very good companion in labor – one who will stick to the text. I stayed in the rem. of day.

Oh for the touch of a vanished hand
And the sound of a voice that is still

April 13th

The Rubicon is passed. We cut the rope – we are adrift – on the sea of study. God help us to win the day. The morning was fair – we had had a good sleep and felt ready to begin warfare. Went to Dr. Fowlers office he told us to go down to College that Dr Depuis would be there to give us his first lecture. We went but being late found he had left. Went to his office & he returned with us – gave us a short lecture on the bones of the back –

showed us over the College, the chamber of horror i.e. the dissecting room and was very agreeable. Dr. Fowler came down also – we had some talk & then after appointing hrs for lectures tomorrow we returned with Dr. Depuis to his office where he gave us a scapula & some illustrations of it. We returned with book & bone & there they lay for my digestion. I have learned somewhat of them & must learn more.

He is coming my own my sweet
Were it ever so airy a tread
My heart would hear it & beat
Were it earth in an earthy bed.

So I fancy was the heart of Mrs McGillivray singing tonight for her liege lord came home. He is not one to strike the fancy as much as she is & yet he is very nice to be what he is. Mr Knight called on us tonight – very kind very nice is and ever was – yes I can, for all my Gorgon propensities look up to a noble man and am quite willing to without any male *pigmy* insisting that I should. Quite an adventure here. A boarder here for a week decamped without paying board, taking Mr Leeks overcoat & Mr McGillivray's vest & a $ bill. They caught him down town where he owned up – forked out the vest – had sold the coat & spent the $. Made quite a little excitement here at least. ... I shall postpone sketching the characters of residents here for present.

April 14th

Another day has passed & I am still in the enjoyment of good health & life. This morning we two went down to lectures found that we were not alone. Miss Beatty of Farmersville & a Miss Dixon [Dickson] of Kingston were there & a Mrs Dixon to encourage us. Dr Depuis gave us a somewhat lengthy & rapid summary of anatomy of upper parts and gave us the scapula & humerus for tomorrow. I have studied pretty hard today & am yet far from knowing them perfectly no one would imagine for an instant that there would be so much to learn about one bone as there is & such fearful names. Dr Day has kindly loaned us a box of bones and we have full employment for our time. I wrote a long letter home today I wish so much for my letters to come. I may as well 'fess up – one in particular. I wish I might have that parting scene again. I wish. I am quite weary with study tonight & somewhat homesick, but I 'maunna be chicken hearted & I will na. This is a regular boarding house – each bedroom is a home & they make no scruple of standing talking to one another in bedrooms – have first class fare & comfortable rooms – all very nice. There's a boarder here a little Methodist chap in the Divinity 3rd year – good hearted – but narrow minded little fellow – his bete noir a woman who knows more than he – he'd not scruple to kiss or romp with a girl but would be horror stricken at dancing. One of these who cry down education of women on the grounds that if they are equally educated they will not look up to male men. As if any such woman would be likely to marry a pigmy. Such a woman well educated ect would never need be asked to look up to her husband. She would understand.

April 17th

Thursday just the same, lectures in the morning – study – and the day is gone. Yesterday morn received a nice letter from C.R. [Charlie] I was very glad to get it. I replied to it by a much longer one – now perhaps I did not stand enough on dignity but then I know he will not think unkindly of me for that. I rec. a nice letter from Maud on Thursday, it did me good – brought a gleam of the old life. Yesterday we saw the Demonstrator Mr Oldham at work on a subject – it was no harder not so hard as I had anticipated. Slept with Mrs McGillivray & had such a good talk with her we seem to agree with each other perfectly & of course I admire her sentiments. Everyone is very kind to me & why should I not be quite happy – satisfied? In Thee oh Lord do I put my trust let me never be confounded. The Demonstrator is just the one of all the students I wd have selected – more indiff. he

could not well be and treats us as tho' we wished to learn &
there was no joke in the matter. Today Saturday we dissected
from 8:30 to eleven thirty & we did pretty well. One forgets
when at work that the sub. ever had the breath of life in it, or
that it is anything but mere mechanism. The Sub. I may put here
for after merriment was an old schoolmaster in Down Ireland –
died in the hospital & his wife was too poor to afford him burial
& so gave him for dissection. An old man about eighty years old.
We have just the upper part. Today I dissected the side of the
chest. It would have been terrible to me to have seen myself had I
not taught myself will power or even had I not been studying
med I would have been fearfully shocked. As it is I really do not
mind it so much as I anticipated – & ate a hearty dinner after the
orgies. Pluck vs Good Luck.

April 21st

Sunday like a good child I went to church in the morning heard
a very good sermon – on 'The people of this world are in their
day wiser than the children of light' explained as those who
lived for the world & its vanities fought a harder fight & worked
more diligently & well than those who fight under Christs banner – I like the church very well & the minister. ... Finished 'The
Princess' in the afternoon – splendid at the last from where
'Woman's cause is mans' occurs down to 'May these things be'.
In the evening went to church again after taking a walk with Mr
& Mrs Mac. Stayed to practice after service with Evvy & then
went for a walk with her, met a Mr Hubble & was introduced
much to my disgust – for I have no time for such now. Monday
to work – dissecting from eight to 9 9 to 11 lectures – 2 to 4 lectures dissect & home to study. ... Tuesday – Well rec. letter from
Home & Adah Grahame – more than welcome. In morning went
early to dissect – lecture from 10 to 11 & then as Dr Oliver
thought we would like to attend the wedding in St. Georges left
his till 15 to 12. So we came up home got some biscuits & had
some fun – or rather food for laughter for Miss Beatty proves a

fund of wit & sarcasm – just rouses all the mirth in me & makes
me laugh too much. Went back to lecture home to dinner & then
lots of merriment as well as food. Back again to lectures from 2 to
3 & it was fixed in the morning that we were to dissect after that
but the other girls wd not & I was not going alone. So we came
back Miss Davidson or Davie, Eloise Depuis went with us to the
lecture. Well I said several times the Demonstrator will be flying
round here to see what is the matter & soon he came & if my pen
were but half capable of describing the scene that followed I
would try If I could but half depict the trial of me as prisoner on
charge of neglecting to go to dissecting & breaking the engagement with Demonstrator & wasting his time. Of course I was the
most innocent of the parties but let me whisper in your ear – I
honestly believe Holy Al Oliver that that Demonstrator has
either fallen desperately in love with this piece of anatomy or is
trying to feign & does well at it. Now it is quite apparent to me &
I'm afraid to others that he sticks rather closely to me in the dissecting room & helps me do the work & so all this being the case
he must needs do all the talking to me & such a furor. Mr Mc –
my lawyer – bringing counter charges & he keeping to his. Miss
Beatty as judge filling the arm chair with glasses astride of her
nose – acted admirably & supported the dignity of the chair or
rather her person no rather the chair supported her person Well
the lad got telling his stories & did not know when to go. Well
after the tea was done & the accompanying war of words – & we
were upstairs having a good time. Mr Mac wants to tell me
something so – privately – confidentially he tells me Dr Day has
been & gone & went & fallen clean in love with me. Terrible – te
te riri ble ble. Two out of three that I have been introduced to
here within two wks surrendering at discretion & to me who
forswore all such things when coming here – unfortunate – alas
unfortunate me. How shall I bear it all. Day unconsciously dis-
closeded the secret to him but I'm not much of a believer in it.
Well today has been a busy one. Up soon after five – breakfast at
six – went down to Post Office & got a letter from Charlie dear
matter of fact Charlie – sensible honest Charlie your letter did me
good & I hope you will continue faithful. Went to College –

dissected till nine then Dr Depuis lectured till after 10 on Anatomy & then we went down to the wharf where I spent a most pleasant half hour in quiet contemplation of the dancing sparkling waves of the St. Lawrence & saw Wolfe Isle just beyond. The vessels in the harbor, the men at the wharves ect & yet I saw as tho' they were not except the water ever dearest, deepest – sweetest saddest voice of nature to the soul. Oh I was sadly happy, thoughts of – oh a wilderness of thoughts swept over my soul & I was mute in utter maziness of calm sweet thought – back to the gloomy College ...

April 22nd

Thursday – Well may we say we know not what a day or hour may bring forth. The day began smoothly enough – up early – down to dissect till 9 then two hours lectures – fixed dissecting room – home & then & then Dr. Day goes to Mrs Mac with the story that theres a Dr Claxton here to dinner came to be introduced to me – wants a wife – heard so much & such praise of me that he thinks of investing in a wife. He is rich – & a clever Dr. well Mrs Mac comes to me with the story & so we arrange Miss Beatty is to be introduced as Miss Smith & I as Beatty & to delude him – well Mrs Mac goes down first & when we come in does as agreed & he proceeds to take an inventory of as he supposed Miss Smith. I saw him taking a good survey & directing his attention to her. So I began on my own score & cut out Miss Smith alias Beatty. After dinner in Mrs Mac's room – Miss Beatty not being there – we had a gay time – I went in for enchanting Dr. Day according to the moments fancy & to reflect some brilliancy on Dr Claxton. I fear Claxton will be here again Wed for Convocation. Oh it was fun – well we had to go down to the lecture on Materia Medica @ Royal Coll. & then from 3:30 to 4:30 to Queens University for Chemistry & back home again – tea & down to Royal Coll[2] to dissect – stayed there till dark. Oldham

2 Royal College of Medicine at Queen's University

walked up with me – a fine honest clever little fellow – gave me a timely hint of what kind of girl Miss Annie Davidson is. I thanked him for it was a friendly act & not one likely to be performed by a fast young man. Poor little Oldham – I like him firstrate & he takes so much pains with us – but I have seen the symptoms coming on lately & now they are developing fast. I wish he had not taken the trouble to fall in love with me – it will be so well, so *un*desirable in more ways than one. Well might ma say – Be wise as a serpent & harmless as a dove.

> 'Oh cleanse Thou me
> from my secret faults.'

April 25th

So ran the text this morning – thus our sins were perhaps more of omission than commission. Our little sins our secret faults are many & most repugnant to the One who sees all things. It is so hard to judge ourselves rightly with leniency or harshness & oh how hard to all things right & to see what course is best for us when troubles & dangers thicken round us, & we feel ourselves in some degree embarrassed by a misstep. Oh cleanse Thou me from my secret faults & help me to see the way my steps should tend. Friday was much very much like other days as seen in the past. The usual amount of little things – the usual amount of study. I wrote a letter home & one to Charlie that night. ... Yesterday morning Mrs Mac. was too ill to go down to Coll. So we two lone females went our solitary way down to the dissecting room. The Demonstrator was there & the little youth is so unused to dissimulation that he does not act altogether impartially, left Miss Beattys table & sat down opposite me & stayed there in fact did most of my work for me. In the afternoon – Mr Carey D.D. called on me – he is pastor of St. Pauls where I go & intend to go. He was very nice & promised to secure me a seat, asked if I were confirmed & a Communicant. Said he would do anything for me he could. In the evening Oldham came in & Dr. Day & Waddel were in too, in Mrs Mac's room & we had high carnival there 'till about ten O'clock. They then left & we retired. Oh dear the utter nonsense that can be talked – nonsense – utter nonsense. I will turn over a new leaf. I will not lower myself to talk with them in that strain – sympathise with clay.

> Through the deep caves of thought
> I hear a voice that sings;

April 27th

Tuesday & well may the above text occur to me. Ah well – ah well. The days when gone are when called to mind much the same. Monday – the usual routine of study lectures, dissecting & the both of men. Dr Claxton wrote to Dr. Day to see if I would be agreeable to going to Convocation with him & I would not give him any satisfaction for I wanted to play some joke on him. Oldham the little goose wants to be foolish walks up with me – dissects for me & sharpens knives. Today Mrs Mac has been ill so we two lone females have had it all to ourselves. Same routine of lectures for the forenoon, no chemistry this afternoon. Oldham walked up with us & in course of conversation gave me to understand that he had his opinion of a girl who would have half a dozen friends or beaus at once. Said he would be up again soon with his sister & sure enough they came only too soon (She seems very nice) They are both very nice but n'importe I do not intend entering society at their door. ... When I came up stairs here Dr Day had a telegram asking if I were agreeable & if so he would come tomorrow. I was at a stand still for I would so like to fool that man. I would like to make a most egregious example of him & hold him up to the world as a sample of how a woman scorns the animal which could only prompt a man fat fair & forty to wish to marry a girl of my age – to cook for him – Oh for the days of John Falstaff! I bewildered Dr. Day – I do not know what message he sent back nor do I care – tomorrow brings its own events. We had some fun tho' all the same –

April 29th

Yes this is a very April day – rain rain & fitful gusts of windy
sleet that makes one think of the home fireside or loving faces.
Ah well – how our natures change with things around us. I who
at one time would long with passionate earnestness for home –
long with an unsatisfied longing to be where I was not, can now
live, the careless happy – where'er – I may be life that so many
cultivate. I would like to see them of course, but I have learned
the well-learned lesson – 'live today tomorrow never yet on any
human being rose or set' I am I am afraid a sensualist in one
sense of the term for I can let what poets call the 'finer fancies'
have full play &yield myself up to the delights of the hour. For
instance – a green bank neath a tree on the waters edge – a
dreamy sky of azure blue with fleecy clouds – floating o'er it a
sweet warm breath of spring playing in the fresh burst foliage of
the trees – a book & a day dream dream worthy of the gods. Now
is not that the play of externals on our senses & is not that sensuality? Oh I love such & only one thing could add to that happiness (!) Yesterday – the usual routine in the morning of
lectures & dissecting ect. Came home to dinner & lo! Dr Claxton
had arrived. He came in again when we were at dinner but I was
just as gay as a linnet but showed a preference for Day in talking
'just for fun.' After dinner I went to my room & stayed there so
presently comes a letter to me from Dr Claxton – very nicely asking me if I would go to Convocation with him. I wrote back I
wad na – that 'we three' were going together & we went
together. ... Today like other days – routine of study Drs & presumptuous puppies

May 2nd

The Spring has come with nature & my spring is not gone yet
tho' I suppose it is waning into the summer of womanhood. Oh
to be strong in the battle of life to lead to higher – better things &

not be led away from our own to less things & less worthier
'Religion pure & undefiled before God & the Father is this – to
visit the fatherless & widow in their affliction & keep himself
unspotted from the world.' Oh if I could but do it if I could keep
unspotted from the world. Be strong & keep aloof from frivolity
& evil. One of my failings I know is my love of praise & goodwill
of others – to gain this I am pleasant to them & waste time on
them to be regretted after and to punish myself to sit up later
into the night poring over books which should have been
scanned earlier in the day when idle people detained me in frivolous talk & idle dallying. Why do people in this day & generation
get so childish in their talk & so maudlin in their sentiments –
and so blasphemous rather than religious. This morning at Communion there were but a half a dozen young people – that is
unmarried & the majority of the communicants were women
past the prime of life & in mourning. Why is it so – religion is
grand beautiful pure ennobling – encouraging – giving higher
aspirations after a pure & perfect life & yet so many if they do
not scoff – shun it as quite a nuisance & as at the best something
they can acquire sometime. Now I will register here a silent vow
that I *will* do better tomorrow than Saturday & see how I shall
succeed. Saturday forenoon we dissected from 8 to 11 & then Dr
Fowler 11 to 12 – home – dinner – ect we three sitting together by
Mrs Halliday talking & sewing. Secured a wash woman – went
shopping with Mrs Mac, had the Normal Group framed and
hung it over my bed where waking I can behold it. Friday Mrs
Halliday a friend of Miss Beatty's had a tumor cut off her face. I
stood watching four doctors standing round & fixing the ugly
cut & I acknowledge I left – for a seat for I turned miserably
ill – & when I went back was white as milk. Now I must get over
this – cultivate nerve – I see that the living bodies will effect me
more than the dead. Sat night Oldham came in – I excused myself & went to study at Miss Beatty's table because there was a
fire there & but merely commenced when the whole array were
there & so there was more conviviality & nonsense than anything else & I quarreled with Dr Day & did not make up till today at dinner. Poor little Oldham. I am sorry for him! Wrote

Myrtie & Alice letters today & went to the Presbyterian church tonight with Mr & Mrs Mac did not relish it so much as my own.

May 9th

Why just think a week has gone since I wrote here. A week much like the one before – a week in which I have found much to learn – have learned little. Have read new lessons in life. Have seen new phases in life – have found new traits of character. Have been glad & sorry, good humored, & cross. How much we need discipline. How much we abuse our stewardships. I want to be good. I fain would be a noble woman as I am nobly formed. Would like to be as nearly perfect as humanity is capable of & even in my own sight – how miserably I fail. I try continually to train myself. I hope I do & yet the animal & the weakness of human nature are strong enemies against that of pure reason & religion aspirations & yet I will overcome them as I may – not wholly I know we cannot but in part as we may. ... We finished our extremeties [of the body] last Saturday & it was quite a relief too. I wish we were as well over the other's. We work well together we trust – & like each other. I feel such a happy sense of freedom of speech with them because they are no carping squeamish little minded beings who try to magnify or belittle what is said to suit their ideas of gossip or slander. They can understand without explaining in 'minutiai' Received a dear long letter from Charlie Tuesday & I answered so he w'd get it Sat. I hope he wrote again today.

> He will hold thee when his passions
>   shall have spent their novel force
> A little better than his dog
> A little dearer than his horse.

These two verses we were discussing today. We agreed that it was true in some cases but there were happy exceptions but Miss Beatty does not seem to be much of a believer in men. Little Oldham still proves kind although I treat him badly. I told him I did not wish him to walk up from Coll. with me – & I ran away from him tonight at church – altho he brings me flowers continually – a lovely boquet of wild flowers today. Dr Day is soon going away. I do not know what would be the best thing to be done with a young man who if he is as bad as he tries to make men believe is a most consummate villian & yet to the casual acquaintance would seem *very nice*. A very aimable lovable young man. Ah! me can such things be. A man or the semblance of such – whose way is paid through Coll. by weary days of toil of mother & sister – who schemes & cheats thro' his course & shortens it to 3 yrs. Who by cheating hopes to win his way – without an unselfish feeling in his breast who glories in his shame –

May 12

Oh it is May it is May & all earth is gay! I rec. another letter from Charlie yesterday – a real nice one just like himself & I sent a reply today. One per wk for each & yet they seem far apart. Oh how weak we are. I am I mean. Today for the first time we went to the hospital to see an operation. An old man was to have his foot cut off. Dr Depuis did it, some other M.D. & students were there. The hospital is a nice large stone structure – very clean & neat looking indeed. The ward where the man lay had about 10 or 12 beds some in their beds – some by them, such fearful mishaps. This old man had gangreen foot. They had him brought into the operating room. Mr Mac & we three ranged ourselves into the observers seats & prepared to see the performance. They gave him chloroform. This was hard too as he groaned & struggled so hard then bared the lower leg & tied rubber tightly round it & cut off the foot by the metatarsus bones left enough skin & flesh for a flap to cover the bare end & sewed it over it. Just before the finishing of it when I heard the joints parting company & the foot go spat on the water, I felt kind o'sick & Miss Beatty & I left. I did not faint but was *very* white & weak. Soon after I went out – Oldham & Day came out to see if I had a fit or

anything as that & out comes Mr Mac & drops on the bed, dead
sick. He did look bad to say the least. Dr. Day introduced
Chown – B.A., M.D. to us. They took great satisfaction in staring at
us & were glad I think that I was sick. I seemed quite an interesting monstrosity tho they were very kind. I'm bound to get over
this – but oh it did leave me less strong than before. They say it is
common for the men to faint – so I'm not so very bad. Oldham
wanted me to go for a boatride tonight but I refused tho' he
coaxed like a – girl ... I like him firstrate as a Demonstrator to
admire his genius but he's too presumptuous to unfortunate me
to descend to his circle.

May 14th

About the same old story of lessons & desultory duties & time
passed in some unaccountable manner. I would I could work
hard enough to be satisfied with my work at night. I keep pretty
busy but yet seem to accomplish little. Today I was much surprised to receive a letter from Claxton – a very nice letter desiring
me to correspond with him. Now Charlie said that even with the
persistence of a man he would hardly try again but he did & so I
will have to decline honor No 2. Have had my patience tried
sorely this week by not getting a letter from home. I was expecting a registered one sure, but it has not come yet. Four Methodist
ministers here now for a week & bless you what four queer,
conundrums two of them – regular oddities – & somewhat hypocritical if I may judge. It is somewhat diff. to keep down ones
risibility when there's so much comicality even in their religion.

May 21st

We have just returned from the R.C. Cathedral – a magnificent
building externally as regards size & structure, internally as
regards trappings. There seems a solemn impressiveness about
their rite that holds you passion bound. The solemn way in

which they perform their rites – the white robed priest in the distance in his monotone way of chanting – the faint odor of incense pervading the air – the pillar & arches with figures of saints in often repeated niches. The surpliced boys lighting candles in grotesque shapes & above all & through all the grand weird strains of the massive organ. One good voice singing alone for a while, first in sad slow, but sweetly pensive strains gradually reaching the glad triumphant tones of one who rejoices in victory & then the grand solemn glorious crash of the strong voiced organ & all the choir of voices. Here one could imagine life on earth to be passing away & the soul to be ascending to a higher sphere. The Catholic (R.) religion may be said to be one of *grand* superstition & real sensuality for it is greatly by the play of externals on their senses that lead them to be so devout. They *are* devout because it gives them a certain feeling of self satisfaction, not only because they have done their duty, but there is always more or less pleasure in doing solemn things – there must be the 'bumps' corresponding to this as well as when the senses are played upon by music a certain pleasure in awe the result of participation in these things – just as 'Laughing' Gas prod. risibility. The papers ect are all making great ado about the death of Hon. George Brown[3] – as tho' he was more than common clay – but then I suppose it is due in some extent to his tragic end. Well how the days *do* go by – here it is Friday night again – how glad I am. Yesterday I rec a letter from home, & wrote back a very long one – I & Miss Beatty came round by the Post Office I told them if I did not get a letter I would go home & cry – so Mrs Mac said she would go the short way home & get a basin ready. So when I arrived here, with the letter too, lo! over my room floor were scattered many vessels such an array of white earthen ware & that mischevous one in a chair, laughing gleefully & clapping her hands over the performance which now was in vain. We often have fits of merriment & act quite infantile in fact. I feel younger than I did last fall, oh me how many changes one can experience in a year! On how many stages one can play. And the

3   prominent leader of the Liberal Party; murdered in 1880

more numerous the stages the longer seems the year in looking back. I have at last become settled in the great work of my life – what I had long looked forward to with some anxiety and much expectation. How soon the weeks have slipped away, here today the Profs tell us we have done half a sessions work & may as well take holidays. And they wish us to take June & July. It has upset a good many plans for me mais n'importe it is good fun to make new ones, & so I make some tonight. Charlie writes once a week & so do I. I rec his every Tuesday morning & I'd be very much disappointed if I did not – aint I a goose – a 'dummy.' This afternoon Mrs Mac & I sat some time by the lake shore. What is there that rouses so much of sad sweet pleasure in look-ing at the water? It always puts me in a dreamy pleasant sad but sweet trance & I could just be quiet & let 'my thoughts throng on me as they would' & enjoy it. Oh just bide-a-wee till I'm out on the 'Bay' with Charlie & that will be worth whole years of ill. I do not know how it is to come about but I expect it will & I will be satisfied that One is at the helm who can manage all things alone. I really want to be good & to do good & yet how miserably lifeless is my religion. I like to go to church. I feel that the service does me good & I come forth ready to fight for the right & within two or three hours perhaps fail to be a true Christian in some way. Then too in prayer I kneel down with the best inten-tions & begin perhaps aright & yet in a moment e'en a second I find my mind far away on earthly subjects & then I am ashamed & yet it occurs again. I think sometimes perhaps I would be less wicked to discontinue the habit of prayer which seemed so void of enthusiasm & yet if I did that I should run a chance of forget-ting religion altogether, & then I have heard ministers say that we should use the means of grace at hand trusting it would do us good. It is for this reason I take Communion. I always feel too wicked to take it & yet if I did not I should not feel satisfied & I do it trusting that I shall be the better of it. Well I know I am in some ways egotistic. I think a great deal of myself or rather I want others to think well of me. So in my own way I think I have kept a pretty high head since here. ... You see I feel all the dignity of a requited affection for somebody else & feel as tho' any friendliness with other gentlemen was treason to him – & what have I to build on there, only what many a woman has built on before – – trust. I think I know him so well & tho' theres no engagement in form between us I feel as tho it were continually understood. I honor him for his silence, & love him for his manliness. We both have our course of studies before us, a long road that has no turning but death – his course the longest as he has not started fully. So that engagement is a thing of the future if at all & what may not intervene – what changes may not occur. Some would say, if you have a good chance of marriage do not throw it away for a chance one of mere love & trust. Others, more romantic would say, if you really care for one another you can afford to wait & well wait no matter what chance offers. And there is one glorious result of education. I am preparing myself by independence to be able to marry for love & not for mercenary motives. I would wait for him gladly & yet I have that within me that wants proof of everything before trusting. I could not bear it seems to me – to live on increasing in love & faith in him while he perhaps might be decreasing in his love for me. That would be a bitter, cruel thing – & yet – & y e t & yet –

'Comes the end with rapid pace
Patience is the chiefest grace'

May 30th

Sunday night, and more than a week since I have written here. Last Sunday went with Evvy MacDonald to St. Georges Cathedral ... In the evening went to St. Pauls where I like to go & enjoy the service I feel at home there – & the people seem in earnest. Dr Day left Sunday afternoon to seek his fortunes as M.D. Went away with all a mother's devoted love & self sacrifice embodied in himself with the hearts of the family clinging to him as 'a great boy' a most wonderful person in whom they saw themselves made great. Yes he went away. I think with some love for them in his heart, but having deceived them to the last.

Told them he passed the exam. & knew he did not. He has had their strength used in paying his way at College & he has frittered time & money away, but by some means fair or foul I will not say got his College deg. but not the Council. 'Unstable as water thou shall not excel.' And yet he is one who plays havoc with a certain kind of damsels who can get up an enthusiasm for a fair looking man if he dresses well & can say soft nothings. He is trying his luck at Harwood on Rice Lake. Expected I was going home Friday & went from Cobourg to Toronto by the boat I was to have been on. ... Mr Mac. left at noon & as Mrs Mac. wanted to forget it, we both took wraps & a lunch & 'Molly Baron' & started for the boat. Left here about 2 Oclock & got back about 10. The trip was very fine. The scenery is truly beautiful. ... Was sick that night but got up ready for work next morning & Charlies letter. He wrote as long as usual but there were some things in it I did not like & so I wrote a cross one back. I wonder how he will take it. I am anxiously awaiting his reply. Well that morn we got the decision of the Profs that our holidays would begin now & continue for six weeks. Dr. Depuis said there was a sub. ready for us & we could go to dissecting again. So it was arranged. Wednesday night we were invited up to Prof. Dixons [Dickson's] to tea. We went for once & enjoyed it very much. They are an admirable family. He is the nominal President of the College, but has been ill. ...

June 2nd

Ah! Well many a second of June have I spent but few so far from those at home. For two or three years when away I returned on that day for the usual Grange picnic, but this time I am not home nor is there a picnic. Monday we started for Coll. knowing we were to have a grind & knowing too that we were unprepared & we lived through it & dissected till 12 Oclock. Came home to dinner then I went to get my photograph taken & back to find Miss Dikson [Dickson] waiting for us to go to The Asylum. We took the st car & went out as far as the Penitentiary. Then walked on through Portsmouth, a village in the Suburbs, where Portsmouth bay an inlet of the lake is. Miss Dikson's father Dr Dixon our President was formerly Superdt of Asylum & consequently lived at Rockwood which is a most beautiful place. ... It is the finest residence I have seen in Ontario. We went to the Lunatic Asylum, & oh what a change. A possessor of millions might live there, & yet be humble as the meanest. Oh how very sad to see poor poor humanity in that most pitiful of plights, idiosy, lunacy. To see our fellow beings, yes of our race, our brothers & sisters such animals, such caricatures of the brighter kind of the species. All grades of society represented one common herd of animals & showing in their way the predominence of certain traits of character, lunatics from so many causes, & of all stages. ... Tuesday morning down to Post & received Charlies letter. A nice one too, & he did not seem to be cross a bit although I was in my last letter. Am I imposing on my own credulity or are things what they seem? I often doubt myself, & yet I think I am much interested in his letters, not much of a confession eh? Well I will not write my thoughts here for I might regret them. Came back, answered the letter saying I would come on Saturday, back to Coll. to work in the afternoon & back again to dream for awhile of the future & of persons in the present. What queer grotesque visions arise before one in day dreams.

June 7th

Here I am at home again, just about the same thing all round – & yet I do think I have a little more purpose a little more energy than I used to have. Last Thursday noon we finished up our work at College & not at all sorry were we to leave that 'cadaver' or its abiding place. In the afternoon Miss B[eatty] went out to tea, & Mrs Mac & I went down town did some shopping ect. I enjoy going shopping with her, she is such a very child of nature, & does things so innocently. That day she wished some paper & Mrs Stacy recommended a special kind & she did not know how much she wanted, asked him how much she should get. Bought it, started off without it, went back for it & then we went on trading & she left it in some other store. We came out again after tea to get it. We did not get it but walked about till about dark, came home & had a nice pleasant quiet time in Mrs Mac's room. Miss B came home & we talked a little more & then packed or started to pack our trunks when in came our Demonstrator. He stayed the greater part of the evening, said goodbye, which was hard for the 'little fellow' – I am almost sorry he cares so much for me for I only like him & tolerate him. After we finished packing, we went to Mrs Mac's rooms & had a comical lunch of crackers, water & dried beef which we chewed for about an hour, then retired. Next morning down town, down to the College ... In afternoon went down to the boat with Miss B & saw her commence her homeward journey. Went back, had a chat with Mr Knight who called an early tea, & off for the wharf. Mrs Mac going with me. Went on board, out on deck when who should I see but Oldham I avoided him however & do not know whether he saw me or not. ... Stayed on deck for some time. After tea, I was seated complacently reading thinking & observing in the saloon – & observed these diff persons – a no of young men rather good looking, but no apparent distinguishing characteristics. A family consisting of pere, mere, mother in law four 'enfants terrible' with their nurse. They seemed to have a fat purse, the father look quite 'comme il faut' as regards 'ton' but the wife & her mother some how suggested 'rich peasantry' & soon after I heard 'my daughter' mark to ma mere 'Mother do you notice the water has a peculiar tint just like a moire antique dress' This last prounounced 'moray an teek' this settled her beyond a doubt. Then there was a divine & his spouse, both ancient looking people, affable & so careful of one another, it is said they work algebra for amusement. Innocent diversion, as innocent as reading 'Night Thoughts' so sahib said to me. Then there was an old English lady with white hair, who could talk & play with out end, who had taken a fancy for live stock & had with her three bird cages – a couple of canarys – her son had sent

her from Canary Isles & a couple of parrots he had sent from
Africa. Then too a young lady who aped affectation & a poodle
'Flossy' my dear. She was a speciman of what a girl might be
who had no aim in life & no need for exertion, beyond keeping
herself 'a la mode' & talking in a certain sterotyped twaddle
peculiar to her class, whose greatest trouble was ennui – &
whose soul revolted at science & all its learned fraternity. Well I
was sitting there taking in the surroundings when a young cava-
lier settled himself beside me & opened conversation about the
book I was reading. I found him more than nice. I admired him
for his knowledge. He was bronzed as the natives of the land he
came from *India*. He was a Scotch Presbyterian by birth, had
been in India fifteen year – was traveling now to see Canada. He
knew so much of the world, & had seen so much of it. We talked
long & exhaustively on many subjects. I shall not soon forget
him, it was such a real pleasure to talk with him. There was no
bombast, no twaddle, no aping superiority, but an easy frank
congeniality about him, that was quite irresistable in its way. We
enjoyed ourselves there till about ten & then I bade him good
night & retired. The waves sang their lullaby, & the roll of the
vessel rocked me to sleep. I was only awakened by the vessel
stopping once in the night, & then dosed again till 5 Oclock
when the boat took on some soldiers ... for Toronto. They made
such a noise that I arose & dressed opened my door to look out &
if I had been a little more sleepy I might have thought myself on
a lost battlefield however they were only soldiers curled up to
sleep. I retreated to my stateroom layed down again & slept till
the bell summoned me. After emerging from my room & settling
down in a corner 'sahib' again made his appearance & we went
to breakfast together. After enjoying the meal spiced with a social
chat, he betook himself to the deck & his pipe. I to my book &
the saloon. Soon after he again sauntered up & as he again made
some allusion to my innocent book I read him a good extract.
Soon after we reached Toronto where he bade me goodbye.
Neither aware of the others name but mutually satisfied with out
short acquaintance. He said 'he wished he had time to become

better acquainted with me for I had greatly raised – lady doctors
in his estimation' ect. As I looked from my stateroom window he
smiled bowed & walked away. The boat stayed two hours in
Toronto & then we sailed for Hamilton. ... Poor Charlie had gone
down as well as Cecil to meet me as I had said at 11 but being
told the boat would not arrive till 5 went home again & so I
missed the delight I had anticipated, & I have not seen him since.
The best layed schemes of mice & men gang aft a gee & so I have
learned not to fret over it. Cecil came home with us, to spend
Sunday, which we did in the old time way. The country is beautiful now, *very*. In the evening we went to Stoney Creek to
church & again as of old I listened to our loved pastor Mr Whit-
combe, in the dear little country church. Today Monday the first
day of my work at home, studied from six to seven then helped
with the housework till eleven studied, practised, wrote studied,
practised, got tea & washed the dishes studied & am now finishing the daylight writing here. I have been very busy & not much
time for dreaming the day & so may I continue to pass my days
in usefullness for I am far happier so – I am content & feel better,
than when drifting idly on a sea of pleasure.

June 14th

Now indeed there is not much to copy here. Many days are very
similar. Last Tuesday there was a little variation. Went for
Charlie's letter rec it but it even made me regret more than ever
that I had not seen him on my way home, oh I want to see him &
want to talk to him. I do. ... Friday J.H. Smith was here for dinner, we had a very good talk what there was of it. I expect him
again tonight Sunday Chet was here. I like him more than I ever
did. I forget to be spiteful 'for memory shifts from the past its
pain & suffers the glory alone to remain' He stayed all day, so we
did not get to church. I do not believe in Sunday visiting. It does
not seem like the sabbath at all. It spoils two things, the rest &
peace of the Sabbath & the visit in some ways for we can not

entertain them as we would on a week day. Today I was up soon after five, studied 1 hr & a half & then did house work & then study & so the day is gone, & I am here in my den.

If I am not worth the wooing
I'm surely not worth the winning.

June 30th

Here goes for a resume. Continued my programme of study & housework with but little interruption. J.G. Smith was here twice & I had a nice chat with him. Then Friday Gertie & I drove into H[amilton] did some shopping, called on Maud. Yes she would return with us, so we were to call at 5.30. Went up to Coll. Inst to see Cecil but he was not there, but I saw a number of the old schoolgirls & had a most lively chat indeed. In fact I was almost ashamed of the hilarious times going on around the buggy. Just as we drove away Charlie appeared. I was the cooler of the two. The meeting was short, quite unsatisfactory in one way & yet satisfactory in that he promised to come down next day. ... we reached home about dark & I found a sagacious droll interesting letter from Miss Beatty awaiting me & her photo. We retired early that night & had a good schoolgirl or mahzhap I may call it womanly talk, so very pleasant after such an interval. Next day we began reading David Copperfield & with a great deal of zest too. Lived very quietly, thought of going for a drive after tea, but while we were hulling strawberries & complacently talking of it who should arrive but Charlie. I was real glad & was merry as a lark for the rest of the day. Of course we did not go for a drive. Ernie & Maud played croquet against Charlie & I & won too, but we didn't care much. Then again in the evening they won at euchre against us. After retiring, I gave the girls a performance, which immensely amused them. They had hidden my nightdress & I pretended to think it had been left under Charlie's pillow. Gracious patience! Next morning were all late getting up, after breakfast. We sauntered in to the drawing room & hall & soon I

found Charlie & I were in the hall alone & so we had a good
long talk. Of course there were many interruptions, but we made
the most of it. It was something like that for the greater part of
the day. Then Gertie & Maud went to church & we had another
talk on the doorsteps & then the girls soon came back & we
retired to our chambers where I again gave them rehearsals to
create a laugh which concerned the 'enfant terrible' keeping her
eye on me. Next morning Charlie left. I was up betimes & helped
get an early breakfast. Scene 'Breakfast table' – Charlie on one
side – mon pere & mon mère sanchioning & I at the head of the
table in blue wrapper but no curl papers, pouring the tea. Then
he bade them goodbye & I saw him off. Did not take him to the
station Mrs Grundy would never allow that, where as if it had
been a 'female woman' of as good friendship I had been in duty
bound to take her. 'Qui male soit que male pense' ...

'That time cannot steal from memory
 That absence only endears.'

... In the afternoon I went down to see Alice & to take tea
there ... Had quite a chat with Alice, & yet I could feel there was
not the same close sympathy between us there had been formerly. I regret it and yet I feel it is there. After tea Maud & Mr R
came for us with a double rig & Alice & I went according to promise for the drive. We went up to the Ocean House, had ice
cream & returned about 10 Oclock. ... Next morning quiet. Cecil
called & I went with him to Mrs Lawsons, had a long talk with
her & Cecil walked back with me – poor child. I fear he is sometimes unhappy. I feel for him indeed. Where trials have to borne
alone they seem so much harder than when shared with another.
'Where trifles light as air are to the jealous confirmation strong
as Holy Writ' There is apt to be unhappiness. I know the lad has
been besieged by small worries wh. altho' they may be nothing
they are all enough to make one miserable. I am glad he is coming home for a time it will do him good I'm sure. In the afternoon Gertie came for us & we returned to Mountain Hall & to
David Copperfield. ...

July 22nd

I am not myself at all today rather too much myself & not at all like what I would be. Have been ill, & in consequence am irritable & nervous & have been guilty of tears & anger this day. Anger from being crossed, & given way to from nervousness & then tears of regret that I had been so weak. It makes me feel miserable to record it to even think of it because I make so many good resolutions & then see them so easily broken. Oh dear dear dear I want to be good & I can't. I wonder if it is my pride that causes me so much trouble oh dear, dear. I *am* miserable and gloomy, just as a while ago I was in good spirits & vivacious, such is life. So much depression follows just so much excitement & vice versa. I feel like writing a long harangue merely of thought & moods but have not time as I wish to record the last week or so. Until last Friday the programme was little disturbed & since then it has not been in force. Friday afternoon Kennedy called, stayed for tea. I learned from him that Charlie was at Woodburn & so directed my letter there – 'fiasco' Next day Ma Vi & Cecil went to town & brought back Myrtie & Jennie. I showed my housekeeping proclivities that day & did a great amount of it. Slept well that night & as we were dressing for breakfast about nine Gertie came in to inform us that Brosie was below to see us. Well as it was Sunday of course we spent a very quiet day. In the evening Brose Jennie & I in his buggy, Gertie & Ernest in ours drove to Church. Not many there but an excellent sermon & an excellent drive. Brose stayed the evening & was loath to go. Next day we spent quietly & sociably. ... Next morning Dan & Mary came & I was very glad. We expected Mary but not Dan & I like him so much. We had a *very* pleasant day. Most of the afternoon we spent at croquet & had an interesting game. ... In the evening we had charades & good ones too. They were acted so well & we were highly amused. ... Yesterday, morning four of them played croquet. Ernest Dan Mary & Jennie while we did up the work then I changed with Mary & played a game, & then we took to books till dinner & after that sang choruses, read talked ect. till toward night we we had two more

games of croquet. ... Retired to our respective rooms the others to
rest but we girls for more fun & frolic. Had a ghost scene, a pillow fight, a scrabble ect & at last closed our weary eyes till late
this morning. Soon after breakfast Dan took his leave & when
shall I see him again I wonder. Jennie, Kennedy & I went to the
drawing room, sang songs & had a chat & soon he too departed
then being left in our own hands we had a dance, one play &
two of us dance, then books, a short sleep waking up very miserable, & remaining so for a good (?) while. ...

July 27th

Here we are alone once more, but I expect visitors soon Roberts
& Shields anyway. That night on which I last wrote was wearing
late when the girls returned Egbert & Jennie with them, then it
was hoity-toity, for some hours however I did not put in an
appearance. ... Saturday Ernie & I went over to Nelson. ... Next
day of course we had to [be] deep preternaturally solemn as Mr
W[ilson] is such a dreadful religious man. His religion seems to
have a depressing effect not at all mirthful they sing the hymn
'Him serve with mirth' but there are many incongruities in this
world. Oh consistency thou art a jewel. After breakfast we Ernie
& I went over to Spences & were most cordially welcomed. We
enjoyed our visit here very much. Their religion is a beautiful
one. It shines forth not only on their lips but in their lives. Had
some conversation but not all or nearly all we wished. After dinner went up to Sunday School – saw a great number of my
pupils, some of them I very much liked to see & it all brought
back vividly to mind the time when I ruled there & was occasionally miserable & happy. Went back to Wilsons – had tea &
then to church, Jim & I in one buggy, Janet, Mary & Ernest in the
other. Went to Burlington to church quite unimportant, unless I
should try to portray Jim's feelings & so I will not nor how
amused & indifferent I was. Next morning we had a game of
croquet & some talk & set off for home about eleven. Such a
lovely drive, beautiful beyond words to describe. Such a long

delicious drive. When I arrived home, Agnes & Barbara Geddes
& Jennie Wood were there & so a quiet kind of day was put in.
Next morning took Jennie to the station. ... About tea time
Charlie came – I was so glad ... Spent a very pleasant evening did
not have a chance for confidential chat till next day which was
one long delightful day in which we talked as much as we
wanted to, & came to a better understanding of one another. Oh
tis well that I should be away, that I should not see him often,
that I should have my studies only, else, else I should become
perfectly infatuated quite maudlin, & go mooning about my
daily avocations in a quite novel manner. Next day he left me. It
was a necessary act & yet we were loath to do it – bah what am I
saying, but yet I missed him after he had gone & wanted to see
him again. How one person can grow into anothers life, filling it,
making itself essential to happiness is a mystery. After he left, I
commenced packing my trunks & this occupied my leisure that
day fully. As I had not much about dusk Ella Lewis & Miss
Moore called & just after their departure Mr Jarvis & sisters,
Grafton & Gussie Kerr & Lyman Lee called for the evening & we
gave it to them. I had a very agreeable talk with Mr Lee, he is
quite a talker, is through his first year at the university, I like
him very well, not for any brilliancy but for his good moral
qualities & then too he can talk more & better than those
'stick-in-the-mud' young men who have never been beyond the
rooftree of home. Retired about 2 Oclock that night & left for
Hamilton at 6 Oclock. Jennie Wood was at the boat to see me off.
Had a small chat, & then Ernie & Jennie drove away & left me to
my Kismet, Kismet I was so very sleepy that after trying to think
& to read, I gave it up & went to my room & slept till dinner
which was a quiet affair, enlivened by the snobby talk of a
stuffed young Englisher who by his persistent upstart twaddle
addressed to sedate 'Scotchy' Captain Sinclair made me think of
'Dignity & Impudence' After another attempt at rationality I
again withdrew to my room & slept till I was roused by the
stewardess who asked me to share my stateroom with another
lady – an American from Cleveland, a very nice young lady, with
whom I became quite friendly. After tea we adjourned to the

deck where I had a glorious think. At first I amused myself by
noting human nature ect & listening to the lively chatter of two
Frenchmen. So strange that there can be so many types in one
species, so strange that we are so near alike & yet so far – far different in nature in everything but form. She retired early & I
muffling up myself leaned over the railing, looking at the water
rather through the water into myself. When I am between sky &
sea two such pure things I can as it were think more clearly can
read myself. I tried to summon self before the bar of my own
sense & try to decide its future course, its future line of feeling &
of acting, to insist that all mooning propensities should be found
guilty & consigned to a watery grave, & that my energy should
be stimulated to a better future. In short that merrier & lighter
days should have been a thing of the past & that my future
course was one of study earnest study & not of schoolgirl rhapsodies over a boy or if you please a man. No, now is a time for
work the pleasure must lie in that. 'The work we choose must be
our own God lets alone' Well I tried to become enthused with the
line I was about to follow, but believe it as I might it was not
with the same vim that I take up my oars now as I did not long
since in the same cause, but I am bound to 'stem with steady
stroke the tide of my own passions' & do my duty & rejoice in
the doing. Arrived at Kingston four next morning secured cab &
arrived here before they were stirring. Mrs Reynolds let me in &
I slept till the Christian hr of seven before making my arrival
known – then after breakfast Mrs Mac & I went down town,
bought up stationary & home to dinner. After dinner the horse
& carriage were sent round to the door & calling for Abednego
[Elizabeth Beatty] we left the city behind us & drove out along
the lake & spent a very pleasant afternoon. I like Miss Beatty so
much. She has so much decision of character & to use Samantha
Allens words 'ketches right hold of her cast iron principles' &
stands herself. Miss Reynolds an invalid at present, is boarding
here & is being doctored by Dr Fowler, a nice person very, will
probably become one of us. Retired early & had a good sleep
which I very much needed. Went to church next morning –
Communion Sunday, & I stayed. Sometimes I do not know

whether to take part or not. I know I am not worthy, & yet if I neglect those means I have, it would be wrong, & so I do it, trusting it is best. Well Mrs Mac & I took the carriage, rather the carriage took us & we took books & victuals & set off to spend the afternoon according to our own notions, not I'm afraid in a very orthodox manner, but I thought I could do so & do no harm. We drove out about three miles – under a clump of willows by the shore. Sat there enjoying a delicious cool breeze, while our citizen sisters were stewing with the heat, & enjoyed ourselves, read some in the Bible, & then we read a couple chapters of 'Bleak House' & about four jogged on about three miles further, then we led the horse & went down & the rocks behind the cedars, spread out our supper & indulged, such a lovely spot with the spray dashing at our feet, & splash splashing against the rocks. We arrived home about 2:30 tired enough. After church the Demonstrator called what shall I write of him – perhaps silence would show greater discretion. He was undoubtedly glad to see me & I like him very well if he would only not fall so far over the precipice as to break his organ of life ... He did go away & we retired. Up betimes & to College. Dr Fowler was there but none of the other Profs. There are breakers ahead I fear but our kegs of gunpowder are in reserve & I'll be bound we will yet obtain our degrees at Queens & not go in with the gentlemen either. Well here tis dark & we have just ended a sad romp & are going to work. How foolish, childish, nonsensical one can be at times. Mrs Mac & I just go in for the whole thing while we are at it & have fun, think we were almost as noisy as male students tho' not as vulgar or low.

August 7th

Here we are again, after more pleasure writing that I have been led from overmuch study by the mere pleasure I took in pleasure. Now for a Retrospect. Tuesday morning lectures as usual, & study & copying lectures in the afternoon, & for a drive Mrs Mac

& I. A good long beautiful drive, called at Prof Depuis & inter-
viewed him, had a chat with Dr Fowler & two excitements about
the horse but arrived safely home ... & soon after Mr Oldham
came in, gave me his photo & let me see for myself that he felt,
all over, actually called *my* photo pretty & that was proof positive that he was far down in the scale. Stayed till Mrs Mac fairly
told him to go. ...

Not enjoyment, & not sorrow
Is our destined end or way
But to live that each tomorrow
Finds us farther than today.

... Next day the forenoon passed about as usual & so did not the
rem. of day. I copied lectures till time for Chemistry lecture & Mr
T[urnbull] going down with us treated us to ice cream by the
way & left us at the Coll. after calling at several bookstores to
settle a dispute about Innocents Abroad & New Pilgrims Progress. After chemistry came home to tea & after went to Barrie-
field for a drive a delicious drive, talk, ect. Sang Juinata coming
home. Reached here about nine & then spent a pleasant evening
talking of books, their writings & their effects. But paramount to
this was a discussion we had about the right of women to study
medicine, not only the right but the fitness of things in so doing.
I tell you now I was roused & I think I fairly did myself justice,
the red spot burned upon my cheek, my neck was defiant in its
curve & I was lost to surroundings & the words came ready
formed. I guess I rather surprised & on the whole delighted Mr
T. for I do not think he holds the absurd ideas he brought up. I
like him very well. He is a great improvement on what I expected
he would be from Mrs Mac's description. This morning Mr T.
bade us goodbye & I missed him the rest of the day for he made
it lively. Lectures this morning by McGwin, Oliver & Fowler, &
this afternoon by Mr Gibson. This is getting rather droll, when
we find three young men have worked their way to acquaintance
with us by means of playing substitute for the Profs occasionally.

However they are all very nice & we do not rage. After tea we started for another driving expedition. The triumvire – & we had a good one & a good time generally. I was I think on the whole the quietest one of the whole. I was thinking of the absent & the future. Oh if I could but clearly understand myself & be what I wished to be. I want to be good. I want to be a christian & a noble true hearted woman & oh – human nature is *so* weak. I feel when looking at myself, how far I am from my ideal. What can I do, what shall I do? Gentle overcoming faith & love God's best gift love. Oh that we were what we would be. Oh Charlie I do not know myself.

Live for those who love you
For those who know you true
For the wrongs that need resistance

August 7th

Sunday night near eleven here I am ready for a good nights sleep, before taking up the burden of life for another week. Life is so hurried that we scarce have time for reflection. 'I would that my tongue could utter the thoughts that arise in me.' Am I doing what is right in being led from my intentions to play civility to those in my path or am I mistaken in the share of civility which is their due? I wish to be good, & which is the proper thing to do, to be led away from the plan I purposed, to please others, not in evil, but in mere pleasure or rather to please them even at self sacrifice. Is it right? How can we resolve what is best? I pray, I wish to do right. From the bottom of my heart I want to be what pleases God best, what I to the best of my ability think God would have me to be, a woman nobly formed 'unspotted from the world' and yet, I am so weakly carried away by the current, as tho' I were a straw on the tide, wh. ebbed & flowed & I powerless as to my actions. But now I must to sleep rather than to soliliquizing ...

August 13th Friday

'The day is warm & hot & sultry
The fresh wind blows & is never weary'

Here I am spending the afternoon writing to my friends & to you
also my friend who never tells what is confided. There is a
strange feeling upon me, of the room being filled with friends
who let me feel the quiet joy of their presence but whom I do not
have to entertain in the sterotyped way. I think it is a misfortune,
either attached to people at birth or else acquired that they think
things are not going on amicably unless there's a constant flow
of talk, no matter whether sense of nonsense so long as 'talk'
continues, then they are satisfied of our friendly intentions a
most annoying instance of this the other night. Coming home
from the excursion about two O'clock in the night, tired so tired
& sleepy, with Mrs Mac & Mrs Turnbull, & do you imagine for a
moment that the last named could cease talking no, oh dear no,
every thing attracted her attention & called for query or com-
ment. She worried me but I left Mrs Mac to do the agreeable by
answering & I only did when directly appealed to. ...

'For to will is present with me; but how to perform that which
is good I find not For the good that I would I do not; but the
evil which I would not that I do'

Aug 15th Sunday

Yes it is just as I heard this text tonight, it expresses my condition
exactly. I would do good, I would walk in the strait & narrow
way and when some fresh resolve has just been made I go forth
to converse with others determined on watching & praying lest I
fall into temptation, then so sure I have cause for regret before I
am again alone. 'I would that my tongue could utter the
thoughts that arise in me' Oh fear not in a world like this & thou

shalt know ere long, Know how sublime a thing it is To suffer &
be strong. ...

>'Blessed are those
>Whose blood & judgment are so well coming led
>That they are not a pipe for fortunes finger
>To sound what stop she please'

Yesterday for instance, when I went for a boat ride that I had settled in my mind I would not go for. Friday evening Mrs Mac & I
went up to see Miss Beatty, soon after we were in, who should
arrive but Mr Oldham. We chatted till nine & then returned. He
accompanied us & asked us to go for a row next day. We had not
the least intention of going, but he still persisted in saying he
would call for us & did, but Mrs Mac being ill I said I would not
go alone & so he went after Miss Beatty & to my chagrin,
brought her over to go. We went how could I help it. We had a
very pleasant row, & gathered some water lillies. In the evening
pretended to study. Today have been to church twice. Heard an
excellent sermon this morning. 'Thou God seest me' We have
just returned from a walk. Mr Mac & Oldham, Mrs Mac &
I – *Poor me.*

Aug 30th

Aye how many times have I wished oh, *so* much for somebodys
hand to clasp mine, that is not here. I am a very baby and I think
the example of seeing another so infatuated has its effect on me.
And then I say to myself, you foolish girl, how do you know but
his love is on the wane, wail you, let him take the initiative & if
that be, infatuation, then there's time for you to 'dream & dream
& be a baby' I do not know why it is but I seem to have fallen
into disregard of you, old diary & have quite neglected you have
had no taste for writing here & so have not. There seems little
out of the usual order of things going on, one day varies but little

from the one before it, and so I think there's nothing worth
recording true there's one day of the week that's better than the
others, i.e. when I get a certain letter, which I look forward to, &
get as usual but when I get it & read it, I'm in despair for several
more days must pass ere the next one comes. To make an entry
once a week & say I rec. a letter would not be interesting in variety. Yesterday Mrs Mac went away & so I have been quite alone,
on this flat & have enjoyed it in a sad, happy kind of way, as I
have a severe cold with it, it is somewhat diff. Last night I
studied till midnight & then wrote some, retired soon after one.
This morning & day I have spent principally in sleeping, this
evening went to church. There was a funeral sermon. I cried
quite copiously, not for the dead or for the appeal in the sermon
but merely & solely because I had a bad bad cold & could not
help it. ... 'As thy day is so shall they strength be' oh may I be
one of those the Lord loveth, & receive the strength in every
hour that comes laden with its round of duties. I do so long to be
better, purer, nobler & I begin the day, steadfastly purposing to
'watch & pray' & live so that I may not regret the day, & then I
cannot tell how or when or in what way I am just back again in
the easy groove, led, enticed so cleverly that I did not nkow it,
but looking back upon the day I am heartily sorry it has been no
better. I think sometimes it is harder to overcome small obstacles
than large because if they were great wrongs or temptations I
would know them to be so & could avoid overcome them, but
when indecision bars the way, when a compromise seems a
means of getting over it. When the ends seem to justify the
means, & then we know, 'he who hesitates is lost' & often I do
not hesitate bec. I do not see it at all. Now in this case what is the
best that I can do. Mr Oldham will persist in calling about twice
a week, & I have been frigid as I well could be & not be uncivil. I
like him very well, he's a thoroughly noble little fellow & seems
to be in love (I may as well say it) with me. I really do not want
to encourage him. I do not wish to hurt him, & I certainly don't
care for him in that way. I like someone else only too well & if
that same some one could hear that the Demonstrator called so

often & see him tonight as he sat in the drawing room gazing at me, while I was patiently waiting his departure, would he be well pleased? & I would despise myself if I were unfaithful. 'Oh for a closer walk with God' when I could see the way. 'There seems to be a wall around me.'

Sept 7th

And the years go by. How many varied moods and occurrences may arrive in one day. Received a letter a satisfactory long one from 'the dearest boy in the world' ... Went to lectures & read it before work began, enjoyed it. Went through the lectures home, to my room reread his letter & just had a good laugh right from the heart, peal after peal, went down to dinner in excellent spirits & then Edgar gave me a piece of information not at all to my taste i.e. that Oldham had told Creggan that without exception I was the finest girl in the world & a lot more ... that *he* shades of my Ancestors! was going to marry me when through College & he'd like to see the man capable of getting ahead of him, such unparalled presumption, & from such a boy too. Clever as he is & good, he's wanting in some bumps or he might have seen ere this that he was only tolerated because he had been & is our Demonstrator. Somewhat conceited too for if he thought me a Goddess, what must he thought himself to be worthy of possessing one. Rec. letter from Mr Dickson very kind & holds out encouragement that I may get a situation as teacher & also get satisfactory chemistry lectures of Dr. Hare. Then tonight I hear the Faculty have decided to shut down on us if we have no new additions to our ranks in the Spring. However of this I'm not sure. 'Sufficient unto the day is the evil thereof' I am not in a studying mind tonight. My thought are wool-gathering. Miss Beatty says in estimation of Mr Oldham that boys are more apt than girls to make confidents of one another. But even if it was a plan he might have had the grace to add, get if he could, but such presumption.

Sept 18th

I wonder often if this will be my case & am sometimes afraid I am liable to such a fate. Even in my love of someone, some days I seem totally devoid of all the tender passions and am a sort of happy comfortable machine that keeps in running order but lacks feeling, seems 'to be forgotten by the world & the world forgot' is the description of the state then again I awake from that and all my soul is filled with longing longing for the May. 'The May' being indicative of many untold ideas that seemingly are the sumum bonum of human life. What I want to put down today is a description of last night, as that has been the most important part of the week to us. After pressing invitations from Rev Mr Young that we would read at their Fruit Festival we consented & so we prepared for it. The papers contained notices of it for two nights before it, that Mrs McGillivray & Miss Smith were to give readings. Well when the night came we were ready. Mrs Mac dressed in a silk lace fichu, chain & a small pink flower in hair & at throat. I wore a black cashmere with velvet trimmings, silver buttons ect. Honiton & lisse cuffs & collar with a large bunch of scarlet geraniums at neck & at top & back of my head, with hair in braids. I was quite well satisfied with my looks, & so did not feel concerned on that point. When we arrived we were ushered to a cloak room by Rev. Young, then came back & watched the crowd. Mrs Young was very nice. The fruit was served first, was quite satisfactory & the tables looked beautiful. The first speaker was Dr Depuis our Prof of Anatomy. Most of his speech was about Mrs Mac & I. Indeed it was quite comical to us that we should be the theme of adoration & plaudits the entire evening. The singing was very nice. The speeches had little of interest to us but what immediately concerned us and that was the burden of both Revs Young & Joliffe & Dr. Mrs Mac read first, 'A Allegory by Samantha' wh. was encored & she responded with 'The Christian Slave' wh. did not take so well. After more singing I came on. Gave Mary Queen of Scotts, better than ever before. I was entirely at ease & held them in rapt attention, when I finished there was deafening applause & a persistent encore wh. I responded to with 'Entertaining her big Sisters Beau' which fairly & completely to use the usual phrase brought down the house & I never could wish warmer fuller laurels than I received. They were very persistent in the second encore but I refused to comply & Mr Young with some difficulty quieted them telling them that probably they would have an opportunity at some future time, & then followed such praise as would delight any one. One things said by Rev Mr Joliffe said very nicely what the majority if not all thought that he felt like a little boy who said to his father – 'I say the biggest rabbit I ever saw in my life this morning but five minutes ago I saw one larger.' Mrs Mac. did not relish this simile. He also said that the Med's would have to look well to their laurels, for one of that mental calibre entering the lists ect ect. & that I recited Mary Queen of Scotts better than he had ever heard it before. More much more of that nature was said & we received congratulation on all hands. Mrs McIntyre presented us for the 'Ladies' each with a beautiful boquet, & we came home accompanied by that persistent shadow of mine Mr Oldham. I was well well satisfied with my part of the evening. Rec. a nice letter from Dan last night & a partnership one from Dr Trout in which she invites me to stay with her for a few days.

Sept 23rd

No one knows what a season of tumult there has been in my heart. Have I just awakened, would that it had been but a troubled dream, but oh my woman heart. I have been reckless, I could not realize what I was doing, and tho' I have been quite frigidly cool, & snubbed him often yet, yet he would rush on his fate. I cannot realize yet that those burning words of love were poured in my ears, that all his eloquence in words, earnestness eyes soul were for me & meant me, to think that the I love you & will you be my wife were really & truly earnest, words from him to me, & I what a mixture of feeling swept over me, but not one

answering throb not one pulsation faster my heart for him. Not a
tremor or thrill in my frame & he so passionate, so intensely
earnest, a boys love truly ... When he first approached it it was
only what I thought a queer way of expressing his good intentions toward me, but before I knew what had happened I was
dazed amazed by such a torrent of words, that I asked him not to
be foolish & please to talk sense, but it was only adding oil to the
flame & so I told him he had no right to talk so, & oh I cannot
remember the wonderful waste of words he vexed me with,
begged, entreated me to give some hope, some straw to hold to,
some hope to buoy him up during the winter, to let him write
me but I said *no*. He pressed me to tell him was there another I
like better – ah, had he known, & I told him he had no right to
ask that question & consequently I did not answer it. He would
not take a final answer then but said the 22nd of September 1881
he would come for his answer. I let him off at that and really, I
believe he *has hopes*.

'The woman's cause is man's
They rise or fall together
Dwarfed or Godlike, bond or free.'

Oct 10th

Ah me, ah me, the days come and go as a dream that is o'er –
as a tale that is told. Why looking back over the time intervening between this and when I last wrote, If I could write all that
has occured all the talk ect of that time I should have a volume –
To try a synopsis – The next night, after lectures I packed my
trunks ... Mr Dickson secured our staterooms & I found I would
have the extreme felicity of rooming with Mrs Dickson. So we
retired & I was oh, so glad, to rest my tired limbs, even in the top
birth, with much twisting & turning I was at last settled for the
night – & dreamt of — Well next morning I was awakened by a
faint voice calling me & I found Mrs D. was sick so I clambered
out, & got on deck as I too felt qualmish but the fresh air soon

revived me & I ate a hearty breakfast. Went below & got 'Bleak House' & when not bored with the Dickson's enjoyed myself at that, writing & thinking. The day was faultlessly beautiful and I enjoyed it much. We reached Toronto about five and found the Hamilton boats were laid up for the season so instead of going to Dr Jennie Trouts per agreement I just had my trunks brought over to G[reat] W[estern] Station & set off for Hamilton where I arrived about 7.30. Went up to Myrties & found they had all gone out for the evening & so I had a very dreary three hours wait till they arrived, & 'they' proved to be Myrtie, Aunt Hester & Mr Oile. I *quite* astonished them as they did not expect me till next day. We spent a very pleasant hour or so in talk, retired till late next morning, then we went down to a meeting of the Weber heirs, such fun as I had, in taking notes, such queer specimens of the 'genus homo' I looked & found several of the characters of Bleak House, if Mrs Mac had been there it had been a still greater treat, to see Miss Flite, Gridley ect. Uncle & Aunt were both with us to dinner & the afternoon, then Myrtie & I saw them off, and returned about dark, *tired*, but what of that to me, somebody was coming, somebody came, and the only check on the purest happiness was that we could not talk unrestrained when a third party was by. He said he would, of course with my permission call & go to church with me. Next morning it was raining, and at night too, alas Mr O. & Mr R both came & stayed the evening as we could not go to church.

'To meet; to know to love to part
Is the sad sad fate of every human heart'

...

7

Aldershot and Hamilton, Ontario
November 1880 to March 1881

In Aldershot and Hamilton Elizabeth resumes the teaching which
is so essential to her finances at medical school. She is no more
satisfied than usual with the occupation but finds compensation
in new and old friendships. Far and away the most important of
these is her love for Charlie Roberts. As the entries indicate, her
feeling for him has now become a major emotional mooring in
her life.

'That one day out of darkness they shall meet
And read life's meaning in each other's eyes'

November 1st, 1880.

Ay, so so it is; I have read the meaning and it is very precious –
the old, old story and yet so new to us, so unlike what the best
imagination could portray.

The first week at home was very commonplace. I took part of
the house work in hand and tried to do my duty.

The next week was more busy. ... Saturday ev'g the Soiree at
the schoolhouse. Some pleasure & vastly interested. Had been
quarreling by post – & had just rec. a most angry letter when
who should appear but the knight in question – We scarcely
spoke during the ev'g because I knew we were watched by curi-

ous eyes but after it was over I told Ernest to ask him home with us – he did – not much was said going home nor that night but I contrived to slip my answer to his letter into his hand before we dispersed for the night. Next day Sunday was so happy – made it all up again, figuratively speaking 'kissed & were friends' only figuratively we are as far as form goes just friends, but ah! the countless airy nothings in themselves are 'confirmation strong as Holy writ' ... Monday morning before dawn Ernest, Charlie, Gertie & I started for H[amilton]. Gertie to attend H[amilton] C[ollegiate] I[nstitute] & Charlie also to school & Ernest to attend Court as juryman & I for Aldershot! Ernest drove me out, reached here about 1. Went on to Mr Moores & deposited my baggage then returned to the school house No 1 E. Flamboro bade Ernest goodbye & entered the thraldom 'On Heaven & on thy love call & enter the bedeviled walls.' Mr. M. taught most of that day for which I was glad as I was horribly sleepy, returned to Mr M's per invitation till I could find a boarding house. Was miserably put up as regards bedroom, but bore it by taking plenty of sleep for the few days necessary. Tuesday night with Miss Harrison (my assistant teacher) started out in search of board, after much difficulty we found the desired article and of a very superior quality for which I am *very* glad. It takes away somewhat from the defects of other things, such as dirty youngsters & school house & a long walk, but all together makes a very good medicine for one who I am afraid was affected with lassitude and wanted some stirring up some 'Agilitine.' Walked back through rain, mud & darkness which left me a token in the form of a lame back which hurts still. Thursday night same here. Friday morning strapped up my ulster & rubbers and after school went in to Hamilton to spend Sunday with Alice – my golden haired Alice – who is much the same as of yore.

Nov 3rd Wed. Thanksgiving Day

Yes & it has been a glorious day – most beautiful in many ways, and yet too I have been disappointed, but to begin where I left off. Went with Miss Harrison up to Mr Moores to tea, after went down to Mrs Dixons & waited till train came in. Arrived in H. found my darlings Maud & Alice waiting for me, greeting me in the most approved style they triumphantly carried me off, happy, as possible, my own self – 'Beth' not the country school-ma'am. ... In the morning Alice & I went up town, did some shopping, saw some friends, & told Gertie I was coming up to tea. ... It is so very pleasant, such talks, & so very pleasant to know, for they have all vouched for it that among all women I hold first place in their hearts. It is such a good thing to have true friends, heart friends & I thank the Giver of all Good that He has so blessed me.

Went up to Gerties & spent a very pleasant ev'g to what could have been expected when I found Don Carlos [Charlie] had made a mistake & had called in the afternoon instead of ev'g. Went back to Alice next morning & for a walk with her & Maud in the afternoon, beautiful day, happy day, health strength & love, beautiful weather ... Went we three in ev'g to Central Pres. but did not see Carlos there but have since learned that he was. Monday's dawn found me up & off – for Aldershot. Took up the burden of life again & lived that day through & at last got to my boarding house so glad to rest & yet as it was the first of Nov. I started studying. Next day the 'daily round the common task' & a letter from Carlos saying if I w'd answer in time he w'd come to me today

Nov. 4th

Well yesterday was a queer, queer day. I wish I could paint it all here. All my endeavors the night before to get my answer to Carlos posted, proved abortive & so I trusted he would come anyway. Of course when they knew I expected a friend & called it 'he' all was settled at once. Well to add to the 'fiasco' what should occur but we must all be invited to a Thanksgiving din-ner & on me saying I could not go, why then the story must be told again. Well they could not be induced to go without me &

Mr Ross offered to go to the station for him. We went but no 'he.' I went with them to Mr Pearts and fared sumptuously, but made my excuses & returned soon after dinner. The whole company being seemingly interested in my return and each having their say. I came laughing away & had a beautiful walk of about a mile, sat at my window & watched & waited that beautiful afternoon but he came not, & I fancy he thinks me angry with him, but n'importe he'll have to learn better than that, he must learn to trust me implicitly, in face of all odds, & know I will not be doubted, no – never. Spent a very quiet evening – studied, ect. Today taught the usual round and found the weather had some effect on my spirits for I was not so buoyant in spirit this afternoon, tho' as soon as the scholars were dismissed, & Mr Ross had given us a very brisk ride home through the rain I felt all right again & quite myself. They are kindness itself here and set a table fit for an epicure – too good for the liver I'm afraid – & are *so* kind in every way. Not many men w'd have gone up for us through the rain & we comparative strangers ...

Nov. 7th

At last at last I can be alone at ease. He came – let the birds sing it – my own brave boy – he came despite the rain and word of weather. Hoping against hope Friday night that the morning would prove fair. I gladly laid me down to sleep on Friday night, glad that the weeks work was done & so glad to think the morrow would bring Carlos, my Carlos. The morning was not worst at once but gradually become superlatively so – but when we were at dinner there came a knock that brought the warm blood to my cheeks & it was he. He had not finished his dinner when Spencer Douglas came in & so it was rather embarrassing for a time but at length Spencer departed, but darkness had not come when Lorne Book from Grimsby put in his appearance & stayed all night. Charlie went away about seven through the mud & rain & darkness, but yet I do n't think he was sorry he had come.

'But let the stream grow wider, and Philosophy
Ay, and Religion too may strive in vain
To stem the headlong current.'

This day although Sunday, has been but one scene of exertion –
oh dear if I could only have been left at home to my own devices.
I would have enjoyed the day so much more, but it is only
another instance of being killed with kindness. They of course
enjoyed it as only Methodists can, a Quarterly Meeting. Mr Book
drove me to church in his buggy & I know I entertained him to
his satisfaction if laughing is any criterion. ... I adapted myself to
circumstances till it came to the – well the latter part of that 'love
feast' when one after the other got up to distinguish themselves –
a noticeable fact that those women who had egotism enough to
be heard all dissolved in tears. One woman would get up – say
how can I tell all – then a gasp & a general swelling up another
gasp as tho' someone had poured cold water down her back –
how can I tell all the blessings another gasp & after a few more
words she's plump down & make folks miserable by her groans,
gasps & tears then a man in all his pomposity would get up – for
instance, one who had lately come to the place (I thought of
Charlie Reay's & his 'good for trade boys, come on') & who said
he was a stranger to most there, but he hoped to spend his days
happily among them as he loved the 'house of God' – the Love
Feast – & enumerated the list in a jocose manner as tho' 'now
you see I'll join in the performance if you'll enliven trade' Oh
dear I can't begin to tell all the remarkable things that were done
& said. I do n't know that I write this in a spirit of evil but there
were some obsurdities that struck me & such comical asides &
quotations would come to me. Some did appear to be really &
truly in earnest, but some I could not vouch for. I had been
observing a woman who from appearance, would like to be
President of a Ladies Aid, or sewing Society, who would make
her light public or die in the attempt. I saw that she took the
opportunity to start several hymns, & then she at last got up to
say her little say but she belonged to the modest buttermilk kind

with the uplifting & down drawing of the eyelids kind & we did
not catch it all but it was the manner in which she tried the hysterical or affected ending, of looking bad, decidedly bad covering
her face with her hand & sinking gracefully into estatic convale-
cence, it was such a comical failure to me that she restored me to
equilibrium, from the preceeding tears. Then too a woman one of
the excruciatingly namby-pamby-meek ones, that butter would
n't melt in the mouth of. I just drew another picture of which
she was the centre-piece viz – a kitchen she making pies, her
back turned an instant a youngster of the house, passing the
table, overturns the pie on the floor. Question – would she have
that senseless exasperating facial appearance? ...

'Resolve shines ever on the front of victory'

Nov 12

What possesses me? I have just awakened seemingly. I feel all
energy all enthusiasm, all purpose today. Was it Dr. Trouts letter
received last night that inspired me or was it that in part, &
Mathews 'Getting on in the World' in part. Howe'er it be, so it is.
I feel as one who has taken a new lease of life. I have a good
scabbard to the sword of my intellect if I may use so egotistical
an expression – Yes I thank Heaven for a good animal life – a
good healthy case for all they be of brain & energy. 'A good
stomach & mediocre intellect' Mathews tells us may accomplish
great things then why may not I with continued health, perseverance, patience & a right method of concentration accomplish
my hopes, my ambition. ...
    We *are* queer machines with queer engineering powers in our
bodies, we are each a sufficient study for ourselves & yet I suppose if we study others too we are better able to judge ourselves,
& certainly I have found a clearer insight to others by a previous
study of self. Now for the last few days. I have been in an undesirable state of mind, disgusted with myself that in order to hide

my overweening tendency toward Carlos I belittled myself
enough to flirt with others and in trying to make them believe
that one nice young man was as much to me as another, & also
I'm afraid, in thinking of my letter from home. I began to doubt
myself, whether I did really care as much for a certain individual
as I formerly thought, so weak am I, so unsatisfactory even to
self. Now I feel as though that was entirely secondary, my one
particular object being to concentrate all my forces, mind & body
on my one aim, a successful career in my chosen profession –
ended – crowned by a happy domestic life far in the future. There
it is, I am so vain, it is foolish pride that is gnawing at my love
for my hero – because all expected me to make some great match
as regards a worldly view, because he has his name to make & is
neither landed proprietor, nor blooded spendthrift, but is only
his noble self with all the future before him – the golden future –
& his fair fame, his purpose, manliness, his souls strength his
all – they do not say much but yet if he had been half so good &
wealthy they had congratulated me & I am so weak as to miss
laudation even here. Girls with only two ideas, but well dressed
& possessed of a quiet imbecility or mock innocent air – whose
idea of an excellent book is that it will make you cry – meet an
uneducated but landed man and the thing is done. 'She did well',
'she has made a good match' While they would say of me if they
knew of any entanglements 'what good did her education do her
or her travels she might as well have stayed at home & married
better' but then that I hope is not all I was born for – viz to be
married – even then if I am happy, why should the 'on dits' of
society disturb me or even the speaking silence of friends. Then,
after all I do not intend to be a poor man's wife. I know myself
well enough for that – that I would not be angelic enough to
always 'smile & smile and be a darling' on four hundred a
year – oh no but then you see no one intends for me to do so. He
is to be a successful lawyer some of these days & what if it will
not be for years – why I will not have proved my profession ere
that & so God overrules all for good & even when in the darkness I cannot see the wherefore or the way – I will trust him &
follow on.

Nov 13th

No letter from Carlos this week the first time he has missed for
more than six months. Rec. a paper from him today & a letter
from Miss Beatty the dear girl – but if she does not flatter me she
must have a good opinion of me. I have no doubt tonight about
my feelings toward Carlos. I have recovered from my indifferent
state & wish he had written, or rather that I had received it for I
cannot think but that he has written. ...

Nov 22nd

A whole week gone to return no more forever. 'Whether we eat
or drink or what so ever we do to do all to the glory of God' so
our bibles teach and to put Christian zeal in all our deeds, to let a
golden thread of righteousness of life, be woven in the daily pattern of life. Ay so may it be, to know that in all things we should
use the 'gifts of this world' & not abuse them. 'Rejoice in thy
youth; & let thy heart cheer thee in the days of thy youth & walk
in the ways of thine heart, & in sight of thine eyes: but know
thou that for all these things God will bring thee into judgment'
So ran the text of Mr Francis' sermon yesterday & it was a good
one. We are to enjoy life but to use it for the master, to be thankful for all & to be sure that where much is given much is req. &
to know that the whole duty of man is 'to fear God & keep his
commandments' The whole duty ay and a greaty duty – to fear
Him to make Him ever a pervading presence, to feel that the All
seeing eye & the *all* hearing ear is on us – near us and to keep his
laws even in *all* things Such sermons I love – I need – God knows
how much I want to do that which is right and yet how often
there seems to come a deadness of real feeling in regard to religious things that makes me feel so unsettled so uneasy & yet like
a disease upon me. Then when I *happen*, it seems to me sometimes as tho' that was the word – to *feel* again really & truly the
responsibilities & possibilities of life I am more purely happy &
feel more energy to push forward in the race. How helpless we

would sometimes feel – nay *always* feel if we had no rudder, no strong tower of defence wherein to trust.

Last week glided like others slowly sedately into the 'has been' but all the week was cheered by thinking of Saturday. Oft I thought 'be the day weary or be the day long at length it ringeth to evensong' & thought Sat. would be a blithe evensong to the week. Sure enough I had not completed my toilet when about noonday he came my own brave boy & stayed till evening. Such a happy quiet afternoon as we spent

'For watchfulness in love is good
  But trust is better still'

Nov. 29th

Here I chronicle that another week of my life is gone and I am a week nearer the 'bounds of life where we lay our burdens down' 'nearer leaving the cross nearer gaining the crown' How each day may be big with events that we dream not of, how each day holds new ideas, new fields of labor, new opportunities, new incidents, that are all unknown before ...

Dec. 3rd

... Time flies apace and study seems out of the question. I am very tired tonight. It is a struggle to keep up till four Oclock sometimes. Oh such a constant struggle with those dreadful rampant obstriperous boys. I was really quite ill this afternoon & would have preferred quiet or going to bed, but had to sing talk play recite to please the others & so the ev'g has gone ...

Dec. 6th

Monday ev'g, Another hard days work done, sore throat added to other ills, making it laborious. Had a ride to school with Mr

Gibbs & back with Mr Read. Sat. Carlos spent the afternoon with me, the dear boy, I have reasoned, fought ideas, conquered & been conquered, renew the battle & again give up to irresistible Kismet which undefinable as it is makes me love him, perhaps too well. Not even here could I put in words, could I unveil the tenderness between us, as Mrs Mac quoted of married life 'Who so lifteth the veil of married life to others gaze defileth the sanctuary' So I could not speak of feelings existing not even here, not even here.

Yesterday went to S. School in the morning & was requested to take the Questioners place next Sunday wk. the future will tell how ect. Ella Easterbrook & Mr Emory here to dinner & then to church in the afternoon & back, after dark, When I did steal a few delicious minutes by myself to rest & to think. In the ev'g Mr Summerfield Douglas was in & then retired.

Jan 21st [1881]

'So time in its relentless way goes on
and brings us nearer the end, the end.'

I cannot in a retrospective glance pen here all the occurrences since last I wrote but will but quote those that I can.

That following Friday Mr Spence came for me & took me up to Nelson, where I spent the hours very pleasantly till Monday morning when they brought me back. There I became acquainted with Miss Appleget & she spoke of giving me her school for 3 mo's sometimes. A queer overgrown person, a specimen of what overfeeding & under exertion can do for any one.

The next week was the usual round of visitors, school work ect & Friday night came at last. Geo. Townsend drove me in to Hamilton. ... He took me to Jennie Wood's where I found Myra Van Slyke & she ready to demolish me with pleasure had another tea, dressed & then sat embraced by those girls waiting not like McCawber[1] for 'something to turn up' but for Charlie.

1 Mr Wilkins Micawber, good-hearted ne'er-do-well in Charles Dickens'
   David Copperfield

We waited till the last moment & he came, had been at the station to meet me. Was I not glad, happy to be once more arm in arm free to talk with Carlos. Oh was I not! T'was but little time we had to talk for soon after we got there the programme began. I came on later & received a hearty welcome to the platform & a lusty encore. I was gratified & yet I know I have given it better.

We had a short quiet walk back & as Sutherland & Jennie were at the gate we bade good night & it seemed so unsatisfactory after all the anticipations I had builded.

Next day was a busy one as not going to sleep till late after midnight we did not rise early. We had a real good talk, a very good one. After a busy days shopping I left on the ev'g train. Carlos was down to see me off & the parting there was more satisfactory. ... I had my lesson for next day to get up. I dreaded it too but had to face it, just of me, so unexperienced in such things to dare to do it before those old accustomed teachers. T'was the lives of Jacob & Joseph. I lived thro' it but was quite modest over my success & the superintendent was all the more warm in his praise because he saw that I was not proud of it. ... Carlos skated over on Monday & chatted with me till about dusk walked home with me & then skated back. Again on Wed. he skated over & Mr C. Smith too had a jolly talk & he took his final departure from Aldershott.

Thurs. twas over, that scene closed, the curtain was down. I was free to go. I was happy & yet not happy. One can endear themselves too a few grains of gold in tons of dross it seems. Ernest came up just as I was dismissing [the class] & drove us to Mr Rosses & then we went on up to Helen's wedding. Arrived there to find them waiting for us. I hurried & soon the knot was tied. There were present about 40 guests very nice, a well assorted assembly, a cultivated one the dejeuner was elegant, the presents costly & numerous. We gave a silver dinner gong. The bride looked lovely in white tarlatan & satin, as did the brides maids in pink & blue. ... Came away that night back to Mr Rosses & next morning turned our faces homeward. ... So all was merry-making till Xmas was a thing of the past. Monday ev'g we were disappointed because of the storm & cold our expected guests did not put in an appearance, however Wed. night Carlos (the chief of them to me) came & I was happy till he went away on Thurs. & I have lived without him since, without his personal presence but still he pervades my every hour with being present in my thoughts. Friday ev'g was one entertainment at Stoney Creek, a success, the best we have had there, a very pleasant time, Mary & Clara & Mr Irving went with us home for the night & part of the next day. Sat. Myrtie left us to commence her duties as teacher at the Beach & I have not seen her since tho' she has been home. ... Thurs. Gertie & Ma came to town & began prep. for our transit. For two days I had the work on my shoulders & the packing too, & getting Cecil & Vi off to Agatha's party. I was glad when Sat came & Pa Cecil & I came to the city. Such a day, work of settling & not finishing then, but getting so we could live. Agnes came too, as did others & Sunday quiet & rest was soon over & I entered on my duties at Victoria School as teach of ... 1st Grade – a beautiful class of 27 urchins ranging betw. the interesting ages of five & eight. So life here began, a long walk, housework & study & I am busy busy busy Truly mine is a chequered life, a quiet country home, reared in a homekeeping circle, taught in the common public school in summer, by governess in winter, all unsuggestive of the tumultuous afterlife. No shadows of coming events except in a lively imagination (which was fed by much reading of romance) which pictured many a glowing scene, in which I was the principal actor. I the heroine always. Then a change came o'er my life I was introduced to society & school life in the city at about the same time.

A full dress party at home, my coming out party, in which I launched on a sea of party going for a short time then to Hamilton boarding among strangers & attending the Coll. Inst. I was as miserably homesick & forlorn as any country girl transported into a new sphere, among a new type of girls could well be. Strange it must have been, one among others of her age & sex yet, so far asunder tho' I felt second to none in capabilities and in general knowledge thro' & of books yet I did feel, & keenly the difference in the outward person. They all grace & taste, with nonchalance making themselves, felt & seen. I with some taste yet meagre means & timid gait & air living among them & gradually making many friends & good progress.

Looking back now I can smile at the sagacity & persistency of a child in its first energy of what was self termed 'love'.

With all the its characteristic, fervor, I had made the object of getting acquainted with his sister as equal to the acquisition of knowledge. Ever uppermost was that idea, to plan our friendliness to *make* her my friend. I was not long in succeeding & little did she dream of the cause then while I as little thought of the end. He [Dick?] is nothing to me now & she [Alice or Maud?] is. To make our idols & to find them clay & then bewail their worship – is a sad, sad truth Time passed on, many pleasures, many pains were known to me then & yet none of so great a magnitude as to be discernible at this distance. The end of my allotted schooldays came & then I was to choose for myself whether I should enter an active continued field of work by choosing the medical profession or would I return to my quiet country home, to live a quiet commonplace, to rust mentally & wear out 'physically' in the drudgery of *all* work on a farm.

I chose the first & as a preliminary step returned to Hamilton to school. Studying yet living more happily than formerly I remained till the following summer. When on a visit to Louth, I passed the 3rd class cert. at Milton & consequently went back there in the Autumn to the Model School. Here I formed a new set of acquaintances & had a fully occupied jolly time the 3 last of the eight weeks out every night, tableau, Oratorie, Parties, rehearsals, school, picnics. This ended. I came home for two months at Mountain Hall With the new year, new scenes, were opened to me. A new & untried unread page to me was before me. With all the energy hope & fear that a diver takes in his first plunge, so may, so did I take with me in this first step of independence. I left home for an entirely strange place [Speyside], to go among total strangers & teach a country school. Who shall tell of the desolateness of the time. Who shall tell of the bitter tears of loneliness which soiled my sense of duty. Who of the gladness when day was done that told of a tomorrow soon to be gone.

This at first but after the worst had worn off, by the time I returned after the holidays it was more pleasant than otherwise. The foolish love I had so desperately clung to had vanished & I was happy. Dear kind Mrs Moore where I boarded made life

pleasant. Jim Dunn, Mr Campbell ect. appeared to brighten the
Autumn sky & I was happy hearted in the loves, esteems, &
kindnesses of the people I sojourned with & truly I thought kind
hearts were more than coronets. I left them with many good
wishes & good friends to go back to the H.C.I. This was a happy
happy time to me. One of the most active & prominent member
of the L[iterary] S[ociety] on every committee, head of the boat
club, manager in picnic's, officer, editor, student, a happy time &
in this six months passing the A[rts] A[dmission] exam of the
McGill Coll. the Matriculation in Med. at Toronto & the Intermediate [Teaching Certificate]. Then home for the holidays & then
teaching again at Nelson for four months. Here again an entirely
new sphere, a new circle of friends and an active busy life. I
enjoyed some of this very much, especially the long rides over
the country roads, at eve, with all the mellow glory of an
Autumn sunset, over the landscape. Home again for a short holiday & then to a new & important part of my life for so it is like
to prove. So it has proved.

I went to the Normal in Ottawa. Went to Toronto for Sunday,
& Monday ev'g started en route for the Capital, Charlie &
Shields going with me. We had a happy time down Such a
strange three mo's but I have chronicled it elsewhere & so need
not detail it here. The latter part of the session was full of pleasure to me & when I came home for two weeks & only saw him
once in ten days & knew not whether that I endured I could not I
would not, but oh it was awful to live so & be mute to all. Soon
tho' I knew that he was not satisfied to be a stranger. I was with
Maud for a few days & he came & since then we have corre-
sponded.

I went down then to Royal College Kingston to enter on the
real business of my life, the study of medicine. Went to Kingston
with all the honor of leader & foundation of the enterprise, to
find a path of roses, a new circle of friends & lovers. Here lies I
suppose the path which with energy courage enthusiasm perseverance all the catalogue of virtues requisite to a successful career
I hope to work out a useful destiny. After the session there with
a short happy busy holiday intervening returned, to home &

Hamilton for holidays. Then again teaching, for two long dreary mo's at Aldershott. The teaching was more than laborious, irksome very, yet out of that sphere I had pleasant hours. Mine host & wife were all the fancy could paint. I hope I shall have more like them. I hope I shall never forget them nor their unnumbered kindnesses.

Home for a Merry Christmas time, after going to Helen Wilsons wedding & a short visit in Hamilton. Reading at the H.C.I. entertainment. In the holidays Carlos was down. Aunt Hester, Colborn & Sara, Jim & Mary Wilson, a busy merry time & soon over. Myrtie away to teach & one transit here where now I find myself more busy than ever, teaching in the Victoria school, doing the housework, studying, all my time fully employed, fully, fully. Last Sat. Miss Harrison called, gave me the news from Aldershott ect. Mary Smith was here to tea. Yesterday Mr & Mrs Ross called & Monday Mr. & Mrs Carmichael, & here it is Fri night. ... Cora Coventry called one ev'g & we had a lovely talk we are passing through the same deep waters & have similar feelings & thoughts. ... Friday all day was dreamy for I was wondering would he come & how could I meet him. Maud & I walked up to H.C.I. but did not go in. Came home & waited.

[February]

And looking back upon thy life
Thy one regret shall be
That thou hast done no more for Him
That did so much for thee

During the last few weeks there has been much going on. Many chats with many friends. Two sleighing parties with much merriment. Parlor Socials at all of which I read, etc. & enjoyed much praise. Met some new friends. ... Have a Plum colored silk making at the dressmakers for Mauds wedding wh. is to come off Wed morning, of wh more anon. They are going to move away to St. Boniface soon. ...

[March]

... Maud married – J.B. Rankin 2nd March 1881 at their house no.
2 Duke St. quiet affair. Maud sick & altogether unlike a happy
bride.

March 14th

Such a grandly truthful sermon tonight by Mr McDonnel of
Toronto. I wish so much that Charlie could have heard it.
  Last week was as ever a busy week, & I so tired, so tired, & I
had a happy surprise too in a letter from Charlie which came
before I expected it, dear Charlie. Is it wrong to love him as I do.
May Heaven be kind to him May Heaven guide me always! ...

'And the sun comes up & the sun goes down
And what is all where all is done!'

March 28th

Ay so it is, we weary ourselves with tasks often self imposed, we
climb from the cradle to the grave, it is ever ever striving & what
is all when all is done – ay – what. 'A noble deed is a step toward
God.'
  I am working harder than my strength great as it is allows, & I
feel so tired, as though, a little more & I would 'go to pieces' all
at once, just as bubbles do when they burst. Home last
Saturday – & since then no lull – no rest & I foresee but little
while here. Oh for Friday night – Friday at the gloaming – will
he come – I doubt it. Girlish dislikes are just as predominant as
they were. Pride is a budget of some size. It really goes hard with
me. ...

8

Kingston and Winona, Ontario
April 1881 to March 1882

Soon after their arrival at Queen's in the spring of 1881 Elizabeth
and the other women discover that the female program has been
cancelled and they are to join male students the next fall. A few
brief entries from Winona follow and the diaries resume with
the coeducational classes. Elizabeth's initial optimism about her
fellow students and the medical faculty are in stark contrast to
the anger which later colours her memory of medical education
taken with men. This is the best year she will have at Queen's.
As the excerpts from her letters to Charlie indicate, the seeds of
disillusionment here are also sown with the revelation of his
religious doubts.

'Oh for a heart that will not shrink'

April 7th

Here I am in Kingston been here since Monday & am now fairly
settled & well with Mesheck & Abednego [Alice McGillivray and
Elizabeth Beatty] at Mrs Shibleys at the College Gate. Well my
entertainment was the best ever held by the L[iterary] S[ociety]
& I am glad such a crowd, & everything well – Costumes players,
music funds, & one all Charlie came down & I was happy, oh so
happy that Friday night, but what misery next day to say good-

bye & only to shake hands because others were by, oh forlorn, forlorn. Monday morning bade goodbye to Hamilton & the many friends. I left there & went to Toronto. Called on Dr.'s Trout & Left ...

April 24th

So it has all come about, what I long ago foresaw. A winter session. After asking & receiving promise of all necessary privileges for the winter we gained our wish. The Prof's all but one wished for a winter session & we coaxed him over all that annoys me is that they did not do so six months ago – it would have saved my trip down there & given me the chance of getting through a whole year sooner but we have to be satisfied with what we have, & all are in a measure.

Had three pleasant weeks. I do really enjoy Abednego's society & when we three Hebrew children are together we just do have a good time.

Got through some work too, practical anatomy, like our new demonstrator very much indeed, quite enough.

July 14th 81 [Winona]

Although the other members of the household have sought solace for the labors of the day in the embrace of the drowsy god, yet I cannot contentedly follow suit until chronicle this day 'To make hay while the sun shines' is a proverb very much in vogue just now & comes readily to my mind after this memorable day. Why memorable you question? Thurs or so, Ernie wrenched his back & could not drive the hay rake, So I was pressed into the service a making hay. Hear Miss Beatty on the subject 'didn't I always tell you you were a flirt' What do I catch you at now? Making hay? Maud Muller! Ever since I received your letter I've been sighing for the poor swains whose hearts you will drag that merciless hay rake over. Of course you will be in duty bound to prove you can be very womanly, even on a hay rake & as you

will wear the prettiest broadbrim in the country & then your
'kerchief' round your neck in the most becoming style a bunch of
daisies & buttercups fastened in your dress will look so pretty &c
&c (tears) Could anything be more disappointing. After having a
programme in detail to feel such a humiliating contract Report
said it was the easiest thing in the world to, well to to 'upset' the
hay, & I was not expecting to use any gt. strength. Alas! My
fallen hopes! Considering that Old Mr Ready, Vick & Ernest all
stoical to the last degree as far as Maud Mullers are concerned,
were the only spectators I had a monopoly of the picturesque
side of it, which, the irony of which made me smile at least. My
distracted gaze wandered from horse to hay, ... for it was time to
pull the affair to upset, & it was a pull, had to take both hands
& rise on my feet. Perhaps you wonder what the horse was doing all this time. Ask of the winds, as for me, he was trying a
Mazurka, at any rate he seemed to have a great tendency to turn
round. By the time he was straight again, again the rack was full,
shall I ever forget, you see the hay was so very heavy, blisters are
nothing ...

Aug. 24th

Cannot write all, to summarize – Jennie Wood was down for a
few days. Mary Todd for more than a week. Ella Lutz for a while,
Myrtie & Gertie at St. Kitts for some days. We had a Garden
Party successful in every way. Enjoyed it because it was exciting
at the time, because I had to play such a heavy role. Charlie was
here & I wanted to play 'indifference' Jim Wilson was here & I
had a difficult part.
    After it was over, & the next days business over I collapsed
into hysteria. Just think – having 'historicks.'
    Charlie was here twice during the holidays & we had such a
happy happy times, oh those golden days! I should be happy
gratefull good with so many blessings. Last night such loving
hearty letters from Charlie Maud & Abednego & today all the
ripe peaches I could eat (!!!)

College, October 28th [Kingston]

I just feel as tho I were really living these days, what with so much interesting study, so much knowledge presented to us, such labyrinths of thought, excited so much to do so little done & such splendid company, really life is active, life is real. Much we have to do & yet we have such rollicking times, of few minutes duration either between lectures or at table. Do not think but that I tire sometimes, when the Prof get enthused with his subject & rattles off at a line a sec, & ones hand is unable to sweep downwards in time. Just to write steadily as fast as the muscles will for an hour, it makes my hand ache to think of it. But that is nothing to the pleasure of it all. The dear old Profs how kind they all are (This line proved to be facetious, as a med would say a little previous) & the meds are wonderfully serene to us. We hear there sonorous voices in the Den. sometimes making day hideous with clamor & their elephantine tread in the mazes of the dance as they whirl their partner with a handkerchief, to the music of a violin. One student a U.S. Dr by name Hicky, our bete noir, the butt of all ridicule & almost the fag of the Coll. is a noticable feature among disagreeables. His first attentions, his self introduction we passed over, as his gray hairs & portly style might be indicate of some worth or respect due but we soon came to regard him as a Falstaff & today & we gave him the coldest of shoulders & the other day, after Physiology (The Prof had the skeleton of a horses head for illustration) some students were standing round the desk looking at specimens & we had kept our seats in the front row, when lo! Dr Hicky wheels round c the horses head in hand & opened its jaws at Miss Beattys & oh! were we not indignant & I did not raise my eyes from the speciman I had in hand tho' report comes round tonight 'Miss Smiths face turned just as red as anything.'

Our first Prof. in the day, is Dr. Depuis a real jolly good friend of ours. I guess I may say mine in particular, the others say so, make it a chief pleasure of his life to show how much he considers us. He told Mrs Mac when she corrected him for calling her Miss Smith that he wanted to distinguish Miss Smith (it was a hard question) The janitor is 'Tom' Coffee Tom Coffee, Mr Coffee seldom, Tom generally Coffee occasionally, is another champion of ours. He comes to our waiting room to inform us he is going to ring by saying 'Yesse can be goin in now leddies!' & we go in grave, sedate, various, Mrs Corlis, a small featured little matron of mature years, the mother in years of the flock, Miss Beatty largest in size, determination in every feature, good nature sparkling in her eyes casts a protecting shade on us in her stately size something like the fighting editor. Mrs Mac the wonder, short haired, fearlessness in her wide open eyes, with a reputation for dislike of housekeeping, & a great ability for study &c Miss Reynolds an interesting girl, the youngest of the flock, a reserved damsel, wrapped in impenetrable reserve & self confidence, with a character capable of being changed greatly in time. Miss Dixon or I beg her pardon Dickson, the good girl of the family of meds 'most too pure & good for human nature's daily food' her week is all Sunday somewhat prim, verging on that ridiculous time, an uncertain age, the self sacrificing, quiet almost sorrowful looking one of the company, & then your truly, who I am afraid will be spoiled by comparative flattery, as they designate me the 'pretty one' ... Next lecture is Prof Fowlers of Queens on Botany, there Arts & Meds are together (we always get dreadful cheers if we go in after the boys & make it a point to be early) The Arts answer Ad Sum & the meds 'Present' to the roll call. This Prof. is so good natured & the boys bother him so sometimes it is really laughable, if he mentions fruit as peaches, they smack their lips if he uses an extra number of long words, there'll be a groan or a very surprised long drawn oh oh that makes us laugh in spite of good resolutions. One day the shower of long words was too much, one boy took refuge in flight through the window. The lectures are very interesting & the specimens fine. Last week we lived on protoplasm, molecular protoplasm, 'we dined off' we supped off protoplasm we slept with it in our minds, it was almost a waste of Protoplasm & I agreed only in part with the Boston girl who said 'molecules were just too awfully sweet to live' & she doated on Protoplasm, 'That depends if its cooked' well I don't mind doating on some kinds of it, depends greatly on the kind, nuf sed.

Next hour comes Prof Depuis, on Chem. (Brother of Dr. D.) &
this also we take with the Arts. He is just my beau ideal of a Prof,
cold, clear, small, wirey, automatic, I can imagine Huxley like
him, by the way last Sunday evg we read aloud from Huxleys
Basis of Life[1] & there from rose a lengthened earnest discussion
with Miss B[eatty] & I on one side & Mrs Mac on the other. Mrs
Mac is not much of a believer & we do not agree on politics or
religion at all, & so it is in some sort tabooed Next from 12 – 1
Oclock, jurisprudence wh. we take in separate rooms & really the
meds are worse behaved there than any other time, tho' Dr Irwin
is gentlemanly to us. From 2 – 3 we have Dr. Fenwick on Physiology, a very nice young looking handsome gentleman (this was
decidedly previous)

[excerpt from letter to Charlie]

Don't I beseech you, because men deem it their perogative to
float round in a sea of loose ideas take that perogative to your
bosom, else I warn you it will prove worse than the most veno-
mous of serpents. Even should all come to the worst should reason, argument, feeling & all good prove abortive, should all the
countless millions that have lived & died happy in the faith
prove to have been misled, deceived, & the small handful that
have created this furor in mens minds prove only wise, then
should we have believed, trusted loved & feared the Great Father.
If you believe in His only Son & his death for us, believed His
teaching & lived accordingly then even tho atomicity be our ori-
gin & our end we have lost nothing, but if we believe otherwise
when we think of the fruits of a rebellious unbelieving life, think
that all eternity awaits us & so soon, think that no ill that could
befall could be more than punishment for such presumption, oh,
it's awful, terrible to think of. I hope just as truly & as confi-
dently that as you expressed it 'you will get over it' as I do that I
shall see you again. ... [end of excerpt]

1 Thomas Huxley, *The Physical Basis of Life* (1868). Huxley was the leading
  scientist of his generation and an outspoken defender of Charles Darwin.

[excerpt from letter to Charlie]

You say you believe in an All powerful Father, after that all things should be easy for you. The Hereafter you believe in, a Heaven of joy & that eternal, but you say you do not believe in eternal punishment, that no man could deserve that, my dear friend *who* of the human race could deserve eternal happiness? That however to me is of but secondary importance as I can trust Heaven for that if I do *my* duty while I may. That we die, we know, but after the dissolution of the body no one knows, no one can know. And if we believe in God & that He is God of Gods King of kings, we can trust that to Him.

I was most sorry to hear you say that you did not believe but what there was enough will to conquer the evil in us, implanted in our own minds. I cannot agree with you. I am very sure God's help has ever helped those who asked for it. If you believe in an omnipresent omnipotent Father, how can you doubt His hearing us when we speak to Him? Just as children aske their mother for what they want, & she gives according as she sees best for her children, so the Good Father in Heaven hears & grants our petitions. It is hard to open the inner doors of ones heart, it seems almost a sacrilege & only in such a cause could I do so, but I avow to you that not once but many times time after time, I have had prayers granted. What do you think sustains & strengthens poor weak humanity in the hour of trouble? Is not that peace & resignation born of Divine comfort a thousand fold better than that fierce doggedness which shrinks back into itself & defies all things. Oh I tell you, thousands on thousands have borne trouble sickness adversity death, with meek & noble resignation because they clung to Him who alone was capable of helping them when all help on earth failed utterly, when friends & fortune left desolate, when the very foundations of things seemed tottering beneath their feet. God's hand upheld. His hand led them safe through all in peace to lifes end.

Don't dare to think that what I say is all & only a pretty fancy, a fiction fit for women & boys, don't dare it would be purest sacrilege.

I tell you, for all some men think in their high & mighty
wisdom that their broad views & comprehensive brains are so
capable of grasping great ideas & that women can see but in the
light. I tell you they can see clearly through some shadows &
that their clear sightedness & keeness of instinct are more trust-
worthy. I do not say it egotistically, but with all the knowledge of
a full heart, that tells me it is truth.

I sympathise with you because I can readily understand why
you doubt, & there is no subject so near my heart as the eternal
welfare of those I care for. I am very heartily glad that you
believe in the great fundamental truths of orthodox religion & I
hope & pray you may hold fast to them with all your strength
always, not only at this present time when gazing out in that
chaos of doubt, you feel dazed, distracted as what to credit what
you are sure of. I don't think it is any evidence of more than
common talent or clearsightedness to doubt, & yet to believe
nothing & I do not feel at all belittled that I have strength
enough based on what little I have learned, to hold fast, the
simple faith, that has made countless men & women noble
almost divine. I feel as though untaught & feeble & yet *sure* on
that solid rock, I held you & others back, tried to hold you back,
from deep dark waters, waters worse than Lethe. That I held you
not by force, nor argument, nor regard, but by drawing your
attention to that religion akin to the souls implanted in you. That
I held you back from the impossible depths of that dark sea of
doubt & tho' now wading in, you would yet return again to the
better plane, to peace & trust. [end of excerpt]

[excerpt from letter to Jennie Wood]

Kingston/ 81   My Dear Jennie. You can just scatter all those
congratulatory thoughts which arose when you received this, because of such a speedy answer to your tardy letter. I was just certain I would pay you up for it by not writing for a while but now
when I want to tell you something new, I just write at once. Now
you know the usual performance necessary to prepare for a great

shock, so proceed to prepare. If you are anywhere but in your
room you had better put this in your pocket till you get there. By
the way I'm glad I'm not nervous else I had thought you were ill
& could not write, when it was so long coming. Oh yes where
were we? Just at the prepare, well *have* you braced your nerves
in readiness? Miss Beatty has gone to Toronto to try the matric
exam. I *hope* you haven't given way to a sense of relief because I
have not told the news yet, & you know fatal consequences
might result if you allowed too sudden a relaxation of nervous
fibre when the tension has been severe. What a lovely day! I
hope you are not cross with those 'cherubs' ... now because you
have headaches, Don't you think, well do, that both you & Maud
deserve reprimanding for trying to be ill. Maud could nt think of
anything else but Chill fever & is kept continually trembling
with it & you, well I hope you have parted company with that
distasteful ill bred headache. Oh yes I'm coming back to the
'news' presently. Do you not appreciate the consideration I have
for your nervous system. By the by *have* you a nervous system I
really dread the effect if you have & if I were by to see such a
dread result as the demolition of said system I should be haunted
by a life long remorse. A remorse that would bring my hairs
(what few are left) with sorrow to my last impression.

Mr Mac is going away this afternoon & so Meshack will be a
lone lorn 'widder' all but me. We pride ourselves on our correct
phraseology. A lovely day, the sky is blue the buds are swelling
& Mrs Shibley is winding the clock. Oh I say, if you write & tell
me whether you think you can bear it or not, then I will know
whether to write it or not & you might mention too, whether
you are just the least little bit provoked or not, just so I would be
sure of the regularity of your pulsations my dear. Had three
hours work over at the Coll this morning & this is my rest before
going to work again.

Prof Fowler, pericarp, is so good natured that the boys bother
him to great length, & one cannot but laugh sometimes ...

Then the other Fowler, Registrar, sober stolid Scotsman the
most influential man of the Coll. weighty & very Scotch our
champion too, but one of the kind that has to be managed, & led

round unconsciously. Could nt be driven, no way. Next lecture we take separately Obstetrics & the Prof in that is my especial friend Dr Lavall, a Christian gentleman. Next Senr Chem over at Queens, I must go get get some sleep, so bye. ... [end of excerpt]

[excerpt from letter to Charlie]

There is not one among those I call my friends & know them such, but I could trust implicity in their honor, virtue & sterling uprightness. Knowing many such, many such true men & women, is it but charitable to think that a large percentage of those who are nominally only my friends would prove to be of good metal if I knew them.

Cynicism is a bitter fruit. I have seen its sad results to fully too nearly not to know. It not only embitters & dwarfs the current of ones own thoughts but sheds its drear shade on those around. Rather to be true to your better self believe your fellows capable of better things, believe them *men* & *women*. There seems such nobility in the mere names rightly applied, that I could use no stronger term. Believe them, many of them not only *passively* good but alive & the fact that life is a serious business & that each has a wide spread influence & that they have *no right* to neglect the God given opportunity to lift up their voices like trumpets in the cause of right. You smile at what you call my enthusiasm. Enthusiasm. I am glad it is & I pray Heaven it may never grow less. Enthusiasm & Energy are two wheels that are good to bring us on our way to success. George Eliot says 'I love the souls that rush along to their goal, with a full stream of senti-ment that have too much of the positive to be harassed by the perpetual negatives, wh. after all are but the *disease* of the soul, to be expelled by fortifying the principles of vitality' I hope my enthusiasm may not decrease. Even if the species, being blind to their better natures should pervert them into gross principle & become false & weak, then all the more need of those who have enthusiasm, all the more need of exertion on my part, that I should not sit passively down & 'thank the Lord that I am not as others are' You may think I overrate my influence & capabilities but I do not think so, nor do I think mine greater than others. Formerly, some years back, I had all the modest mistrust of my power or influence, that the most humble could have but as day after day showed me some unexpected influence I had had in this affair & that or this character or that denouement. I began grad. to awaken to the fact that there were glorious possibilities for good within *my* girls grasp & when last night an English lady of whom I had often heard but met for the first time spoke in such a solemn way of the vast responsibilities & noble work possible for me & said she was glad to know such a woman & that she had a great veneration for me for undertaking it could I but feel that girls as I am I have some power for good. And as day by day the circle widens, that is watching for my ultimate triumph or defeat, do you wonder it heightens my enthusiasm. I think it would move the most phlegmatic to some life, some person. [end of excerpt]

[excerpt from letter to Charlie]

Just let me tell you yesterdays programme. Study from 8–9 just all it was possible, lectures from 9–12 then study from 1–2 then lectures till *six* oclock. Practical Anatomy from 7–9 study 9–11 & get to sleep at 12. Is not that terrible, really had not time to go to the P.O. We have a great deal of anxiety to arrange our studies for Council & College & there is such diversity of opinion among them all, Profs & student, that we can not depend on any of them but have to rely on ourselves.

If I saw you I could chat by the hour of our little College experiences & our own jolly moments between lectures when we seem for the moment to throw off care, but I get tired sometimes & we liken ourselves to the Pitcher Plant wh keeps receiving materials for food but can only retain a certain amt. ...

Meant to have gone to the office tonight after lectures but was so tired that they made me lie down & Mrs Mac read us a story, then I could not bring myself to study so, hurrah girls! let's have some hickory nuts & down we went to the kitchen & meeting Mr Gibson on the stairs we pressed him into the service by making

him hunt the hammar. Soon they were all down the four gentlemen, & Mrs Shibly & we four & we all & ate ate, hickory nuts,
apples, candy & had a jolly time for a couple hours & now I
must study till midnight. Really, I wish you were enjoying yourself in such a hearty manner as I am. I am more jolly, merrier
wilder than you could imagine. The girls wonder what possesses me & I do myself & I wonder more how I endure so
much study & with so little sleep as I do & can run up those
long steps at college ten or twelve times as I have today. I think
the abundance of animal spirits, the fun, the hearty laughs we
have, are the preventitives of all sickness & all that sort of
thing. I hope I shall find my voyage on professional seas, as
pleasant & prosperous.

I am so glad for Sunday & I make good use of them, sleep,
sleep, sleep & would you believe it I only go to church once as a
rule & that to convocation hall, where we have able Divines of
diff. denoms. I am getting vain, oh very vain these days, when so
much flattery & so many kindnessess are current especially
among the gentlemen. Still I have not forgotten how to blush, all
over my face, heard downtown, or at Mrs Leslies where I met an
Arts Student that I blushed that day wh the Botany class saluted
us with much clapping on our entrance, dreadful! Its cold today
& more over the coal stove is out & we are loaded with shawls.
Mrs S. says she is going to start the coal stove early in the morning, & we vow we won't get up till she does. Breakfast well we'll
have a number of spasms tomorrow morning. Am I not a self
denying being when I resisted the temptation of the requests of
three, several gentlemen to go to Madame St. Remyo last Tues
Evg but I dutifully stayed at home & pored over the books. [end
of excerpt]

Feb '82 [excerpt from letter to Charlie]

Am desperately awfully wicked. Just think I accepted Mr Halls
gallant offer to escort me to church tonight & whats more, did
it of malice aforethought, because I wanted to disappoint

Williams who did call after I left & presuming I had gone
to my own church as usual followed to St James but she was n't
there
  I hope you are feeling better than you did & feel 'youth's
bright wine' welling up in your veins as the poets say but I know
better it only creeps along & is venous old at that, but there are
two grinds tomorrow & six lectures besides & I have not 'read
up' yet so goodnight. Have been dissipating, Mr Shibley & Gibson hired a lovely double carriage & teams & took Mrs S. & I to a
Select Assembly at Centreville. Left here about 2 Oclock Tues. It
was very select & nice & I did enjoy myself, of course this was
against the rules of the nunnery, but I did not see anything im-
proper about it. Had the most lovely drive coming home, saw the
dawn break & the sun mounting in the Eastern sky, so beautiful
& calm.
  But after tea that same day, I collapsed into lunacy & scared
the girls out of their wits did not study till I went off to sleep, but
have taken the lectures today. ... [end of excerpt]

Feb 26

Have been very studious & quiet this week till Friday & then lecture first thing, then as we did not care about the next lecture wh
was to be a 'grind' (classical name for oral exam, instituted by
Act Parliament – 1900) we went to the hospital Dr Depuis giving
us a sleighride over, back again & as Mr Mac's rig was at the
door he took Miss Beatty & I for a drive, or rather I drove them
till chem lecture at eleven wh we dashed up to Univ in great
good spirits. Was introduced to Miss Fitzgerald who is *the* topic
of the hour, a third year Arts student who having passed the 2
first year exams at Toronto without attending & cannot go there
was compelled to come here. She is 'divinely fair & most divinely
tall' ... Pleasant evg, met Miss Machar[2] the poet, author. After tea

2 Agnes Maule Machar (1837-1927), a feminist poet and writer; a lifelong
   resident of Kingston

went to church & after to Evangelical services wh. Oscar Owre
held forth. ... Next day worked at Anatomy till after 12. The pro-
sector going is good drill on the brain. After dinner Miss R[ey-
nolds] & I called on Miss Fitz & we are the best of friends She
came with me to the hospital. There was an operation, poor Tilly
had to have some more of her ankle taken off. Miss F. stood it
sans a shiver & her talking to me kept me up, the best I ever
stood it yet. She thinks maybe she will study medicine after Arts
course. After that I went to Mrs Leslies for tea & spent a pleasant
evg there. Mr Herald was there & walked home with me, that
half hours agony ended he said *goodbye*. Came home, early as
had an engagement for a drive, had been in only few minutes
when Mr Anglin with lovely double rig & spare dashed up to the
door & away we went, for the folliest lovliest drive you could
imagine with glasses coleur de rose. I had the pleasure of driving
too, till my arms were limp. He is one of the nicest manliest fellow you could meet. They say he is engaged. I do not know, but I
do know is is most kind always & we all thoroughly enjoyed the
drive unless some little monster c green eyes worried the others
as it sometimes does because I get the preference shown me. I do
have the happiest times, only an occasional blue spot when
something serious like that half hours misery c C[harles]
H[erald] disturbs the 'sweet' serenity of my dreams. Today is
Sunday. Miss Beatty & I went over to the hospital after dinner to
fix on Susie's apparatus (sequel – ran away c married man) she is
a nice girl, been there long time hip disease, wished us to come,
bandaged her up & brushed Tilly's hair & came away leaving
them grateful for the time. ... Monday evg, this has been blue
Monday. Yesterday Miss B attacked me about reading novels on
Sunday & left me angry at something I said, & I was not in the
best mood at dinner. Mrs C[orlis] & Miss R. at tea began exercising their wits over me & of course I spoke up for myself, & Mrs S
& Mr H. for me, but I do hate rows with all my heart & I've felt
like 'nobody's child' ever since, too proud to cry & miserable not
to & so have carried a stone in place of a heart all day.

Heu me miserani! We've made up again but I am blue still. I
know I too was to blame. I might have been wiser & better & I'm

sure I've felt like the most wicked disagreeable person alive, for the last 24 hrs, as tho' I must be unbearable & altogether hateful & life has not been rosecolored today. ...

Mar 1st

Such a queer life is boarding house life & we are perhaps a distinct type ... after our good friend & landlady retires, Miss R & I with noiseless steps & lamp descend to the place where the culinary operations are carried on, both as to manufacture & to consumption. We forage, & where she bestows the finer foods, any dainties such as pies or cake is a mystery to us however bread & butter, syrup & meat, suffer tonight. When we went down last night we found two chairs barricading the pantry & two the cupboard & over the bread can was a tin pan placed so as to bang & the bell on top, but we are obtuse to such gentle hints & gained access to the bread & studied very innocently after thus 'doin nothin'.

March 7th [excerpt from letter to Charlie]

... a general jubilation over coming home, at the close of 2nd Session of Coll, when the Co-education was in its most pleasant stage. Tons of oyster supper we girls gave Mr Mac on his departure for the North West. We four associates of Mrs Mac bought oysters coconut dabs cakes apples, & lemons & we had a jolly time not alone in the gourmand style but we grew festive & waxed eloquent wit graced the festive board, & hot lemonade was imbibed freely. Mr Hall Chairman, we laughed incontinently & sang as parting ode And be he gone And am he went, And am we left He to lament Oh cruel fate to you unkind To take he gone & leave us 'hind'
    Miss Reynolds & I are 'the girls' I told them. Mrs Corliss was 'ma' Miss Dixon & Mrs Mac the married daughters. Miss Beatty the eligible one & Miss R. & me the 'hateful girls' – I like to tease

Mrs C She is over 40 & is a very independent kind of a 'Ma' but we got her laughing in one of the lectures & she really looked apoplectic, we were in the separate room that time, we have to preserve our dignity by being sedate & grim when 'the presence.'

Thurs evg No lectures tomorrow except chemistry & *our Botany exam* which is enough in prospect to make cold chills play tag up & down ones spinal marrow. ...

Awfully hard to keep down tonight & go to study my Botany & if I just take off brakes for one instant I shall have set them all by the ears, so I will have to postpone my ebullition till tomorrow. ...

I must tell you Dr Corlis is here has been since Thurs, & this being Sunday & no other evil at hand to fall into, religion fell to our lot. Believe me – you have my sympathy about peoples religion – being so dogmatic, being hurled at one in such a bristling way, one feels anything but angelic toward them or their religious views. If there's one thing more than another that locks up the good of Christianity it is bigotry, prejudice & their kind. They are so 'I thank the Lord that I am not as other men are' & 'If you do not stand on my base you are not on safe ground' They were not attacking any pet dogma of mine or I theirs but after church we went to the R.C. church to hear the music wh. was par excellence & so then..... & people came into discussion. Dr. & wife held that no one sans 'change of heart' according the their views could enter the kingdom of heaven & that all the countless heathen would be condemned. I think it is a strange thing when people who could not help themselves from being what we call heathen, & living clean lives according to their best knowledge should be punished everlastingly. I retorted with 'Blessed are the pure in heart for they shall see God' they affirmed no one could be pure in heart sans a change of heart &c while I that a pure heart is one unspotted of the world the flesh & the devil as far as a clean life can make them. Then too the poor abused R.C. is he while believing the essential creed of God the Father, God the Son & God the Holy Ghost ... to be eternally punished because he has some minor beliefs wh. have been inculcated into him from birth. I get out of all patience c such nar-

rowness & tho I don't profess to know what is going to become
of them I can't help but believe some of them are as deserving of
heaven as there would be censors

Friday evg we had a Taffy party & euchre after it. Sat. the
whole party of us visited the Penitentiary & Asylum & in the evg
danced & talked, we had a jolly time but are going back to hard
pan tomorrow. ...

If a description of the various employments, the great walls,
the lone dungeons, or the happy looking convicts would make
you smile, or a few narrations of the 'inner consciousness' of a
few individuals out at Rockwood as portrayed in their particular
types of lunacy would make you hilarious I would forth with,
hold forth, but I *must* tell you one melancholy phase of mind
seen there. Mr Hall, a medical you know, my escort during the
trip in particular & the girls in general, was the hero –

A golden haired nymph glided up to him pounced on his hand
& anxiously asked when was he going to take her away, & before
any of us suspicioned such a thing she gave him a lightening
kiss, just think of that.

Now look here, don't you go abusing Valentines, cause why, I
was the recipient of a handsome mass of painted flowers, white
satin & cupids, & tho' it had a 3 cent stamp on, I discover it came
from our own house?

I must confess I like dancing sometimes & the fever has been
on me strong, however I did not go to the Ball last night c Mr
Gibson.

Yes I believe that an excellent criterion for right, when we
have the sanction of our inner conscience, but sometimes I cannot for the life of me tell wh. thing is the right & proper one or
which will have the best results then if I do rightly, I ask for help
& believe then that the outcome is for the best & rest satisfied. ...

You need never be afraid of tiring me with what you call a sermon. Your innermost thought, your truest prompting. I think
there is no trust more sacred than that, soul speaking as it might
be termed. My heart is light to think you have reverted to more
religious feelings, have owned your allegiance to the kindest
Father of All. I am sure you are happier, there is so much com-

fort, so much happiness in the thought that there is One ever present, who really cares for us, who helps us in every good, & to resist every evil, Who comforts us in grief, & trouble, Who is ever patient & ready to hear. Indeed one never quite knows how much more than all else a trust in Heaven is. I know of times gone by when most despondent when friends had disappointed or any other cross I have taken my troubles to Him who ever hears & have found peace & been comforted & resting satisfied that all would come right, it always has. Many & many a time when it seemed as tho' it must be wrong, as tho no good could possibly result in time I have been grateful, most grateful that things had fallen as they had, the end resulted in better things than I could have foreseen in the fondest dream, & if we cannot always trace the 'far off divine event' we can trust.

It is hazardous to my vanity, the way in wh. it is excited here, & if I look to the right or left Mrs Mac's eagle eye follows me to see if I return any of the smiles on the wing. Really it amuses me, last night in Chemistry in looking if I caught Mr William's glance & smile fastened on me & unconsciously returning it on bringing my head to right about Mrs Mac pounces on me c 'were you smiling at him' & on asked who 'him' was she said 'Mr Cumberland' (who sits in from of Mr W), 'I saw him smiling at you' so I was guilty of a double offense. One of the Meds' has just left me a book but tells me he dare not look in my direction for all the boys would know it. I shall begin to think I am attractive, when I hear such remarks are made of me as she 'is the pretty brownhaired girl' &c as distinguishing me. No use denying it – this chile is cleare gone spilt. ...

Cook calls it an Infinite Oughtness, which is to all men who think clearly not merely a Some what but a Someone. 'It is incontrovertible that man often hears a still small voice within him saying "I ought" It is incontrovertible that man often answers the voice wh says "I ought" by saying "I will not" It is incontrovertible that instantly & invariably after saying to "I ought" "I will not" a man must say I am not at peace c myself. It is incontrovertible that he who is disloyal to the voice wh. says "I ought" must also say "I ought to satisfy the injured majesty of the law I have thus violated."' [end of excerpt]

Perhaps Mrs C. & Miss R. will come here to board. They do not get on as amicably together as Mrs C. & I did. Nellie says she guesses Mrs C. has thrown me at her head about five hundred times, by telling her what a peacemaker I am & easily get along with individuals.

Rec a letter from Cecil at McGill today. The dear boy full of energy & success & a bit of sound advice to me his grown up sister, to be careful *not* to impress the tender hearts of my gentlemen friends here. He speaks so soberly as tho' their hearts were universally free & guiless as his own & that unless I was reserved they might suffer largely the dear fellow. I took it to heart too & went over again for the hundredth time everything I do & say, & really wonder how I am to know just what to do. Truly a woman has her own trials & as much need of Heaven's help as man ever could. Just now has come a letter from one of my gentlemen friends C.H. To know what to do & say & how? I want to do right. I would not hurt anyones feelings purposely, & how to reply to the very inner heart it seems to me of a man one respects & likes & not harm, one to whom I would do good, seems more, is more than I know unaided. He is no flirt, no boy, but a man of good heart, a man I respect, & how shall I answer him best. I have not the least remorse to suffer for & was most commonplace whenever I met him & only had one private talk with him during a walk. I wonder anyone could be so suddenly dreadfully in earnest. ...

Mar 11th

Heard Rev Ramsford today in Convocation Hall, he argues so broadly & so feelingly, his sermon goes home to individuals. It is to each he speaks & to the heart. One of those grand men, whose great heart is all aglow with enthusiasm wh. never dies, whose life is a sermon, whose soul yearns to do his fellows good. Heaven bless him & those like him, who are able to stir us out of our apathy & make us long to do good, make us for the times at least capable of noble things, who make us long incessantly to enter on a new life, to cast behind us the petty things that encumber

our better selves, to make as he said 'our lives a pulpit from wh.
should emanate the truth of Gods love to man.' I wish with all
my heart I could hear such, more often especially these days for a
selfish drowsiness seems to have fallen on me & tho I want to do
good, evil is present c me. Oh I wish there were more like him, to
lead us to purer air, to enthuse us with grander aims in life, to
make us feel & know 'the individual withers & the world is more
& more.' That we could sacrifice self to do good to others, to
make our *lives* our true honor, not other mens opinions.

To see there before me, in the choir, among the hearers, those
who in week day life, jest at things pure & Holy, whose own
lives are not all unstained who are so greatly out of joint with
purity of purpose, & cleanliness of life, how strange that they
should go forth tomorrow & be even the same they were yesterday, how strange & to look at them & believe them each the object of family ties, mothers love, mothers & fathers hope. How
strange that they so very few of them at least should bow the
knee to the Great Lord of All or even try to please Him in their
walk of life. Where *is* the root of it all. And when I think &
think, I feel so much of a mans life is traceable to the mothers
moulding & then why will they not leave carping at 'womans
sphere' & try by all means human & divine to mature, expand
enoble the mind of every girl to try to lift their thoughts to better
things than the petty foibles that so enwrap them, & men so flatter. To educate them in the broadest sense of the term & make
them grow in compass of thought so that when the fuller promise of the next generation shall blossom for mankind, the
young men may not be the weak morally, the tainted physically
or the dwarfed intellectually, but a race of *men* & the young
women not the puny creatures whose cramped physique can but
support a cramped mind. Indeed I feel strongly on this point. I
see gross evils & no attempt at remedy. So many fine dames in
jewels & idleness raise their pretty white hands in horror at
women who do act & live in reality because they overstep their
notions of 'womans sphere' because they do not subscribe to
their sense of the fitness of things, of dallying in the primrose
path of fat idleness, & leave the children out, out on the street to

play with whom, when & how & where they choose, whose delicate ears are disturbed by the voices of these same children who
are sent to school at day, as soon as old enough, & to bed at
night, to get rid of them. Who when their ungoverned, untutored
passions rise & they fall out & chide & fight 'are punished indis-
criminately' right or wrong all round for the offence of one. A
saving of time & patience on the parents part? wh. dwarfs the
childrens sense of right, justice, tenderness, love & care, oh these
same women, these censors of wrongdoers? these 'I thank the
Lord that I am not as others are' These monitors of christians,
these blind, blind women, raise their voices in loud depreciation
when one of their sex so far betrays them as to long for more
light, to seek nobler things than the creature comforts, of idleness
or the inactivity that nonentity brings.........

Mar 13th

One of the superanuated Profs died today & so we will have a
holiday & tomorrow. Miss R. left this morning at four so it has
disturbed us some what.
   Today Miss B & I had an operation with Dr Depuis & Mr
Stewart (a final man) taking off a frostbitten toe. It was a severe
strain, & for two hrs after I felt very queer. Did not get him properly under CHCl$_3$ & he did groan so & yell so, it was dreadful. ...

Mar 17th

Exams announced for next Wednes. & study now for everything.
Sunday had the pleasure of listening to McDonnell. Afterward
went to Mrs Leslies to tea. C. Herald happened there also. We all
went to hear him again in the evg & was more pleased than in
the afternoon. *Monday* very busy, shopping in the morn'g & to
hospital to say goodbye. It really did me good to see how much

they cared for us. Miss Beatty & I were the only two lady medicos left for the last week. Took dinner c Mrs Lesslie & bade them
adieu, the dearest nearest friends I have in K[ingston] & held
highest in esteem a noble women, a pattern wife, a beautiful
mother. She seems to purify the atmosphere wherein she moves.
... Had a very tiresome wait at the station of nearly 2 hrs. T. Bertram was my fellow traveller up & very glad was I that he was.
We had a very lively chat & it made the otherwise irksome trip
less so than it would have been. He is so young & fresh looking
& so merry withal, he was quite likeable. Arrived at H[amilton]
went to Jennie Woods & waited for them to come for me. ... Next
morning went out to Dundas & stayed to dinner & returned by
the 2 Oclock train to find E[rnest] & Gertie waiting for me &
Gertie returning to school after being absent a week c mumps.
They invited me to come home & have mumps but contrary as
ever, I have not taken them. I know in fact that I don't take
things readily, never did much in the pilfering line & have never
accepted gifts that would place me under obligations, if I could
help it. Here I am at home, & feel as tho I had been here weeks
not merely days, mud, mud on every side & bleak gray skies,
howling winds & frequent storms, stagnation point as to the
outer world, & since I have been home Mother has been away at
Bartonville, Aunt 'Lisbeth, Mrs Lacy in part for whom I was
named, died Friday morning. Mother's Aunt, & always to us
'Aunt 'Lisbeth' Such a terrible winter so many passing away,
poor human weaknesses, breaking down c the little extra weight
of unfavorable weather. I have applied for one of the situations
vacant at Easter in the P[ublic] S[chool] in H. I think I can study
better there than here. Then no household cares will cause me to
divide my attention & then too I'll have the advantages of the
city, which one particularly misses at this time of the year. I have
been reading 'John Halifax' & like it very very much. Alice lent it
me ... I made 80 per ct in Botany in the exam. I have a gt. am't of
studying & reading to do this summer if I only can have resolution enough to keep my mind to it, for next year will be a hard
year.

9

Winona, St Thomas, and Sheffield, Ontario April to September 1882

After an arduous session at Queen's, Elizabeth retires to the family home for a rest. The death of her old Hamilton friend, Mrs Lawson, brings this comfortable period to a close. The next series of entries from St Thomas are much less happy. Plans for Elizabeth and Alice McGilivray to take practical training with the doctor husband of another medical student, Mrs Corlis, soon fall awry. As the excerpts from letters to Charlie indicate, Elizabeth finds the situation both personally and professionally intolerable. Her escape to work with a physician cousin in Sheffield proves her salvation. However, the letters to Charlie document the persistent strain under which their relationship is labouring. Its survival has become more and more uncertain in face of Elizabeth's dismay over her lover's moral lapses.

April 1882

The end of the second session in medicine is past. Two years ago now Mrs Mac & I were together beginning our medical studies. Well do I remember when two years ago she & I learned the scapula as the beginning of our professional work & maybe! we learned it well. I only wish I had as vividly impressed the other ossa on my mind as that first scapula, marked 'Betsy Carr' died at hospital 1871 & their own subjoined disrespectful epitaph,

copied from somewhere. 'Poor Betsy Carr her's gone away. Her
would if her could, but her could n't stay. She'd two bad legs & a
baddish cough, but her legs it was as carried her off' Have been
thinking & planning to go to St. Thomas to study c Dr Corlis, in
June for two months. ... Rec. letters from Herald, Lawson & Williams & Dan who wants to take up the subject. The Future of
Canada & debate it with me, was amused at first but am going
to do so & am reading Marshalls Canadian Dominion with that
in view. I argue for the bright prospects the great future of this
fine Country!!

Rec. a circular from Mrs Mac her husbands. He is General
Manager of a Land & Loan Co. at Grand Forks ... hope he will
not be worsted in the speculation, rife there at present. ... Have a
notion to read one of Dickens stories am getting hungry again
for fiction. Ernest has about half a dozen men & boys at work
now. Mother is out tying up some grapevines & Pa is trimming
the orchard so that I am 'monarch of all I survey', my rights
there are none to dispute (i.e. when Ma's outdoors). I see Mary
Todd has passed successfully at the Normal. Mary Lavall is
teaching down this month at one school & such teaching. It puts
me out of all patience, seems such waste time, not only that for
some things wrongly taught will take such a long time to un-
learn. I do not think the youngsters of the day are suffering
because those like her can not get a certificate, but I beg her pardon I should not judge

In a letter received today I read this extravaganza. 'There is one
lady in whose light all others fade away into nothingness. I don't
care to know any other' What a luminous body, must be kind o'
phosphorescent & consequently poisonous. I fancy he will be at
least chagrined by the reply.

Rec. letters from Maud & Alice, both pressing for me to come
& see them. 'The earth is full of messengers that love sends to &
fro' How well & yet how little we can realize life to be earnest, to
be real. There is a great happiness in feeling that within one lies
such a power for good in the world. One even one poor mortal
has so much within, is capable of producing such untold results.
Like a stone cast in the ocean, tho' the 'spot' whereon it falls is

small in comparison to the whole, the motive power small, yet look at the widening ever widening circles of waves that roll away whither who shall tell? ...

Rec. word yesterday that Miss B[eatty] & I came first in Chemistry – no percentage given. I was agreeably surprised ...

May [and June] '82

What a beautiful sunny day it has been. I have been to the Mountain for a ramble with Ernest, Myrtie & Vi. for flowers, & ever & ever what memories of flowers, & woodland walks & birds, sunshine & youth, that same woods will recall. ...

Was at church today & heard a good sermon by Mr Whitcomb 'Ask & ye shall receive' as simile he said what child but felt pleasure in asking of its father if he knew he could give. Said 'some say' of what use is it to pray to God for things we wish when we believe him Allwise to give us what is for our good. Viewing it in that light he said of what use were many things, nay half the things of life were based on mere sentiment. Nations have gone to war with nations, peoples striving c peoples for a mere sentiment. Soon he said all our land would be disturbed for a mere sentiment. All social moral & civil laws were based on sentiment. Take sentiment from our lives & we would be but little better than the beasts that perish &c &c. ...

Cecil leaves in the morning for Thorold to assist the Engineer on the new Welland Canal, he does not know how long he will be there. Am going to stay most of next week with Edith & Georgie. I like writing letters when I have anything to talk about & one of my gentlemen corres. takes politics as his main topic, often another practises his sermons on me & a third his debates – heu me miserum! Rec. a 20 page letter from the divine, which annoys me, worries me & altogether exasperates me, till I'm doubtful whether I'll answer. And Dan has written me a long article contra Canada's Future greatness wh. as yet I have not appreciated I'm discouraged that I'm never free from un-answered letters & every time I'm away more petitions for me to corres. till I do not know what to say. Next wk sewing, dress-makers, Alice coming on Thurs & 'haps Cora on Friday & I want to go to St. Thomas soon. Gave Victoria her music lesson this morning & in the afternoon Frank Lawson was down & his mother is very ill. Next day Ma & Vi & I were down to Geddes. The girls are as blooming & nice as ever. I always liked Agnes. Ernest & I started for Hamilton Wednesday morning. He to attend the Synod & I to go on to Aldershot. How well I remembered then those few weeks that I taught there. The schoolhouse, the roads recalled forgotten hours, that no doubt with all these little things make the sum total of live & its results. I notice how much more vividly *place* recalls incidents because names I could not possibly recall away, when there came to mind uncalled. Just as naturally as the place to the eye. My spirits did not soar to any extent on the way, for it rained sans intermission nearly all the way, but I thought well this is a sort of introductory practice. I do look as tho' I had been sent for, & felt altogether quite professional. Of course I found my friends the Rosses as nice as ever & as happy. They are another happy instance of contented & peaceful marriage, it is good to see. Mr Flatt the teacher boards there ... Ernest was to meet me there, come out by the 5 train & we were going to drive up to Wilsons that night but it rained & he did not come, got on the wrong train & got off at Copetown & stayed at Uncle Isaacs that night & went next day to Guelph to see the Model Farm. I drove to Wilsons alone. ... That evg was the entertainment & Kennedy (Jake) came home with George. He is a brick, so quick witted, carries himself c such sang froid. The load of performers from Waterdown stopped there on their way. Then we in two good loads went o'er to the schoolhouse. The programme was fair had some good songs from Misses Galloway of Burlington & Harrison of Milton, but as is often the case, the most, the majority preferred the comic songs. ...

That morning was occupied chiefly in trying to keep our eyes open. In the afternoon Janet, Mary & I went calling, drove, it rained but still we went on, rain is so common now, getting used to it. Made five calls to see my old friends & indeed I was glad to see the children my former pupils. I saw them the night of the entertainment. The dear children, passing into the lobby among the crowd, the litle arms were stretched out toward me to see which could have the first shake of hands. Many kind things were said & I'm sure their present teacher could not have been pleasantly surprised. They tell me she is very — but I would likely be the same under the same circumstances. How the children change, out grows their former selves. One little fellow I liked so much, with great big black luminous eyes, little Charlie Sheppard came to me after the programme was finished & stood mutely before me with those great eyes fixed on my face & he even forgot to be bashful & gave me a kiss. It was something dreadful now I look back over those two days to think of the number of kisses given, 'enough to weight a royal merchant down.' I don't mind the children. I like to have them like me. I don't indeed mind them, but when we were calling, one house there was Mrs D. two grown daughters & 3 of my onetime pupils, which made six all round in & six all round out – twelve. I detest the way girls have of kissing every other girl every time they meet friend or foe all alike, till a kiss is nothing more than a shake of the hand to me it is. I have been kissed by some girls that I would a thousand times have preferred the coldest hand-clasp & then too it would not be quite so objectionable if out of public, to me a public kiss means nothing, it itself, but too often an index of empty heartedness. Sat. morning proceeded to Hamilton ... About 4 I went on my homeward way (it was raining still all the time) & when I reached home my feet were almost floating in the bottom of the buggy. I was pleased to get by a warm fire & get dry. Am glad I went tho' come back with healthier spirits, more myself. ...

June '82

What a truly awful sermon I am reading in Mrs Lawsons last hours. To think of her a dear kind friend, a woman handsome & strong, ambitious & clever with the pride of life so strong within her at one time & now now she is dying. Her life is ebbing out &

she has no power to stay it, with all her iron will, no power to stay, no power to further her mothers plans, or guard her sons future, never no, more. All the life she has known ended & what is all when all is done. Surely oh surely she will find rest hereafter. She has labored so long here & yet thro' all her struggles her hopes, never quite fulfilled, her projects not complete 'so bowed so broken' it makes me weep to see her, only the shadow in every way of what she was, & to think it is even so with all, when all is done, we must all pass away sometime, perhaps soon, we shall go back to dust & *be* no more as we are.

[excerpt from letter to Charlie]

Do you know you talked of something as being of a psychological nature, that is bordering on the 'soulful' is it not. Now I have it, you went to hear to Wild Oscar,[1] did n't you now? You spoke too of 'live factors' which suggest to my infantile mind, something with limbs & an appetite..... Do you never feel sort of homesick on dreary evgs, especially about dusk when a bright fire & a cheerful room are necessary to keep one from the depths of despondency.

    I'm sure I'm very much obliged to Miss Bertram for her praise & am very glad she likes me even as I am very sorry the others did not. ... I am sorry because for one thing, if they do not like me they of course ascribe it to my course of study & it is such a mistake. I'm sure if they knew me, they would not say so, because tho' I am well aware of many faults in myself, yet I am very sure they are in no way due to my studies or my College life. It is such a sorry mistake & it affects me much, for if after knowing me they prate about the unsuitability of the course & all that cant, why it goes sans saying that I must be obnoxious, for in me they have seen a speciman of the type. What makes people so stupid & talk about things they know nothing about take up such & such an idea & keep harping on it. When there is never

1 Oscar Wilde (1854 – 1900), British playwright and author

any outcome of the system to justify their hobby. As instance my
Rev. friend who does not think it fit & proper &c for ladies to
study med. & yet forsooth he would like one for life, as wife. His
objections could not be based on very solid ground or they
would not get over it so easily. Ah well have to take a great deal
as we find it, I suppose. I often forget all about it for a long time
& then some uncanny creature resurrects the subject & awakens
me to a momentary sense that I must be doing something un
ordinary, but still it does not seriously trouble me. I think it worries me more for their sake, that they are such people, & the
popularity of the project than for my own for I am one of the
happiest of mortals. Expect to go Monday noon from Hamilton ... to St. Thomas to Dr. Corlis. Cecil is home today & really
the house seems twice as lively. [end of excerpt]

June 15th

Mrs Lawson is *no* more like as we are. I cannot say how dreaful
it seemed at first, when I looked at Mrs Lawson's dead face I
never realized it fully till then & it swept over me with such a
rush I broke down utterly, it seemed as hard to realize death, to
understand that no more in this life will we see & know her, &
when they had gone to the cemetery it seemed harder still, to let
them put her down in the earth, why should they, she looked so
like herself asleep & who would tomorrow talk to me just as
ever, alas! ... Monday, dawned bright & clear as tho there were
no desolate homes & hearts, & the noise & hurry of life ebbed
cityward, growing louder & louder still, as day advanced ...
    Left Hamilton about One, & beguiled the time with 'Her Bright
Future' as we sped on our way. The view is very beautiful as the
train ascends the Mountain & when we left all that behind, &
were passing thro' the farms I could not but think of the difference between the lives there & in the city. How many pleasures
denied the farmer who worked hardest of all. Never at least seldom becoming wealthy enough to surround themselves with the
comforts & tasteful things so plentiful in the handsome suburban

home & even if by hard striving & dreary economy they have gained the means, how many lives retain enough of their healthy freshness, their early tastes to make their surroundings beautiful or their lives useful. No doubt it is a very happy circumstance that there are those who are content to remain on the farm & whether it is acceptable or not, they have my sincerest pity. I could n't endure to be always at the mercy of wind & weather for yearly success & never at peace because of it. ... Of course there were many observable types, travelling, & I had my book, but without the slump & tall bare trunks of a fire swept swampy land was not calculated to cheer, when my thoughts were often turning back to our late lost friend. Arrived about five & found Mrs Mac & Mrs Corlis to meet me. Holidays I find have improved their looks especially Mrs Mac, ever so much, & more comme il faut than when I saw her last & I like her better than I did almost my old admiration came back, indeed quite till some quirk or more expressively some 'kink' in the smooth running hours destroys the perfections, as for instance politics. It 'riles the old Smith blood' to hear wholesale denunciation & vitupertion of either party & when I hear people whom I know to be ignorant of the political science take upon themselves to denounce the opposite party as wholly corrupt, it certainly does not seem to me to exalt the speaker, especially when the people of Canada are pretty equally divided on the question & now at least the majority of an opposite opinion from Mrs Mac's wisdom. I believe there are good & bad in both parties & that each have principles worthy the enthusiasm of its disciples & I think it blindest egotism in anyone to say anyone is less worthy of respect in the smallest little because an upholder of a policy opposed to theirs. Dr C[orlis] is also a Reformer, so I am surrounded but the 20th will soon be here.[2] I suppose it will be a Bedlam in the matter of confusion & noise & worse in the matter of drink, &c &c. It does seem strange that men who eulogise the principles they stand by as purity, honor & truth, whose oratory or the copied phrases of

---

2   date of federal election won by Sir John A. Macdonald and the Conservative Party

their leaders would have us believe them to be men of great
nobility of soul, can so contradict every such sentiment by losing
their ideas & principles 'pro tem' in what they are pleased to call
the convival bowl & yet I doubt not there will be countless such
Tues. Heaven help us its 'a' a muddle when we know what
human nature is capable of & yet see what a grand persuasive to
change sides election day is the gratification of a taste. See the
brain superseded by a few small glands & nerves in the tongue
&c. For it is uncontrovertible that many men will vote sans brain
determination for a drink. We have been going through a severe
exam, grind in Anatomy, & Mat[eria] Med[ica], we three, the
whole evg & now I can sleep sans rocking I fancy.

Friday Morning, beautiful morning, the Dr. out. Mrs Corlis
doing housework, Mrs Mac playing & singing & I am here in our
cool room writing. The air is still full of politics. I'm glad I'm not
in the melie & can wait patiently to see how the different parties
conduct themselves Tues. This has been a lazy day. I'm quite disgusted with myself, for doing so little study but intend to do
some tonight. This is the strangest sort of life & certainly not a
laborious one. ... I like the Dr. very much & am sure I shall spend
a profitable summer. They are *very* kind indeed, & make it as
nice for us as they can, but what makes it so strange is taking our
meals out. We go down the side st (we live on a corner) nearly a
block to a widow lady's (Mrs Bentons) for our meals, we are the
only boarders & take our meals alone in state. We are *perfectly*
satisfied here, but it is odd to march off down there for meals
three times a day. Dr. C. has three sons, the eldest is away at
London, then Philip who is 13 & then little Charlie is about 5.
He is a dear little fat boy. I romp with him, chat with him, rock
him to sleep & feel very glad there is such a person. When I first
came there was a great excitement about smallpox & I think DrC
vaccinated about forty Tues, but now it is quieter. We were all
vaccinated but I am not affected yet.

St. Thomas is a lively place, quite an American element here
... The city is growing & promises to be quite an important city.
I'm sure if the continual puff of the train is any criterion it is
grandly important already. I can scarcely get used to it the un-

ceasing snort & yell & puff of the engines in the yard over by the park. They have a vim peculiar to the line like some great angry giant, it makes me nervous still.

June 18th

Was at the Baptist Church tonight with the others ...liked the sermon very well. 'Holiness profiteth to all things' he said it certainly could be no *loss* to live holily & it would be much gain &c. The preacher was a most peculiar looking man, small & fair & distinct enunciation, destinct almost to painfulness as 'po-ze-shon' & gos-spil. ... The people are waxing hot for tomorrow. Is this a sign of progress?! Men are frantic tonight, & it is a good thing, the bulk of the parties have chosen different ends of the city. It is really amusing. I don't believe one half could tell the principles of their platform, are enthused with some mad idea of party. One continuous procession eastward now to the Conservative band playing horses running, men tramp tramp tramp, the air rent c huzza's. Much repetition in every civic centre, much much repetition down to smallest hint of drunkenness & for the hours present Canada has gone quite mad.

[excerpt from letter to Charlie]

I do not want to be Pharisaical but I wish you would realize how dreadful such things are & hear you have forever foresworn them. It is ... perhaps tho' unworthy of you a fear that men may call you puritanical, pious, &c some such nineteenth century misnomer, but what is anything to you beside the perfecting of the manhood God gave you. Never was country more suitable to freedom to do & be what one pleases. There is no one to say you nay, no one, but what in their real heart would honor you for it. Fallen as any man may be & much as they would like to laugh down better natures to their level, they still must instinctively honor, the man whose principles are something better &

stronger than to give way to ridicule or fear of what such as they can say. Don't talk of heart hardening & smoothly drifting to indifference, but rouse yourself & be what you know you might be. What more eloquent sermon than the wrecks of manhood you see around you every day. 'Act act in the living present, Heart within & God o'erhead'

Dr. C's quite frantic over the elections, quite regardless of the effect on practice & he is smiling & happy because here his Reform man won the day. I do not dislike politics in themselves but what frets me is when two get arguing & then voices get gradually higher & higher & then perhaps there is an angry wordy fight. I do not understand why it is that politics have such a power to irritate perhaps some heat is necessary to inspire one to volubility. I was amused yesterday at an exception. Every man seemed wild c enthusiasm. All were hurrying to their respective goals, bustle, talking, fast driving, tumult, everywhere, but no surely, that is a mirage, delusion or is it a rara avis from another land no, I see before me a real flesh & blood man, the very soul of statuesque reposie seated in a lumber wagon jogging peacefully, nonchantly home, looking over the noisy crowd, passing along the street with mildly wondering eyes, much like Rip Van Winkle. The Dr has just been in c returns & states Conservatives in, in both N. & S. Wentworth. Crises always seem to have so much trouble connected with them. Even when one half is jubilant with success, the other end of the scale is deep in the valley. Man's inhumanity to man. How very cold it is, lucky too, if it had been warm it might have been too much for the fever heat of mens blood. Spontaneous Combustion &c. ... If I had no other knowledge of Sir John than the raillery, the bitterly denunciative epithets hurled at times by the Opposition it would lead me to believe him great, his intellect colossal. This is an intensely quiet life no croquet no boatrides, no drives, no gentlemen, no ladies (outside house) no games, no dancing no nothing but books, medicine sleeping & eating, less than Bohemia, much less Mesheck [Alice McGillivray] & I taking breakfast at eight all alone, at widow Bentons, if early we read, at times eat with a book before us (a story book) then back to our hermitage, & perform our domestic duties which consist of making the bed. That responsible duty over, & being divided between us, has not overcome us, we study till 12:30, then another grub orgie, & return to lose ourselves in sleep, then study till 5:30 then up town to the post office & to tea & study from dark to mid night, except Tues Thurs & Sat which are drill nights & the Dr. gives us close grinds over the work. This is the humdrum day by day. At rare intervals varied by seeing a patient Mrs Mac & I agree daily we are fortunate creatures. Some funny things occur. There's one lingering around the outskirts of my mental works but it the especial one will not come to pen. Meshack & I find abundance to amuse us, the ludicrous side of anything is very striking to us. See an excellent article in Sat. Globe by Huxley on Woman's Rights.

[later] I have tried to coax my imagination into believing we were two exiled femmes soles in a moated grange c portcullos always up. You see our room on its two external sides is parallel c two brick walls, the drug store at the side, the new office in front, & each at about five feet distance so that the avenue (!) between is an imaginary moat, so that we only see the sky by stretching our cervical vertebra out of window & gazing heavenwards, & sunshine by proxy from the stone wall. ... If it were not for Mrs Mac I should be desolate indeed. I am so glad she is with me. Were she one whit less than she is she would become monotonous, like everything here but she is one of a thousand & we are all to each other these days. Sometimes I think I could not bear it if she were not here & even then we are blue sometimes, for we might as well be in the remotest country place for all that we know of our fellow creatures here, or in the desert of Sahara for all the practical knowledge we are gaining. I wish with all my heart I had never thought of coming to St. Thomas, but had gone to Dr. Smith. I have written him tonight to see if he can be bothered with me for a month. I can't get away from here before another month sans unpleasant feelings & there's no use to let them know how dissatisfied I am. I have learned a good lesson to insist on an exact agreement before beginning its fulfilment. I wrote to them before I came several times & thought all was de-

cided but it is all different, that is a thing to remember in itself, but that would not matter so much if I were getting value received but I am not. I never was more disgusted c a farce than this, we have known no more of the cases the Dr has had or the diseases treated by him in this week than if we were home. He prescribes a fee for us – 25 for both for 3 mo. & leaves any further margin to our discretion wh means he would take double if we offered it. I always thought there were two sides to a bargain, but ma foi, there's only one here, & that is his for we receive nothing, unless it be his gracious smiles which however delightful they may be in themselves will hardly further our medical studies. And of course these are very good people & wd be astonished out of their seven senses if they could dream of such amazing ingratitude as this to be unmindful of their efforts in my behalf. Had I never known them in business relations I w'd no doubt have had a more excellent opinion of them. It seems sts as if I could not bear this longer. I can never describe the utter dreariness & misery of this kind of existence. I almost lose my desire of life if this were perpetual I should never remain compos mentis. It is the merest existence, it is dreadful. I know I am naturally a social being & to be so completely exiled for so long a time is misery enough of itself, but to know how much more there is in the world of every soul to be active, how much I must do, how much to learn, & then to feel myself caged here c but *one* single duty & that study, wh is insufficient to maintain mental & physical strength. And when the utter shabbiness of these friends c whom it is not policy to quarrel comes over me c fuller force, when circumstances combine to show *how* shabby & that they are imposing on us successfully are making life useless for the time & all I sacrified to come here for the good it w'd be professionally, no wonder I feel bitterly toward them. They are *so* clever, they are such *good* friends they are doing so much for us, even at a sacrifice. 'These young ladies are studying c Mrs C in *my* office.' And I have been in *his* office twice, once to be introduced to it & again to see a tooth pulled. Then our room is dark & dismal, not as to furniture, but to light & view, *so* dark so dismal, only the stone walls to look at & the shrieks & hisses of the

perpetual engines across the block to listen to. We go for long
walks wh is our brief respite from a most inactive inglorious
existence. I almost hate myself sts to think of it & to remain but
to go away w'd be folly, for we might not get certified & so lose
all. I try it for two wks longer c Heavens help & Mrs Mac's society wh two things have kept me from insanity for the last month.
Mrs Mac feels even worse than I for she might have been in
Dakota with Mr Mac. Seeing so few people we diagnose them
well, our hostess, for instance a most eccentric woman, a reg.
American c all appreciation for her own sex but not much for the
other, her husband alive rec. 3600 a year but dead she earns her
own living. There has been an Am. gent boarding there recently,
a most unsufferable bore, when he attempts to soar out his business knowledge wh he delights in doing tries to make us take
false for true & true for false c a bombastic volubility wh only
leaves him floundering in unknown waters. Dr C never read a
novel in his life & little of anything except what has been com-
pulsory to attain his degree. [end of excerpt]

July 20th

Shall I ever forget the sunset tonight, more than words can describe, was it most beautiful, sublime. I'm sure the soul leaps up
to recognise its Author at such times. I know I am the better for
living the last half hour, in saddest sweetest thought wrapt in the
perfect glory of that mystic sunset. We went out to the country
for a walk & coming back faced the Western sky & we stopping
in admiration & amaze. ... I am grateful for tonight, it makes me
stronger to take up the burdens of life. It makes my spirit leap
within me, to begone before me. Underneath the lights I look at.
In amongst the throngs of men, then my brothers fellow
workers. Ever reaping something new, that wh they have done
but earnest of the things that they shall do.
    Yesterday, the Dr & family were away at Simcoe & F. Scoville
their cousin returning in their absence we three had a talk. ... We
made sixty pills for McKibbon [the local druggist], each. I could

not see such a diff. between rolling that paste, & flour dough. It
reminded me of nothing so much as when we used to make clay
marbles. When I think of the pleasant summers home of some
social life, of 2 mos lost time from the short life allotted & wh I
value too dear to squander, of the practical knowledge I might
have gained, of the value of money spent of the help I might
have been at home, & all for what, a lesson dearly gained, a loss
of faith in two more of my kind, a farce wh I must perforce keep
up thro weeks of a dead blank, a wasted time, such dead sea fruit
is bitter. I am anxious to hear from Dr. Smith for both Dr. & wife
here are daily more distasteful to me & I hate the hypocrisy
forced on us. This life is the nearest to exile I can imagine. I shall
never forget them, truly I am in the valley. I suppose I'll the more
enjoy the hills. We have a favorite walk out. North of the town
where we climb thro a fence, & cross a field to a gorge on the
bank of wh hill of discontent we discourse our talk of woe. We
returned last ev'g more dreary than ever, in a very acme of
melancholy. We felt we *could* not go back to our dungeon, & we
went up town & jostled against our fellow creatures, seeing some
onions displayed, we thought about the most desperate thing to
do was to get them. We did, we bought a bunch came home &
getting bread &c we had an orgie, that would have make the
saints weep if not from pity, from onions. We ate & ate. We went
to sleep & only arose Sunday morning at eleven. If one last con-
vincing proof of our utter forlorness were needed, that would
prove the coup de grace.

Rec. a nice long letter from Miss Fitzgerald & a very kind cordial one from Dr. Smith, telling me to come soon & stay long. Mr
McKibbon is very kind & has been always in giving us free play
in his drug store. ... Mrs Mac is awfully blue tonight, poor girl
she is not so fortunate in having a cousin Dr. ...

Christ Church Rectory, London, July 30th

As the poet says 'things is various' wh I endorse. Mrs Mac & I
left St. Thomas yesterday afternoon. Found Rev. J.W. at the depot

put me in a cab & saw Mrs Mac on her train & I was soon in the arms of the family, who press my prolonged stay & I have consented till Thurs. as there is to be a Garden party here on Wed. & then I think I'll stay a few days at St. George c Meshack. Last evg a gentleman friend of Gussie's took us for a drive a delightful one, all over town & out to Hellmuth Coll. & then the grounds & then to Victoria Park wh was lighted by Electricity. The 7th Band played too & was enjoyable. London is a very handsome place & the Rectory is a large house & nice roomy grounds c plenty of shade trees but I will be glad to get to the Drs & be at peace from watchfulness.

Aug 7th Sheffield

It seems I lived thro' an age wh in London. I can never tell what deep waters of thought I was in there. It seemed a sort of transition state wherein I could see things as I never saw them before & awakened to life with new eyesight & felt for the first time I had closed for a woman's journey, 'girlhoods beautiful gate' It was 'no one' nor 'nothing' in particular that so affected me, it was all that had been, that was, & the 'dimly seen future' I suppose. There tho all meant kindness everybody & everything was a complete bore & my one effort was to be agreeable & yet keep up my train of thought. I am sure that I would not have endured the affliction of visiting & all its concomitant evils if I had not believed it part of the educational system & that I was surveying for future use, & as reward made friends c Dr Street who said I might have been in his office this summer & hoped I would be next summer, he would only be too happy to help a lady studying sans any fee & would give me all the practice possible, together with the hospital wh. he attends part of the yr. He drove over to the hospital one day with me & introduced me to Dr. Wilkinson the Dr in charge who also was very kind & said if I would come next summer he would give me the dressership in the hospital & all the practice I wanted. ... Saw enough of cousins

while in London to last me a lifetime. Whether I am unnatural,
hardhearted or something of the kind I do not know but I do
know that if a cousin *or* any other relative has not congenial
ideas I tire of them just as soon as if they were strangers & alien.
Arrived here Sat evg & found Dr & wife & Essa to meet me. It is
a complete rest to be here. There have the happiest home one
could find. The atmosphere is health, free from deceit & hypocrisy. No one was ever more glad & grateful for healthy surroundings once more than I for it is such a good antidote to
morbid melancholy – the smothering weight of unexpressed
thoughts, often inspired by what one sees of maltreated affections scarcity of honor, prevalence of deceit wh. perhaps may
make it easier to deal with many units that make up the whole,
yet cannot be in any sense exalting to anyone. Life seems
stranger ever day, & the earth a grand chess-board, where there
is unending effort to checkmate, to be victor over others, to gain
the desired ultimatum at any cost. The Globe had quite an extensive on Democracy, the novel that I read in London & wh no
doubt sank me deeper in pessimistic thought. It said it equalled
Disraeli's & spoke very highly of it. The character of the heroine
Madeline Lee, haunts me still. I can sympathise with her. I
understand it all & well. Have also been reading a Day of Fate
E.P. Roe.

Aug 9th

Have had a most delightful day. Dr & wife have just left my
room after a chat after our return. First thing then a.m. we drove
to Wm. Willards. The old man had a bad fit of epistaxis, Medicine aside, the assembled female clan was my particular subject
of interest. Among them the village gossip, Mrs Main better
known as 'Eliza the gossip' Needless to mention, she like all the
rest of the startled saints of Beverly took a sort of morbid interest
in me, much as they would in his Satanic majesty should he condescend to appear in the flesh, female Dr's being to their mind

through dim distance something quite abnormal & fantastical. Its awfully uncharitable but its rich, to see them gaping round c their hands on their lips looking like ghostseers & quite as lacking of ideas. But I beg her pardon the old lady did have some ideas & was not afraid to advance them, indeed I should ascribe that to the good people of Beverly as characteristic. Drove back for dinner & such a lovely drive, good roads, no dust, good rig, good horses. After dinner we off to Branchton to Mrs Buchanan's 'richer still.' I preserved a calm Samantha like exterior in accordance c cast iron principle hard as it was. Behold her after the style of Mrs Rip Van Winkle – Hippocrates aid my pen – a woman of the mincing kind, attired after the most prevailing style some hundred years ago especially as to the head, give it up. Operation, removing Polypus from the nose. Previous to this she thought 'sumthin to strattin her stummac' wd help her tho she assured us she had none in the house, & never took it. The Dr gave her some & withdrawing the empty glass she began 'I think it such a foolish thing' heigho think we here's a temperance lecture bounty gratis, but behold, we are disappointed 'for a woman to study medicine, she will have to see such dreadful things'. The discussion was not entered on, I thought bless her! it would quite put to flight her very light wits if I should tell her just what I had seen. Her daughter appeared, you could easily see a family resemblance. She was a young woman in physique but in face looked as tho' she had just opened her eyes to the light of day. About as much expression as in a mud pie. The mater wanted her head held, the budding flower of innocence looked quite scared & c more gesticulating than speech conveyed the idea that in her city sisters words would be 'she really couldn't she'd faint'. So this ferocious hardened imp or prodigy did the 'holding business' & when the basin of bloody water was to be emptied, the B.F.F. [Budding Fair Flower] turned up her sweet nose, shut her eyes & twisted her cervical vertebra into fearful curves, succeded in getting the basin out sans appearing to have seen it or been contaminated. It was all comical then on paper the comicality evanesces. After tea bore out again. Have had such good old talks c the Dr today. I don't know when I've

had such good laughs or such serious good talks as today. The
Dr talking to Sam Cornell, a local celebrity about baptism, Dr
said 'Well I tell you what Sam if its dipping that does the business, they'd have to anchor you out over night' He had the grace
to laugh ...

Last Sunday wk Mrs S[mith] & Mary were here from Ancaster
& we went over to hear Mr Edwards preach, but I'm so awful
wicked. I was more amused than edified, & made them all laugh
over that & yesterday's too. An older gentlemen preached & I
like him very well. Dr Lundy & wife were here yesterday. Dr is
very talkative blunt & witty but I ween he is a cranky stick at
times. I am not studying so hard now, tho' I did just before Dan
came & was glad of a rest. The Dr & wife are well mated, a
happy family here.

Sept 4th [excerpt from letter to Charlie]

I am sorry, deeply sorry that incident of your smoking, should
have occurred. I could not help feeling as I did & would be less
than I seem if I had not. If you had seen the white set face. I blew
out the lamp to keep from seeing a second time after I ... fled to
my room you might guess something of the dreary thoughts that
kept me waking through the small hours of that night. I could
not help it, nor help the constraint it caused. ... [end of excerpt]

Sept 17th [excerpt from letter to Charlie]

What a lovely country this is for fruit. I have been the rounds for
today. Somehow Sunday that is, the afternoon is always a sort of
Gypsy day, in summer & autumn. It is intensely satisfactory to
have the kindly fruits of the earth at hand in plenty. ... I've been
reading 'Taylor on Insanity' & I'm more & more bewildered who
shall say who is insane or who is not.

You are indeed ill to be so delirious & for such a long time but
then I'm not going to sympathize, you needn't feel alarmed. I'm

snubbed I am. Just find me asking of your chills again, yes just, but then you poor cild. It was so delirious, it did n't know what it said. Never mind I understand all about it, have been reading Taylor on the diff forms of insanity & this is a clear case. Still I hope you will have lucid intervals, tho' here you continue to talk of irrational things as hysterics in connection c yours truly, the prosy practical 'Senior year young girl.' A never fear young girl. Mid floral aroma I'll take my diploma & then I'll be quite pure. [end of excerpt]

10

Kingston, Ontario
October 1882 to June 1884

In these emotional, often tortured entries Elizabeth reveals the personal cost at which medical education was won for women in Canada. The pettiness and vindictiveness of faculty and students at Queen's leave her embittered and angry. The support of families, liberal papers such as the Toronto *Globe*, local Kingston citizens, as well as the influential Dr Jennie Trout in Toronto fortify Elizabeth and her friends in their opposition to injustice. Nevertheless, emotional and academic survival remains precarious. Only two bright notes emerge in this period – the promise, eventually realized, of a separate women's college, indeed two, and Elizabeth's relationship with her future husband Adam Shortt, the Queen's student who helped see her through these critical months. A woman no longer a girl emerges from these experiences.

Kingston Oct 7 '82

Tonight as I sit here alone & think think the long long thought of youth, I cannot but be grateful, thankful to the Giver of All good that so many blessings fall to my lot. What could mortal wish for more ...

Here begins the to me remarkable part of my adventures [on the way to Kingston]. Truly God overrules all for good. It is so very wonderful how through strange adventures trial & adversities He leads to what is best for us. I have often, nay always compos mentis trusted Heaven, that however mysterious unaccountable & strange things seemed, that somehow He was leading me to some good for myself, not that I am presumptuous but I ask & in some way I have always found that good *was* the final goal of every ill. All my life long I have wondered that I should be so blessed. Truly it is the Lords doing & is marvellous in our eyes.

No familiar faces on the car. I received a seat to myself but shortly a gentleman turned the one before me so he would be vis avis, so when his back was turned I quietly turned mine & so brought myself face to face c a mild placid looking middle aged woman of apparently the middle class. We began a desultory conversation, she was very aimable. I found her destination was K. too & she was an Evangelist, a Primitive Meth. had been a Wesleyan but they do not admit women preachers & as she said to her denomination did not matter. She was going to K to preach for an old friend of hers Rev Harris. From the minute she said Kingston it seemed to me that in some way she could help me & revolving many things of all the difficulties I knew of getting a boarding place in K, its many evils, I thought perhaps a Rev. gentleman might know some help. So after we had progressed favorably in our conversation I mentioned it & she was quite sure he could & would, so she kindly insisted on introducing me to the Rev. gent who met her at the depot & he was very kind. We went up in the same cab & to one of his parishioners, Mrs. Lakes. She could not take me, but as I was going to the Windsor she (Mrs Lake) whose daughter I met here once before *very* kindly invited me to stay all night with her. I accepted her kind invitation ... I shall never forget the misery of those succeeding hours I walked miles [in search of a boarding place]. I called at diverse & varied places. I walked till exhaustion & approaching night overtook me & as the Cabman had taken my valise to Rev. Harris I called there for it & under Mrs Watsons (my fellow traveller's) sympathy, kind words & cooing I broke down, weak as it may seem, I actually broke down & for a few

dreadful moments gave way to tears, not that I was purely fainte
hearted but I was so intensely wearied & felt so much alone &
unprotected. I shall never forget the kindness of those people, to
me, a total stranger. They gave their sympathy, kind words &
help for Mr Harris called at some possible place & sent me word
that night that it was all right, he had found a desirable place &
for me to call in the morning. Wh. I returned to Mrs Lakes, she
too had found me a possible place, so that I was quite cheered. ...
I went to both places. One a widow lady of independent means, a
very kind ladylike person wanted me to come for company sake,
but I would have little time for that & it is so far from Coll. The
other place, here, is more convenient & I have a small room quite
to myself, but she wants four more ladies. If everything holds out
as it begins, I think I'll be satisfied. ... Everyone had been so kind
Mrs L[ake] & daughters I had found kindness among total
strangers. The boys were exceedingly kind, all they could do for
me they did not even allowing me to carry my valise down stairs
scarcely to turn sans some kind attention. They seem five very
nice students. Stirling smokes for the whole. I have not seen a
single lady student yet, nor a double me either. I cut all old associations & started afresh & I am *very* glad I did so. Had a kind
letter from Miss Oliver, a new student, intended missionary, saying the Toronto M[edical] C[ollege] wd not come to terms & she
was coming here, but she did not come by the train I expected
her. Met Mrs Mac's brother in law he says she is in the country. I
hear Mrs Corlis is boarding c Mrs Shibley & that her Josiah came
down with her. How my heart palpitates c pleasure at soon
beholding maybe 45 [or 65] freshies in Arts. Met Miss Fitz today
at church hearing Mrs Watson. She tells me of a shark, a female
quack here that fastened on her & told me to beware. Miss Blaylock from New Carlisle on Bay Chaleur is here & Miss Oliver &
they room together. ... Miss Blaylock is a very interesting vivacious clever fun loving mixture, a mixture of many tracts of
many known friends. Miss Oliver is excellent & I foretell a good
student. ...

Went to church this morning c Miss Blaylock & this evg with
Miss Fitz to St. Pauls wh. I like best of all here. Miss Fitz came

home with me & we had a very long pleasant talk. She is tall &
handsome, dignified but not at all assertive, a sweet girl & we are
good friends & board near each other. She says very complimen-
tary things about me, & that the boys are 'raving about me'
hyperbole – . Tomorrow is Univ. Day & the games come off. I
hear Sparrow my once drawing master at Ottawa is now at the
penitentiary here for making counterfeit money. ... He was a very
lenient teacher & kind. The house is all dark & stll, the noise of
my pen & the ticking of my clock the only sounds that I hear.

Oct 19th

Life is fast getting into the old routine, yet as far as I am concerned I am much better satisfied in that I room alone & I can
study or write and dream when & as long as I choose, & using
my time to advantage, I have also more time for sleep. There are
many advantages in having a sanctum where one can have their
own thoughts. I hear Tom Bertram is much interested in Hilda
McLaren. Mr Armstrong called again last evg & he told me Coll
news. I am blue & lonesome tonight. Dr Fenwick our Prof in
Inst[itutes of] Med[icine] wishes to be a power, & when some
ideas of his were neglected & he was 'sat upon' by the Faculty,
why I spose he got mad! I know of no other reason for his having said unkind things of us, not personally but in the abstract
such as 'he had no respect for a woman who studied medicine &
would n't have them in the house' It is dreadful to have such
things said of us, when God knows (I say it reverently) we try to
walk circumspectly & as womanly as woman may. It seems *so*
unkind to be misjudged. Last year he was very nice & it seems
strange that he should alter in this way, after knowing us &
knowing no evil of us. Mr. Armstrong said, in speaking of some
students opinion, that he was often amused that 'those who
thought it w'd destroy our fine feelings were the only ones most
devoid of any such fine feelings, the most destitute of a better
nature,' we have no need to be told that it is on the surface, we

see it & know, those who see everything through vulgar sensu-
ous glasses, think *all* must so regard the most beautiful of works,
while those who have not that low grovelling nature & see
through purer minds, see no harm to us. Dr Sullivan whom we
all dreaded, has proved a pleasant disappointment. He was & is
just as nice to us as it is possible for a Prof to be. The students
behave even better than last year, especially in class, for wh we
are very thankful.

Sunday Evg.

Have heard such an excellent sermon Gandier, of the students,
Miss Fitz & I went to hear him. I have not heard so good since
Rainsford. 'What shall we do with Christ' & he described the
death & life of our Savior more vividly than I ever heard it before. He is one of the cream of divinity students. His face shines
with real manliness & worthiness. How much good such men
can do, not only with words but in their lives. I have known
many noble hearted men & women & I am I hope the better for
knowing them, for I believe Goodness is so real & that 'words
that are things hopes that do not deceive, Goodness that is no
name & happiness in dream' Miss Fitz came home with me & we
have been having such a good long talk & I am comforted for she
pets & likes me, so heartily, that I know no little jealousy mars
her friendship for me. I am so glad we are near each other. ... I
like the study, but I will be glad when next year comes & the
worst of the classes will be over & then the end will soon come.
Why I cannot just tell but I shrink from some of the classes not
because of the lectures a bit, but the boys & the dreadful ordeal
of answering questions before so many. Sometimes I think the
circulation will get such a shock that it will not recover. Seems as
tho' *something would* break & I should die there & then. When a
whole roomful of students in silence most profound (just then)
are waiting for me to answer it is just torture & I guess I always
blush, like a red red rose, but I can't help it. They are all staring

at me & it recurs to me about so much that has been said of my blushings as 'she's the only one that could blush' (I'm sure they've no need I do enough for all.) Especially Dr Depuis so often calls particular attention to my poor self, by starting up suddenly in describing something & asking me if it is so in the book. Perhaps I'll get over it, but I'm worse than I was last winter at grinds anyway. Prof Depuis wife & daughter called & Prof Fowlers wife last wk. Miss Hamilton a lovely girl of Bay Chaleur is here & hopes to study medicine, is studying for matric. My first rival in the way of looks, tho' the very plain faces of the others gave me the palm before I am totally eclipsed now. I do wish they were all pretty for people think them so excessively plain & tho' I've no claim to beauty I'm not ugly for wh Deo Gratias. Alice is going to Boston this winter for Conservatory Music. Thank Heaven for the trait of forgetfullness, so many countless trials, that after a time are as tho' they had never been & the sunny things remain so much longer in retrospect. We commence work in the morning c more than usual zest for Dr Fenwick speaks of having a written exam & we do not wish to bring up the rear, more especially as Friday wh. a question (a hard one) was asked, none of the boys knew it altho' he especially appealed to those he calls the 'honor men' & tho' we knew it, he quite ignored us. It angered me considerably. Read up some 50 pages of it yesterday & today could not help casting sheeps eyes at the forbidden fruit. ... To Chalmers church, McCuay, in the evg. We could see at a glance that the vanities of the table would interfere with fine head work tho' he did commit a ponderous alliteration: 'The impenetrable panoply of Pharisaical prejudice' Kingston is a desert for pulpit oratory like some others! The Freshman *do* look *so* fresh some of them. Our poor youth seems to be the butt of all fun. Ashton wears a flaming red plaid shirt, wh at first sight is the attraction & he walks so mistrustfully, as tho' there were veritable pitfalls. While I doubt his discernment sees the worse, the moral pitfalls, freshmanlike he carries a stack of books under his arm. One morning, Anatomy lecture was fairly under way, when some one turned the door knob, but no one entered for the very good reason as every Soph knows its peculiarity of turning in opposite way from normal locks. Another attempt to open the door, no entrance. A generous Soph or Senior goes to the rescue while a murmur of 'freshie' went round the class. The look of condescension & patronage & 'is it a boy or a dog' look that the Soph bore as he opened the door was amusing, but when poor Ashton entered, with his under lip hanging down as tho' he was about to cry, was too much & he rec. an ovation of claps &c. They say he came one day c kid gloves & a cane of wh he was soon relieved. He all innocent asked a kindly faced student 'Don't you spose they'll give it back sometime?' It is too bad. He's no doubt good & innocent, but he will not long be so, so one can see all the transitions till often they emerge final men in more things than one. Student said wh he thought much over his studies & studied much into his head, it seemed to expand to endanger the walls of the room. I suggested he might put it out of the window. It seems rather dreadful that in Football, there should be so many accidents. McCardel not yet out, Brown limping about and Herald with a broken leg. Rather dreadful to be wounded in amusement. It would be heroic, perhaps if necessary for home or country. I'm busy, & will be more so ... but I'm healthy & happy these days as I can be. Hospital tonight, Meshack & I have good laughs over 'man'.

Nov. 5th [excerpt from letter to Charlie]

Mrs Leslies. Have been here since yesterday. I'm here every day or two anyway. She is such a dear friend. She is not like the usual aged by marriage kind of person, but is so womanly & girlish too. Mr L is very nice too one of those pure hearted kindly men that adorn mankind. Annie & I are keeping house while Mrs L is at church. I've been reading nursery rhymes to her till I'm hoarse. She like Essa even wanted me to sing at breakfast. She is a pretty sprightly little darling & claims me her especial

property & is helping me now by holding the blotting paper.
Rec. a letter from Herald, telling me of the 'accident' & asking me
to come & see him, wh. is quite out of the question & not
answering that as I had dispatched a condoling note, I rec.
another letter saying he wanted to see me very much would I not
come & that he had spoken to Mrs Leslie & she did not think it
out of the way. I am sorry. I would go to see a dog that was hurt
if I could help it but I do not want to do anything that will compromise me in any way. Mrs L & I have concluded it but not tho'
the girls say go with Mrs L. I do not want to be a cruel or hardhearted but I cannot do any good by going & if it got abroad,
there w'd be no end to it. I do not dislike him but we never agree
five minutes. ... We have a gentleman boarding in the house now,
a final Arts man & intending theologue, very nice & quiet[1] & we
are a very peaceable family altogether. Hard work, lecture from
9–11 home, prepare for next 2–3 home copy notes back, 6 home
to tea & then hospital & 8–11 study, & tired out. [end of excerpt]

Nov 11th

The day is dull & dark & dreary & I should be at clinic, now but
'felsh bad' stayed at home. Thanksgiving day was just a treat.
Studied all forenoon, from dinner to 6 went over my wardrobe, a
truly feminine occupation, but none the less a pleasure, then
wrote letters & in the evg the girls came & we spent a jolly evg.
Our landlady is a jewel. She gave us a regular Thanksgiving dinner. Turkey, cranberry, & sauce, plum pudding &c Lovely day
for I was *in* all day. We do not regret the change, our gentleman.
He is a final man, very nice & quiet. ... Principle Grant arrived
home from the Old Country the early part of the week bringing
the new Prof of Physics Mr Marshall, who was installed & gave

1 Adam Shortt (1859–1931), M.A. Queen's 1885; 1885, Professor of Philosophy, Queen's; 1886, m. Elizabeth Smith; 1891–1908, Professor of Political Science, Queen's; 1908–17, Civil Service Commissioner for Canada;
1918, Chairman of the Board of the Historical Publication of the Archives
of Canada

his inaugural address last evg in Convocation Hall. Miss Fitz & I
went & were well entertained. The students congregated in the
gallery & the noise & singing before the performance proper, was
loud & furious. John Brown, Old Grimes & all their fellow cele-
breties made the air ring ... while such choice poems as Moses in
the pool, Buyr Tarin & Saw my leg off moved all present especially the feet of the singers, whose treading & whoops together
with such instruments as canes, tin horns & goose quills, gave a
full orchestra. Once wh Grant was just midway in his first sen-
tence in a calm, there came a distinct lovely sorrowful 'squach'
from the goose quill, wh excited the risibles of all Grant not
excepted who looking gallery ward smiled & said 'he hoped the
gentleman was not speaking in his own vernacular' wh quite
silenced his gooseship. The new Prof is a very fine looking man,
looks like a triumph of *mind* over matter, all brain. Clear cut, fine
features. Has been in Japan five yrs as Prof Physics. Christmas is
near but this will be my first one away for I'm going home with
Miss Beatty I think, it will be odd. I am getting fearfully, awfully
vain. Dr Depuis said this morning to the class! He was proud of
Miss Smith & c which brilliant remark was elicited by my
answering several successive questions, & I heard *a* boy behind
me say to another 'so are we, so are we all' I wanted to sink
through the floor but it was obsinately firm & I drooped. Sunday, I have distinguished myself to myself. I was intensely blue &
nearly collapsed at teatime under the sympathy expressed for my
homesickness & hurried up stairs to cry, but did not, studied till
the middle of the evg & then Mr Shortt kindly read chemistry to
me from his notes & so I went to sleep without giving way.
Could nt for the life of me give any just cause for being blue only
that all the girls were teasing me hard about so many gentlemen
admiring &c. Mrs Corlis comes out often with quite startling
expression of goodwill to me. I really think after all she may have
had & has good intentions toward me tho' I'll never be infatuated with her. ... I believe Fenwick thinks we have cancelled any
chance we might otherwise have had of clearing our names, by
entering med coll. His reasonings are often this wise likely 'Any
good looks a girl may have were given her purely & solely to get

a husband with', & as we were quite lacking in that respect we look to medicine in despair, never dreaming of such a hope in that state of life.

Tues.

I'm just paralysed in a state of collapse, so are we all. For all places for startling adventures commend me to a Medical Coll. Its too comical for paper. At close of lecture on circulation Dr F[enwick] said he w'd like to have a vivisection & he thought as the boys had been so successful in procuring 'cubs' 'our girls' might procure a cat. Wh. he intended as a delicate allusion to old maidism likely. After going to our waiting room I jokingly said 'let's each into class tomorrow with a cat under our arm' never dreaming of such a thing as reality, but they took it up at once & tho' I did not believe them said they w'd do it. I thought it forgotten till in the evg Miss Blaylock asked me if I had any message, she was going down with Miss B[eatty] & Miss R[eynolds] to see about 'cats'. I tried to persuade them out of it & *yet* did not believe them. But they did collect four cats & had them safely housed at Mrs C's. Today I again tried to persuade them not & as they insisted, I stayed away from Lecture, this afternoon, & here is the report they have just made. They put the four cats in a bag & sent them to the Dr's office, & he thinking it 'groceries' sent it on to the house. The servant received it with wide open eyes. At class time the girls went in sedate as possible, noticing a twitching about the Dr's mouth. They had fairly become seated (boys too) when the door opened & admitted Mr Foran (a student) grinning from ear to ear & leading an unfortunate puss by a long string. He heroically led it up to the altar (desk) & tied it to a nail. The storm of applause over this feat had scarce subsided when two students appeared with a bag between them, wh contained another sacrifice to science & wh they deposited before the altar. Another storm louder than before, another approaching calm & the opening door revealed Lorne Cumberland leading a cat by a long string & making heavy exertions not to laugh. He also approached the dread place of sacrifice & tied the cat to a

nail. The thunders were greater, louder, longer, the dust thicker,
the air real with shouts & laughter when oh ye shades of
departed cats again the opening door reveal Burdelle with solemn brigand-like looks, coming slowly & solemnly in leading
another cat. He came up to the other victims in ill concealed
wonder, gazed surprisedly & blankly at them turned his back on
them & tied *his* cat to the leg of the stove. An observer would
scarce believed human endurance could bear more, the Dr. was
leaning on his elbows convulsed. The moments passed & they
were compelled by exhaustion to decrease their risible exertions
when ... the Dr. stooped & drew from beneath his desk a bag,
with *four cats* in it & holding it above the altar informed the students 'This was the ladies contribution' Blocks & blocks away
might the wild tumult have been heard, peal on peal, clapping
stamps & convulsions generally. But the horrible man said also
again 'I see one of the ladies is absent perhaps she is exhausted
with last night's resurrecting.' It has been an awful day. I'm quite
fatigued.

Nov. 22nd 1882.

No one knows or can know what a furnace I am passing through
these days at Coll. A furnace fiery & severe as any could be & not
affect one directly, physically. Not a day not a lecture passes at
Med Coll but something makes me shrink something hurts me,
hurts me cruelly, & why? Not because there is anything in the
whole range of medicine that should make me blush or feel hurt
in the tenderest part of a woman's nature. It is not that, oh no. I
can sit here in my room & study the textbooks with as pure
heartedess & singleness of purpose as moral may bestow on one
subject. No, no, no, it is not that, it is not that. It is the environ-
ments. It is that we are obliged to take it not alone with *gentlemen*
but the blackest hearted roughs, if lowness of nature & baseness
of thought have power to blacken ones nature.
  It is horrible beyond words to tell – I writhe inwardly. It is like
being in torment. Not that they so actively or personally demon-
strate their beastly natures, they dare not so openly. They dare

not be personally rude or obtrusively impertinent. It is not that but that current through the class of whisper – derisive ... ejaculations, turning what never was meant as unseemly to horrible meanings, the thousand & one ways that can be devised by the foul hearted to create a smile on the faces of their fellows. No one else but those who endure can ever understand *how* many ways are possible or how day by day it seems harder to bear for we have borne so much.

And then to know they – *they dare* to judge me immodest, indelicate, unwomanly. To know how we are misunderstood misjudged by most. Oh it is enough to rouse such contending such violent emotions as to make life's load too heavy. That *any* should misjudge, that *any* should have other than sympathy for us for the great sacrifices we make, sympathy for *that* we endure from lesser souls, from ruffianly men is incentive to deepest indignation. Do we desire it, do we like to live this way. God forfend. If we did then it would be our own fault, but if ever there was a huge injustice crying for redress it is this. That there is any sane objection to ladies acquiring the knowledge of medicine, to me there is no question. Granted that we want heartilly & with all our strength with all the power of wishing, we wish for separate Colleges. We want the knowledge that is our due, & we want to gain it honestly, purely, uprightly without harm to any & to all good to ourselves. The good we seek has in itself no dross of filthiness, nothing to scald & scur our natures every day, nothing to make life a furnace, if only they would let us have that & nothing more. If they cannot give us what is fairly & justly ours, then when we, for the sake of humanity and because 'right is right we follow right', are they not bound by every manly trait, by every honest & moral principle to accord us the *best* of the poor substitutes we condescend to take. That it is not so speaks not well for humanity. Injustice, injustice, injustice, rings in my ears & rouses me to bitter thought that sometimes I should dearly like to repay them fourfold what they make me suffer now & I try to crush out every resentful bitter, revengful thought, to believe that I shall know ere long, know how sublime a thing it is to suffer & be strong. I long for sympathy, the sym-

pathy to all my thought & yet I must study & I must go on & at
times be merry, & social, & lonely but for One ever present
friend, but for Heavens comfort I had indeed been desolate.
Friends of course I have, but which of them could *fully* understand. I never think of giving up without completing the course.
I never count that possible only I shall be glad when this years
strain is over & next year please Heaven will be the last. Years
hence perhaps I shall look back & wonder that I should ever
have been moved in this way by such cause. I am grateful that I
have the trait of forgetfulness. for 'memory shifts from the past
its pain & suffers the glory alone to remain.' Time brings solace
in that shape, heals the wounds tho the scars remain. It is late
now, I have not studied tonight. I tried in the early evg. but it
would not do. But as I am too proud to fail in answers tomorrow
I must study yet tonight.

Dec. 9th

This has been a terrible day a terrible day, a day of trouble, of
which little can be said in words. It was all in the shadow of our
disaffected Prof. Dr. K. Fenwick. The crisis that has been im-
pending came. We were in class as usual, & in noting a physiological fact, wh. as such we did not could not object to, He took
unnecessary occasion to enlarge on the subject to the extent of
calling forth applause from the baser minded students, to which
he responded by repeating the fact, *quite* unnecessarily & as it
were by his manner & voice asking their appreciation of his own
vulgar levity & of course they responded by uproarious & dreadful applause, then he began further to expatiate on it by telling
an anecdote of wh. we only heard 'By the by this reminds me of
an anecdote' for by this time we were on our way from class. We
had determined on a former occasion when he had transgressed
his necessary bounds if it occurred again we would leave the
room. Of course this was the gauntlet & we would not go back
till we were righted. Dr. Fowler (registrar) wrote to him but
found it necessary to call a meeting of the Faculty & we put our

grievances in form & sent it in & glad are we to say that every
one of the Profs were staunch as possible to our side & we are
assured that we shall have our rights & have our lectures in our
waiting room which adjoins, so *that* part of it is agreeably settled.
But that is not all. Some ill advised person manufactured a vil-
lianous article wh. appeared in Friday evgs. Whig[2] doing us
gross injustice. So that now the matter is public & in *such* a false
form. Worse still the students have gone against us, at the insti-
gation of Fenwick who has always made himself 'hand & glove'
with them for popularity's sake. He has made them believe that
they are the suffering community by our presence in as much as
he has to garble his lectures on our acct which is *entirely* false,
for altho he never has done so, *we* do not object to listen to any
physiological or scientific truth if it is told to us as such, in due
course of study, in proper manner & proper order in the class. In
no other class have we suffered in this way. If he had some of the
classes we would not be able to stay in the room, one day in the
week. I am so exceedingly sorry that any open rupture has taken
place. I could bear Fenwick's rage without a murmur but to
know the students are pitted against us & that the public are
laboring under grievous mistakes concerning us is like a continual nightmare to me. Day & night, it is ever present & makes the
days begin with dread, for what they may bring forth. We desired the Faculty to print our letter with their endorsing, but as
yet it is under consideration before Princ Grant & Dr. Fowler.
We know how delicate a matter it is for members of a Faculty &
fraternity to come out openly publicly against one of their no. in
this way. The more so as he is quite a popular physician, being
one of those bland smiling men of external polish wh. within is
black as midnight. We do not see the end as yet but in any case it
is intensely disagreeble. That the press in all places will take
pains to copy the pack of falsehoods that appeared in Friday's
Whig, goes without saying.

At present it is a time of trouble but I hope & pray that good
may arise out of the evil, that all will yet be well as it must be.

2 *British Whig*, local Kingston newspaper

Wednes 14th

These are dreadful days, stormy in every sense, now the snow is
blowing terribly a regular whirlwind of snow – & oh such
stormy times at Coll. *We* are passive now, the war has passed
from us to the other students & the Faculty & we wait the issue,
confident for ourselves. Such a fabric of false cowardly state-
ments as have appeared in the papers here, is hard to conceive
possible. They have lost sight of the first issue & now are all in-
tent on having us sent from R.C. [Royal Medical College] wh.
endeavor we may lay to the charge of Fenwick & his aide de
camp – that despicable of all despicable people Jack Herald &
more over it is apparent to not a few that it has been brewing
brewing, waiting something to catch to, to work on & now they
are doing their utmost & are very determined. Sooth to say I
have heard repeatedly from good authority that the real griev-
ance is they are afraid for their laurels in the spring & one Prof
went so far as to say so outside the Coll. Wh. the more surprises
me because I'm quite confident there are many of them able to
out distance me if they tried to. They scarce, some of the least
diplomatic, take pains to conceal the fact which is extremely
ludicrous. I could write much on this head & of interest too, if
only time permitted but the end is not yet & I am extremely worried in that we have our final Senr Chem exam tomorrow.
    These days are days of deep mental waters, Monday I just
broke down but am all cheerful again now. I have promised to
spend the holidays with Miss Beatty. These days of trouble seem
hard to bear, way down in the depths, weighed down by the
constant nightmare of trouble, waking & sleeping & feel crushed
by difficulties, haunted *all* the time by the weight of misfortunes
that have gathered around us. I have sat & stared at the wall till I
seemed stone myself. I have paced my room in frantic thought
have thought till my perplexed brain seemed giving way, all my
nature on the rack, maligned by the Press, wronged by the
Faculty, hated by those who feared me but had yet the power to
wrong me. It seems beyond belief that it was I myself, I who had
thought to live peaceably, on friendly terms, to propitiate their

anti-sentiments to the project in the abstract, who had been flattered & sought after by so many of them individually. It has been
a weary weary time to me & has taught me a bitter lesson & I
could almost hate them individually & collectively for their un-
kindness, injustice, unmanliness, their cruelty their jealousy,
their spite, but now I am worn to the feeling of indifference to
them & to every Kingstonian & careless of cultivating their good
opinion in the least. Those friends I know, I am thankful for, &
they have a little lessened the bitterness of the time but still we
have so intensely suffered. I am more myself now since being at
church this morning & am able to throw it off at times & even
forget. Of course it is not over, when we cannot tell not anyway
till the session recommences. The girls are for forcing the ranks,
it would be hard but we do not think they have any right or
power to expel us from the classes, when we are registered students for the term. We do not know what to do yet, we are trying
to put all thought of it out of our minds till after our exams are
over, Tues to wh. date the exams were deferred by circumstances
& the 'boys'. We have been so very much disturbed we have not
been able to study this last week & it is much to be regretted for
we would like to excel them very much more now they have
shown so plainly & publicly that they do not like to compete
with us. I am sure they are being chastised in a pretty severe
manner by the Press. The Globe in aspecial, to wh. I shall ever
feel grateful for the support they have given us in this dreadful
ordeal. I wonder what some of the 'decorous' young men think
when they see it in print that they 'never could have had
mothers or sisters,' 'that they showed want of intelligence &
good breeding & c'? Anyway & at most or least, they *did not* get
what they desired, i.e. separate exams. Wasn't it paradoxical,
they cry out that women would lower the standard and yet are
afraid & ask for separate examin. The Faculty promised to give
us 'Separate Classes' wh. sounds very well in print but we *know*
what it means, simply what one of the Profs happily styled 'a rehash' Wh. rehash w'd be served up to us in a very few minutes &
we w'd be expected to work up our subjects from books & then
compete with the boys in the spring to whom had been given the

whole proper lectures. It is self apparent that a second hours lectures could not be properly given on the same material in anatomy or surgery as it is necessarily spoiled in demonstrating, & of the idea of us asking for the first lecture w'd be preposterous, & worse than ridiculed since to the boys the Coll. must in a measure look for government in the future. There is not one of the students that can look us honestly in the face. Not one that I have met since but looks much as if he had stolen his mother's coffin & in justice to the better minded I must say I think now on maturer thought, in calmer mood they are quite ashamed of the whole thing. I think so. I hope so, for the sake of mankind. What we have seen from the actions of the students & Profs generally, at this last crisis speaks little for the 'high principles of honor' supposed to exist in the educated &c. The gentleman, Mr Shortt who boards here has been a staunch friend throughout & he & Prof Lavalle are about the only ones who have come out scatheless to my eyes in the whole affair. It all seems like a horrible dream from wh. I must awaken but yet has been long & terrible. Then too the weight of it must hand over us all through this usually merry time, this time of Peace & Goodwill to Men, & yet I feel today that in God's good time out of this evil good *will* come, somehow somewhere, sometime, 'good will be the final goal of ill' I pray Heaven it may be so, for now it is very dark.

We go to Lansdown on Wednesday afternoon, perhaps I will stay a week with Mrs Leslie in the holidays.

Lansdown, Dec 27 '82

Much as I like Miss Beatty & all here yet sometimes & I am very homesick & I think to myself what did I stay for, why did I not go home. Still I am enjoying myself as well here as I could anywhere away from home at this Christmas time as I am trying it for the first time. Sometimes I wonder if I will ever get back again to the perfect light heartedness of a month ago, before the fray began Of course I do not go moping round all the time as tho' life was a constant funeral, but the troubles of the last month have subdued me wonderfully & made me much older. I shall be heartilly glad when we are back at work at K. & the Rubicon of the new regime crossed. I dread it so much. We do not intend to force the classes at present but it may come to that. It wd be dreadful, but the injustice in so many ways that has been done, it is so great & so jarring that it has roused every one of us to that degree, we dare do all that may become a woman. Law & equity on our side, we felt we could so scorn any conduct of *such* men, that we could & we dare force the classes, by being in our places in some classes or anteroom in others, when the classes assembled. Neither Faculty nor students have the power to expel us from the classes. The same plan was tried at T[oronto] Sc[hool of] Med[icine] Dr Trout writes me, when she attended & it came to light that holding class tickets, they had no power to eject them. We have a devised plan tho' in a better way. We are comparatively little concerned as far as ourselves go, for this session, at least. What most worries us is that the girls who wished to come in next year seem cut off. I am glad their lordships are so graciously inclined toward our individual selves as to 'particularize'!! That they should particularize one as being under the ban of their disapproval & that one Miss Beatty is but another instance of their stupidity & inability to understand a character so far their superior they cannot comprehend it, for Miss B. of all of us is I think the soundest most admirable character. Tho' nature made the form less graceful than ordinary she redeemed that by a superior mind. Our plan at present is to give them a try at separate lectures, for we wanted some classes entirely so for awhile anyway & there it will harrow the Profs to such a bewildering extent that it will afford us some pleasure to see it, to get the double hours in to suit the hours at Queens &c. There too we are going to keep strict acct of quantity & quality of lectures & if they do not come up to tune we will have them on the same ground, the boys went over, breach of contract & if nagging is any punishment maybe they'll be punished. Anyway we are indignant enough to push it thro' to the very end, now. I am very glad indeed that the Press generally have so berated the students & Faculty. It's just lovely the way they are handled both in Ont.

& U.S. & I am quite sanguine that in a greater degree than I ever
hoped much good will result, has even now, in one way, in that
it has stirred public opinion & brought it before that far(?) seeing eye so vividly. I had no idea that Conservative Canada
viewed the subject so liberally & I am delighted to find it so. I believe if some philanthropist would step to the front c funds a
Women's Med. Coll. w'd be the result at once, or if any man w'd
canvass for subscriptions in Ont enough w'd be given I believe it
to be quite possible & quite easy if there were only the right & fit
person forthcoming. It makes me feel very helpless being a
woman & so impotent to do what would be such a 'public
charity.' Among other monstrous untruths, the students say
there was no stamping & treading before we left the room that
eventful day. A false tirade c signature of 'student' has appeared
& we guess it to be by his Satanic majesty – J. Herald. It certainly
sounds like him. One student Anglin of whom I have always had
a high regard as the creme de la creme of the med. students, has
gone along with the rest & with him the last shred of respect for
the students as a body. He said at a public dinner, to shield their
late questionable deeds, 'that it was not from a lack of gallantry
they had taken that course, but love of their profession led them
to desire to learn all they could of each subject & that the Profs
were obliged to omit some parts because of the 'mixed classes'
wh was a most stupendous falsehood. Not one of them has & *all
destinctly* so *state* except Dr Fenwick & he had the least disagreeable subject of all & *he* is the only one who ever gave us offence
& much as he may declare, we know *no* science he could give has
been unsaid on our acct, tho he may have been afraid to garnish
his lectures with vile stories as he attempted that day. He has
said he was compelled to garble his lectures. I'm going to start a
rumor that the ladies are about to sue the Prof of Physiology for
'breach of contract' in not giving the *full* lectures our class tickets
pay for. *So* absurd as tho' we did not want all the science they
could give us. Miss Beatty & I talk of going to Glasgow or Edin-
burgh next year & thus escape the Council too. It would not cost
so very much more. Still we three seniors feel comparatively easy
as concerns our future for next year will be final work & I do not

dread it half so much as this year. Oh I am so glad it will be over in a year & a half. I am not the least out of conceit of study. It is only the unhappy hours these boys have caused us, all the time by their presence & now by their persecutions. It has been a weary weary time. I shall remember.

Dec. 28th

It sounds beautiful no doubt to outsiders that we are to have separate lectures but they do not consider that the second lecture will be but a sorry rehash, both literally & figuratively. Indeed Dr. Fowler of 'settled convictions' had the effrontery to tell Miss R. that he would *run over the important parts of the lecture after he had lectured to the boys & tell her what to read up.*' Most striking speech from the Dean of the Faculty!!! Who but a few days previously was loudest in his assertion that 'if mild measures did not mend Dr. Fenwick's ways, severe measures wd be resorted to' & 'you may rest assured ladies your rights will be protected.' I am glad that I have manly honorable brothers & a father, or I should have little faith in mankind after seeing such a mass of them found wanting, even in simple honor. ... I would not wonder in the least if some unversed in Med ways, should think we had reason to thank the boys for procuring us, what under proper conditions, we would most desire, viz. separate lectures. There is generally I believe a wheel within a wheel. Am busy all the time these days, sewing visiting, reading, studying. The days pass so quickly & so little done at study, especially. Thurs we thought of studying, Frid we spoke of it. Sat. I took a couple books down stairs, then Sunday & Christmas intervened & Tues I studied an hour!! Have not been out much yet, twice, & a few have been in but the programme begins tomorrow, to my sorrow for I had preferred to be quiet & stay here all the time. I am glad it is not any gayer & not ultra fashionable else it w'd be a great bore. Rec. an Elgin newspaper. Ridgetown Plaindealer, & Kingston Whig, both c editorials against students & Faculty, the first particularly scathing. Have been laying low my pile of un-answered letters since here & exchanging Xmas cards. It w'd be curious to know how many sheets of them I've sent away & how sick I am of writing about Coll affairs & always cries of 'more' 'more' in the next letters, till it is almost painfully mechanical the way I have to grind over that Coll. fracas. Every letter I read, I think 'Another county heard from' & another hours work & more, no sooner do they read, than they become interested. No sooner interested than their appetites increase for the theme. No sooner so stimulated than they supplicate for more & I struggle on hoping to throw a little light on the subject, in a few cases at least. Maud too writes for more. Maud the matronly, Maud the monopolized mamma. Maud the never wearying slave of sister Ina, & I think I'll write to her fully when I can get my courage to the sticking point & ask Jack's opinion. Mr Mac was in K. before we left & Meshack is happiest of the happy these days. Oh! won't it be something to live for to see Dr. Fenwick lecturing to us alone! We had a comical attempt at it, when the boys were on their strike. He nearly strangled, he raced, he fell headlong over phrases, words, letters, he splashed struggled & away again & was just 16 minutes in delivering that burst of science, while we oh we nearly ate our handkerchiefs in vain attempts to preserve order, but no one felt the ludicrous so keenly as those who were there & tried with great effort to pretend to write down that lecture, a thing impossible.

Jan. 7th '83 Lansdown

Sunday morning & I am writing here in Mrs Beatty's kitchen where Abednego [Elizabeth Beatty] are settled by the stove, perhaps for the last time ever, as we go back to K. tomorrow, to take up the battle of life in an especial earnest. I dread it – dread it. If we were like it was last year it wd not be bad, but c such bitter recollections of all those places of all the people there. With a sense of unpleasantness & of bickerings of diverse kinds, sure to be in this near future. In fact I am not in as good a mood to meet it as 3 wks ago. Then I had my courage & energy up to the sticking pt but a few weeks of idleness & inactivity ... leaves me not much zest to enter the contest again. I have had a very good time here & I'm sure I could not quarrel with anyone but myself. This past wk. we were out every evg but Tues & then a little party here. No dancing parties tho. Nor do all play cards, yet for 'bill of fare' commend me to Lansdown. Its something awful the luxurious tables set & the amt of candies & nuts we have consumed is astonishing. But after all the coming & going, the dressing & performing, I am not 'chirked' up to any great extent. I like them all here, especially in the house, but its a perfect bore to go visiting to go to little parties & worse to help entertain comparative strangers. I'm as sick of society as if I had been thro' the mills for an indefinite number of seasons. I am infinitely better satisfied to stay quietly in the home when I have congenial company as I have here.

It is a dreadful state of mind to be in truly, when everything seems a weariness of the flesh & every days chief value lies in that it is past, oblivious that it also brings me nearer 'the bounds of life' & Death. Ah I cannot but think what experiences the future may hold, must hold for me if alive. What a world it is, only a few years at best & then. I do pity with great sympathy those who do not believe in Heaven. It would be too terrible to bear – too dreary a life if we knew this was all. So many suffer who suffer always, who never know the best of life, & how horrible if 'all *were* darkness at the core & dust & ashes all that is' & Death dissolution. I am glad for that, that there is an Hereafter where we shall be happy & at rest. I do not know how I *cannot* know how, but I *know* we will be happy & I trust the how to Heaven. The press after all are taking our side of the question, & the Globe has come out strong, & The Montreal Witness even better. I wrote a letter of thanks c two corrections 'that no concessions were made in regard to exams & that we were to have the same at same time & place' & also in regard to another paragraph in same paper, about our prefixing Mrs & Miss to our names, wh. absurdly some of the Eastern papers accused us of, because a K. paper saw fit to public our names in that wise. The only way I can see to excuse the boys for adhering to such a rank

falsehood that they were so used to applauding in that class &
were so excited they did not know what they *were* doing. It was
too keenly painful then & now for me not to remember 'oh those
dreadful days, & what is to come 'Godknows' & that He cares is
more than enough. I see in last nights paper they are going to
petition Legislature to hear it. They say too that opposers of the
idea are to make use of our recent troubles as example. While I
regret to be so counted on the wrong side instead of being of
some use for the right yet there will perhaps be such a thorough
inquiry into the fray that a clear analysis of it may be obtained
where otherwise it would have remained obscure. Any ventilat-
ing of the subject is to our benefit. Any knowledge of the true
inwardness of the affair is another impetus to the removal of
prejudice. Two Oclock – the dishes rattling visitors expected &
dressing to do & then to church & next morning back again to
battle. And I am glad to go back to study for it keeps me from
thinking & that is much to be desired. I think I should go mad if
I had nothing more to occupy myself with than the incomplete
days have furnished here, would furnish anywhere, *unless* I had
all I could do to keep me employed. It seems to me till last Spring
I had only 'stood with reluctant feet where womanhood & childhood meet' but now, however, much of bitterness there is in the
doing I must put away childish things & undertake life as a serious business.

Kingston 244 Gordon St. Jan 14th – 1883

Here again, under old rule. Spring nearing rapidly. I am half
gone. Feb. short lectures done before March is & then Westward
Ho! Monday Miss B[eatty] & I came upon the Merchants Express, wh. means a van in the rear of a freight wh. is taken
advantage of between K. & Brockville. It was a little incident that
broke the monotony of travelling & we arrived a few hours before dark for wh. we endevored in order to interview a couple of
the Profs, with a view to get our lectures first. We were more
amused than surprised at the apparent surprise of Dr. Sullivan at

the idea of lecturing two hours a day. It was quite apparent he had no intention of so doing & said we could stay in the adjacent room. Dr. Oliver was slow to understand how could he arrange but did eventually. So with *some* interest in what the morrow would bring forth we were deposited at our respective boarding houses to await the morrow. Miss Oliver returned soon after I did & proceeded to have the general good talk girls, separated for 2 wks consider necessary to a complete readjustment of acquaintance. Next day we were there & ready for battle but all went smoothly & well in the forenoon. In the afternoon Obste. & Surgery were taken as formerly, we took the same lecture in the next room, but Dr. Fowler our Dean & Prof of Prac Med gave Miss Reynolds hers alone. Could anything be more absurd than the Dean grinding over his lecture to Miss R. in our waiting room (She is the only one of us taking his class this session.) It seemed very comical, that it should be & at the boys dictation too. Next day Dr. Fowler found that the other final lectures were not giving double lectures & so thought may be the boys did not object to Miss R. listening to his in the next room & had his class occupy that especial room in place of the usual one below stairs. Wednesday we all went down to hospital to clinic by Dr. Depuis at his request. The boys sent in a remonstrance at once to the Faculty that they were breaking their promise, & so when Dr. Fowler appealed to their sympathies to let him off from giving a second hr to Miss R. they were *not* agreeable. So he wants Miss R. to go to his office for lectures & she will not, nor would any of us. Dr. Lavalle & Sullivan don't intend to do otherwise than they have done & I expect the door will be open for us tomorrow as usual & then more developments. Dr Fenwick ostensibly gives us separate lectures but on no day does he give us more than twenty minutes sometimes so rapidly & incoherently that we could not possibly take it down. I met Mr Knight, Headmaster of the H[igh] S[chool] here & the one who gave me Dr. L's address to open communications with the Faculty & had quite a satisfactory chat. He says Fenwick told him he meant to tell some stories to the class that would make it uncomfortable for us & that he tried to shame him out of it but that he insisted he would & *he* did. Mr. Knight's sister intended to come next year. He advises going into the general classroom & taking our places as before. He thinks it a perfectly wonderful piece of wrong doings inexpressibly so. Can't understand how so many should act so blindly both Profs & students. He is studying med. too, is up at the dissecting room & says he tries to shame the boys & he thinks some of them *are* heartily ashamed. Miss Oliver when home met with almost an ovation, was made a heroine in Stratford, St. Mary's & Toronto & finds we have more sympathy than we ever dreamed of & heard in Toronto second hand from one of the Profs of T. Sc. Med that they would receive us make concessions to us, it may be we will make some arrangements there for next season, but in Kingston we intend to stay for this session at least. She met two young ladies in Stratford who intended to come to K. next session, so with Miss Dickson back & a Class of five new Medico's I fancy Toronto w'd be willing to make some provision for our welfare. Since they cannot exclude women altogether they might as well make a virtue of necessity. Time will show however. I am glad to hear such a heavy petition is going into Legislature in favour of admission of women to Arts Classes in Toronto. Rec. a nice long letter from Lizzie Robertson who is now teaching in Belleville ... Cecil did excellently well at his Xmas exams, of wh he sent me the announcement. I wish I could do as well, more especially now when so many are anxious that we should. Mr Knight says 'I would give 50 dollars to see you scoop the boys out on the exams in the Spring' Alas poor me if I only had more stick-at-it-ness there w'd be more hope. Am greatly relieved tonight to hear that Miss Blaylock is coming back to complete our quartette & happy family. Affairs seem settling without us shouldering any blame. The afternoon, the final subjects we take at the same hr as the gentlemen (?) in th adjacent room. Fenwick we take by himself, he's enough of that kind at one time. Mat Med & Anatomy we have had so far separately. 'The old order changeth giving place to new & God fulfils Himself in many ways.' What at first was very dark, shows glimpses now of fairest dawn & I can feel that altho we have borne the brunt of battle it has done incalculable good.

Jan 13th

Grip had a taking article for us by J.K.L. The boys bought up all
the copies so we could nt get them, but we did eventually. Miss
B[laylock] has come back & we seem pretty lighthearted, considering the deep waters we have been in recently.

24th January. This from the Century:

'Bend your head lower while I say the rest
The greatest change of all is this that I Who used to be so cold,
so fierce, so shy
In the sweet moment that I feel you near
Forget to be ashamed & know no fear
Forget that life is sad & Death is drear'

College affairs go on about as usual, no fresh disturbance in particular tho' I feel as tho we were treading over a mine that might
explode at any time. The boys, some of them continue to pass
resolutions but there does not seem to be much fruit for so much
labor & more over they have broken up into factions & they can
waste some of their surplus energy & oratory on each other.
Heard one say to his hearer 'if the Profs have left nothing out of
their lectures then we have been working without grounds &
have been made fools of before the public'. I should heartilly endorse that last, but as we hear them thro our floor of course we
are reticent of expressing what we feel. Another in his oration
says 'whats the difference, if they won't allow women here, they
will only go somewhere else & we might as well have them here
as anywhere else' &c &c Likely they will do something generous
yet & astonish us, if they are capable of it.
    Dr Oldham has been down from Chatsworth & for the third
time did me the honor &c says he will not give up hope, will
wait five years &c &c. I thought at least I would be glad to see
him, as we had pleasant memories of those times when he was
our Demonstrator, but I wish I had not seen him for now all

pleasantries of him are effaced. He says he has made 4000 since
he went there & it is not 2 yrs. Money may be the root of all evil,
but the want of it is like the whole tree root & branch, he is so
odiously lacking in breeding. Tues Rec. letter from Cecil & am in
high good humor. So many flattering things, sent Cecil my photo
... last week & the dear boy went into rhapsodies over it & tells
me a host of handsome things people are kind enough to say re-
garding it & that one of the 4th year men when he found one of
these Medicos to be Smiths sister shook hands with him congratulated him on having such a plucky sister. Why I almost
think life is rose color after all & not all ashes. Am in a better
frame of mind altogether & have been working more satisfactorily at the studies for the last few days. It is terribly cold weather
now & the streets are a perfect wilderness of ice. I think I am
about as full of moods as Canadian winters.

Jan. 28th

I am stupid. I am tired, too tired to do anything. It is Sunday evg
but I studied too hard yesterday, from 9 to 1 Oclock & from 2 to
4 & when 4 came my head was burning hot & I went down town
for a walk & came back, looking as tho' I had had a fever, & today I am limp & tired. Went to church this morning & slept this
afternoon. Have not read any today wh. is quite wonderful.
There is a perfect wilderness of work to begin at in the morning
& I'm in the humor to do it, if I only can. I have more zest for
work than before this session. Perhaps it is the calamity of coming exams, that have roused me. Spring is coming & so are
exams, sooner, 20th March & the Council 3rd April College
affairs go on much the same as ever. Quite satisfactory lectures in
all subjects but Physiology & that always a farce. The Salvation
Army has marched on Kingston. Tonight I believe they sound
the trumpet in Victoria Hall. How smallest incidents bring trains
of thought. Instance now, my window being open I hear voices
talking on some door step, which brings a summer like feeling of
twilights of breezy coolness wh is so pleasant after a summers

day. Botany exams show Miss Reynolds 2nd & two boys 1st, ahead with 98 marks. We are glad but of course we'd have been 2 marks gladder if she had excelled all. However the boys are angry one couldn't contain himself, would look at the bulletin then fly round the outside of the crowd & swear, then go up to it & look again & then swing off & swear again & said, in indignant words about them putting 'her' up there. Some days I feel as life was machinery sans feeling I go through so much every day & awake next morning & repeat it again. I feel I am becoming stony, don't feel much in anything but go thro each days work mechanically.

31st

Am in excellent spirits. Dr Depuis thought (perhaps) I was going into hysterics this morning. I had been laughing so heartilly at a mistake between Sam Bertram Mrs Corlis & myself & the poor boy by mistake called on *her*.

Feb. 3rd [excerpt from letter to Charlie]

Am quite concerned just now about my eyes, they gave out last night entirely, guess I caught cold in them, after long tension of them. Am going to poultice them tonight & get glasses at an early date. Have not used them today at all. Was at church & Mr Shortt has been reading to me from Harper. He is very kind & we admire him very much. He is like a brother to us, three girls. Miss Fitzgerald is a dear girl & loves me passionately but we cannot see much of each other as we wd wish we could. Dr & Mrs Corlis have just been to call on me, & he was the best of all my friends nearly cut my fingers on my ring so energetic was his grasp. Tom Bertram called last night & was in a very jolly mood, is generally I believe. Dr. Trout writes me that Upper Can. Coll is turned as a future Ladies Coll. but we think too good to be true. Oh for a mammoth brain & plenty of perseverance & eyesight these days. I'm interested. It's a real pleasure to study if I only had all the necessary apparatus. Mrs Mr Mac, Dr Corlis, & the

Salvation Army all in town today & still the walks are not
shovelled & navigation is a matter of difficulty from the snow.
Your letter has made me sober & sorry, do not tire, do not fall
into content so deep you care not to go on, it would be like the
wandered in the snow, a certain death to ambition. If your ambition is such that you mean surely to accomplish a certain height
a certain goal, everything will give way to that, you will make
every days deed tend to that one object. Little things may not
count much in each days course but the total tends a long way to
success or failure, in the course of a year. Do not in retrospect
think that you have fallen short of what you should have done
with the idea that the future can not be different, that any weakness producing part regrets is more than yourself, & will over
rule you, but let it rather incite you to stronger exertions to over
rule it. Do not speak in such ultra acrid phrases of political
events of conservatives not being on the side of *honest* admini-
stration, 'an ignoble cause' 'Not choosing that good part' 'not
being in the right company' such rabid terms in any cause in any
case overleap themselves & fall out other side to me, at least such
strong language always speaks more for the party to which
applied than that of the user. Surely you forget, it is the political
side I have always most respected, if for *no* other reason, than
that it was the politics of men I have ever had cause to respect, of
men of my own home. I am not ultra conservative you know & I
am certain as I am of anything there is much of good in either
party & many admirable men on either side. It must be so, or one
would have outlived the other. I must prepare for a grind. [end
of excerpt]

Feb 13th

I guess it was a false alarm about my eyes & tho I have had several pairs of glasses on trial yet not necessary at all now & I am
glad eno. But it was but the fore runner of worse ills. My eyes
were bad Sunday & Monday & Tues tho' not well I went with
Mr Shortt to see Ragans [illegible – a play?] & enjoyed it hugely
but after I came home was very miserable & next day broke

down entirely, they were quite frightened about me, they worked hard & next morning I was better for their nursing. I was just awful hot & sick. Everyone was *so* kind, I can not say *how* kind & I'm sure enough love & sympathy was tendered me last week to keep several families in stock for a year. I wasnt out till Sat ... & am gradually getting back to a normal state But lo Sat. News had an item to the effect that Miss Smith Med student was seriously ill. Whoever put it in is more than I can guess but my! it caused a drefful sensation. Sunday the sexton went to Miss Blaylock in church for Rev. Cary, to know how I was &c, at St Andrews they were asking Miss Oliver & in the afternoon two ladies called & offered to sit up nights &c!! Miss Fitz. was stopped on the st & asked, Principal Grant, stopping the girls too, all the Profs, Even Dr. Fenwick when I went back to class smiled very benignly & said 'you're better I see' &c. The boys were asking Mr Shortt at Queens & Mr Brown ... gracious! it was a time & the fun of it was I was all better before they found it out. Too bad to lose time now, so much work to do, & it is hard to catch up. ... Lectures close three weeks from Friday at our Coll & woe is me exams will soon follow & 'then & then ye gods! That I had still naught but this shuddering & distracting thought' Guess we will be here next year after all. Rec. a long letter from Dr. Trout with the projects formed for Toronto & hopes are flat in that direction At Histology lecture on Sat the only Med beside us girls was J. Herald, how nice he must have felt. Never did see such a place for snow. Snow & wind. I feel like a perfect rattlebrain in regard to everything but the studies & they hang over me in perpetual nightmare. Mr Shortt has been explaining a little about shorthand to me & I wish I could learn it. He cannot say enough good of it, values it best of his possessions apparently.

Feb. 13th

Am homesick tonight, blue, have not been well lately at all & oh I wish I were for there is a mountain of work looming up before me. I get so tired & sort of discouraged sometimes because I don't feel well & I want to study & I cannot. The girls have just gone, from our weekly review in Anatomy, & as I cannot well sit up longer I will go to bed.

Sat. Evg. – Midnight

Another week gone & now it seems I have done so little compared with what I might. It is no small matter of trouble to us that we do not stand a fair chance with the boys. In any case we would so much have liked to do well, all the more now, when everywhere we are looked to & prematurely congratulated on how we will excel the boys in the coming exams & for us to know we have no ghost of a chance is not conducive to a free & happy mind. I am feeling more like myself today. Had Histology lecture at Hotel Dieu & then home to tea. A gentleman in to tea, a friend of Mr Shortts, Mr Brown. Since tea have been trying to put in the usual number of hrs study. I am trying hard to think of nothing but the hard hard facts of examinations. I'm just getting to hate that old College. It reminds me of that horrid old man in Bleak House that had a cat with him in his old rookery where Miss Flite boarded & how when two men were searching there they found the walls all reeking & discovered the cause in the spontaneous combustion of said old man. Yesterday putting my hand on the bannister, it felt cold & clammy & sticky I nearly shrieked to think of it. I don't know what some of those students would n't do. Someone or somebody broke thro two doors at Coll the other night & stole an armful of books & destruction of something goes on every day. Tomorrow is Sunday & there's a chance to look away from books with an easy conscience & rest, rest. I wonder how many weary bodies & minds hail Sunday with as much quiet gladness of anticipation. I think they will always be bright spots in memory.

Feb. 23rd '83

Every day things look blacker as regards any tithe of justice for us in the future, near or remote. We have given up all hope of making any high standing even if we were allowed wh. every day seems more doubtful. We will have the same papers, but if they will not class our marks with those of the boys the outside public will not understand & the boys will virtually have gained their point. And then the humbugging we have rec as regards lectures & the injustice & calummy we have so wrongly suffered. None but Heaven knows or can know what we have suffered & do suffer daily. I try to shake off the depression, the 'weight' ... & perhaps do in a measure for a time when some new feature some new wound 'tears agape that healing wound afresh' & strikes me back again into deep waters & I believe it is half due to that, my miserable health, of late. Today my head is so queer & hurts & since noon I have not studied successfully at all, but tomorrow is Sunday & rest. It seems to take the life out of my life as it were, it makes me old, it makes me sad & it is dreadful to be so, to feel that youth & simple heartedness, carelessness, spirit, are slipping from me & making me look so different, & feel so different. When we are fighting in a good fight & should have all support to aid us, to be turned on by all, with such mistaken zeal, with such injustice it is hard, so hard If I can only fight it out till I get home I'll be glad. Lectures close in two weeks but after that the exams. Coll. then Council[3] in April. It is midnight now, & I am a watcher, the clocks tick keeping one company for Miss Oliver must take the morning train home as a telegram rec. this aft says her father is dangerously ill & we wd not have her miss the train for anything.

March 3rd

Dear Miss Oliver lost her father & before she could see him again, it was very sad. I have been in excellent health & spirits, this last week & wonder what possesses me to be so happy & so careless & fret so little about my exams as I do. I am rooming with Miss Blaylock now, but she leaves next week, & after that I expect to do the most studying. We expect to pass but still we

3   exams of the Ontario College of Physicians and Surgeons

have given up every hope of making any good stand in the
exams. I've bought a pair of skates. Mr Shortt was kind enough
to undertake to teach me how & I wanted lots of exercise. I've
only been out twice & have not made any progress yet, no proper boots & now there is no skating on our common, but lots of
snow & cold. Lectures closed nominally on Friday tho' we have
Histology & Chem yet for some time. My stay here will be so
prolonged I'll stay for Convocation, as Council exams do not begin till 13th April. We are working away as best we may, but
have no hopes more ambitious than passing well. In order to try
for any prizes, the competitors must make 60% on the written
common exams & I doubt very much if the Profs would credit us
with it if we make it for it w'd be the easiest way of settling the
difficulty paramount among the boys, vide next issue of the Coll
Journal, wh. comes out next week & Grip too. There is a most
satisfactory movement in progress in Toronto at this present the
outcome of which please Heaven will be I hope a Medical Coll
for women.

I believe because right *is* right to *follow* right is wisdom to the
scorn of consequence.

Who struck a jarring lyre at first
But ever thought to make it true

June 22, 1884

It is a hard task this that I have set before me, not the writing in a
diary as a resume of what is almost painful at the least tiresome.
I am a woman now, & so changed from that unsettled irregular
immature young person who thought she loved, & like thousands of others misused the term. Still I believe I did love an
ideal – that I tried hard to believe I had found – & then when it
was no longer tenable by the strongest hope, my ideal being
gone, love was no more then when I did find my ideal[4] – & the
man was more than my perplexed faith drew as such – love not

4 Adam Shortt

only blossomed again, but grew to perfect blossom and in the light of those days, I began to know myself more too. Then the long night of sorrow since he went away [to study in Scotland] has given me time for thought, so life is more & more – is fuller, wider – deeper, thoughts & deeds are more so much more a diary would be irksome to me, so much repetition tho' the measure of it goes across the sea.

The Social History of Canada

General Editors:
Michael Bliss 1971-7
H.V. Nelles 1978-